Atlas of
PHONOMICROSURGERY

Atlas of PHONOMICROSURGERY

Author

Nupur Kapoor Nerurkar MS (ENT) DORL
Laryngologist and Voice Surgeon
DNB Coordinator, ENT Department
Director, Laryngology Fellowship Program
Bombay Hospital and Medical Research Center
Governing Council; Association of Phonosurgeons of India

Forewords

Marc Remacle

Milind V Kirtane

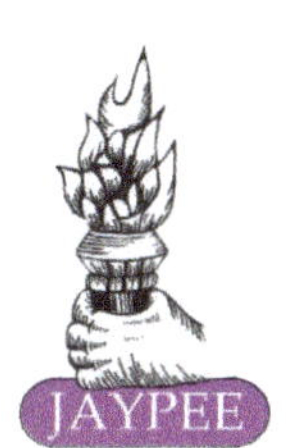

The Health Sciences Publisher
New Delhi | London | Panama

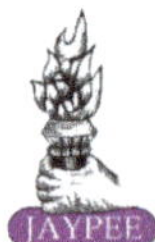

Jaypee Brothers Medical Publishers (P) Ltd

Headquarters

Jaypee Brothers Medical Publishers (P) Ltd
4838/24, Ansari Road, Daryaganj
New Delhi 110 002, India
Phone: +91-11-43574357
Fax: +91-11-43574314
Email: jaypee@jaypeebrothers.com

Overseas Offices

J.P. Medical Ltd
83 Victoria Street, London
SW1H 0HW (UK)
Phone: +44 20 3170 8910
Fax: +44 (0)20 3008 6180
Email: info@jpmedpub.com

Jaypee-Highlights Medical Publishers Inc
City of Knowledge, Bld. 237, Clayton
Panama City, Panama
Phone: +1 507-301-0496
Fax: +1 507-301-0499
Email: cservice@jphmedical.com

Jaypee Brothers Medical Publishers (P) Ltd
17/1-B Babar Road, Block-B, Shaymali
Mohammadpur, Dhaka-1207
Bangladesh
Mobile: +08801912003485
Email: jaypeedhaka@gmail.com

Jaypee Brothers Medical Publishers (P) Ltd
Bhotahity, Kathmandu
Nepal
Phone: +977-9741283608
Email: kathmandu@jaypeebrothers.com

Website: www.jaypeebrothers.com
Website: www.jaypeedigital.com

Atlas of Phonomicrosurgery / Nupur Kapoor Nerurkar

First Edition: **2018**

ISBN: 978-93-5270-224-4

Dedication

I dedicate this book to my parents, my children—Kanika and Anaaya, and my husband Rajeev, with love

Foreword

It is my pleasure and honor to have been asked to write the foreword for this *"Atlas of Phonomicrosurgery,"* written and edited by Professor Nupur Kapoor Nerurkar.

I have known Nupur for some years now and have also had the privilege to take part in some of her well-established courses on laryngology. From our first meeting, I have been impressed by her knowledge of the anatomy, physiology, and pathology of the larynx.

The larynx is a very complicated organ. Beside its major functions—voicing, swallowing, and breathing—it contributes to the expression of our emotions and feelings. This is why phonosurgery and, in particular, phonomicrosurgery is so complicated to master, as the entire personality of the patient is contained in the production of their speaking and singing voice. The phonosurgeon must understand not only the etiology and management of the dysphonia but also must anticipate what the patient expects from their voice after the surgical treatment. This goes far beyond the capacity of performing only a good procedure. There is no doubt in my mind that Dr Nupur Kapoor Nerurkar masters all these aspects of phonomicrosurgery.

This atlas is another demonstration of Dr Nerurkar's teaching prowess. What you have in the hands is much more than a basic atlas with the usual pictures illustrating the various pathologies of the larynx and the vocal folds. This atlas encompasses the microscopic and histological aspects of the vocal fold lesions, the principles of phonomicrosurgery, the tips and tricks for difficult scenarios, and safety during laser use and anesthesia. The subsequent chapters are a comprehensive review of phonomicrosurgery specific to the different lesions. Not only is there a systematic presentation of what must be done but also how to do it step by step according to the pathology. The two major techniques performed today—cold steel and carbon dioxide laser phonomicrosurgeries—are described, emphasizing advantages and disadvantages of each of them.

If this was necessary, this atlas gives us another reason why Dr Nupur Kapoor Nerurkar is a leading phonosurgeon, well-recognized not only by her patients and colleagues in India, but also all over the world.

Professor Marc Remacle MD PhD
Department of ORL-Head and Neck Surgery,
Voice and Swallowing Disorders
CHL-Eich
Luxembourg, Luxembourg

Foreword

Laryngology as a subspecialty of ENT has gained considerable importance over the last decade. With advanced diagnostic techniques and refinements in operating equipment, treatment of patients with voice disorders has undergone a sea change.

The author of this atlas, Dr Nupur Kapoor Nerurkar, is a renowned laryngologist who has received recognition in the field of laryngology and phonosurgery not only in India, but also internationally.

The workshops on phonosurgery conducted by her yearly have proved to be a great learning experience for not only budding phonosurgeons but also for all ENT surgeons who encounter patients with voice disorders in their day-to-day practice. This atlas details a step-by-step approach depicted by high quality photographs which encompass diagnostic, surgical, and histopathological aspects of phonosurgery.

I am confident that the readers will vastly benefit from the comprehensive knowledge gained through this atlas.

Dr Milind V Kirtane
Professor Emeritus
King Edward Memorial Hospital and
Seth Gordhandas Sunderdas Medical College
Mumbai, Maharashtra, India

Acknowledgments

This atlas is an amalgamation of the work I have had an opportunity to do at the Bombay Hospital and Medical Research Center over the past 10 years. I thank my patients for the opportunity to serve them and their faith in me.

I am extremely grateful to Mr Bharat Taparia, the Chairman of Bombay Hospital and the management team for supporting a state-of-the-art laryngology setup, conducive to optimal patient management, teaching, and archiving of data.

The Departments of Anesthesia, Histopathology, and Radiology have been incredibly helpful and cooperative. I thank Dr P Kulkarni, Dr JP Arora, Dr G Mujumdar, Dr K Patel, Dr I Talwar, Dr S Jaggi, and Dr S Shah in particular. All my colleagues in the ENT and Speech Language Pathology Departments of Bombay Hospital have been supportive, especially Dr R Nerurkar and Dr S Muranjan. The Association of Phonosurgeons of India (APSI) has encouraged all my academic initiatives and I thank my APSI colleagues for the same.

The assistance provided by all my laryngology fellows and residents over the years has been a huge help in getting this atlas to see the light of day and the operating theater staff could not have been more accommodating.

I am indeed fortunate to have learnt from many laryngologists all over the world and I hope to be able to teach as generously as I was taught. Professor Marc Remacle has not only been an amazing teacher for me, but also someone who has always encouraged me in my endeavors, and I am honored that he has written a Foreword to this book.

Finally, I would like to thank the person who is integral to the birth of this atlas, my mentor, Professor Milind V Kirtane.

Nupur Kapoor Nerurkar

Contents

Abbreviations

AKT	Anti Kochs treatment
AORRP	Adult onset recurrent respiratory papillomatosis
BLVFP	Bilateral vocal fold paralysis
BMZ	Basement membrane zone
CC	Clara chroma
CO_2	Carbon dioxide
CT	Computed tomography
DNA	Deoxyribonucleic acid
E	Endoscopic
ESR	Erythrocyte sedimentation rate
H&E	Hematoxylin and eosin
HD	High definition
HPV	Human papillomavirus
JORRP	Juvenile-onset recurrent respiratory papillomatosis
KOH	Potassium hydroxide
KTP	Potassium titanyl phosphate
M	Microscopic
MLS	Microlaryngoscopy
NBI	Narrow Band Imaging
NF1	Neurofibromatosis type 1
OT	Operation theater
PNS	Peripheral nervous system
RA	Rheumatoid arthritis
RL	Rigid laryngoscopy
RRP	Recurrent respiratory papillomatosis
SA	Spectra A
SB	Spectra B
SEC	Subepithelial cyst
SEH	Subepithelial hemorrhage
SEIT	Subepithelial infiltration technique
SLP	Superficial lamina propria
TB	Tuberculosis
TLM	Transoral laser microsurgery
URTI	Upper respiratory tract infection
VLS	Videolaryngoscopy
WL	White light

CHAPTER 1

Microscopic Anatomy of the Vocal Folds

INTRODUCTION

The vocal folds have been defined as two fold-like structures that extend from the middle of the angle of the thyroid cartilage to the vocal processes of the arytenoid cartilages.[1] However, these are the membranous vocal folds, and the area including and posterior to the vocal process, is the cartilaginous vocal fold.

The true and false vocal folds were earlier referred to as vocal "cords." The term was coined by the French anatomist Antoine Ferrein in 1741.[2] As the understanding of the laryngeal structure improved, anatomists realized that rather than being a "cord" or a band being attached at either end and suspended in the larynx, these are actually "folds" of membranes which are just lips of tissue covered with mucosa. The false vocal folds or the vestibular folds do not contain any muscle and are formed by respiratory mucosa covering the vestibular ligament. The true vocal folds, however, are covered by stratified squamous epithelium and do contain a muscle (thyroarytenoid) and have a multilayered anatomy, which is critical to its efficient vibration. The point of maximum contact on the true vocal folds during phonation is the mid-membranous vocal fold, referred to as the "striking zone" and most phonotraumatic lesions are found at this site. The epithelium over the anterior vibratory portion of the larynx is stratified squamous epithelium and in the posterior glottis pseudostratified ciliated epithelium.

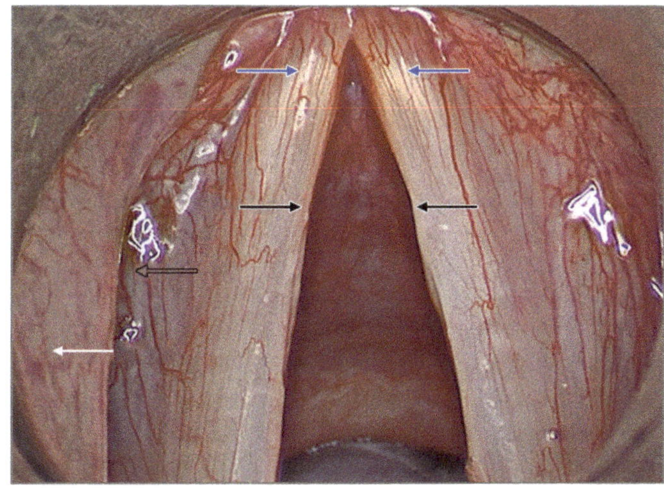

FIG. 1.1: Microlaryngoscopic view of the true vocal folds. Blue arrows: anterior macula flava; black solid arrows: striking zone of the true vocal folds; black hollow arrow: left ventricle; white solid arrow: left false vocal fold. An endotracheal tube is seen in the subglottis. (M-CC)

Stroboscopic evaluation is a gold standard of care for both diagnosis and management of voice disorders. It is essential not only in assessing the pathology but also in evaluating the mucosal wave (vibration) of the rest of the normal looking vocal folds.

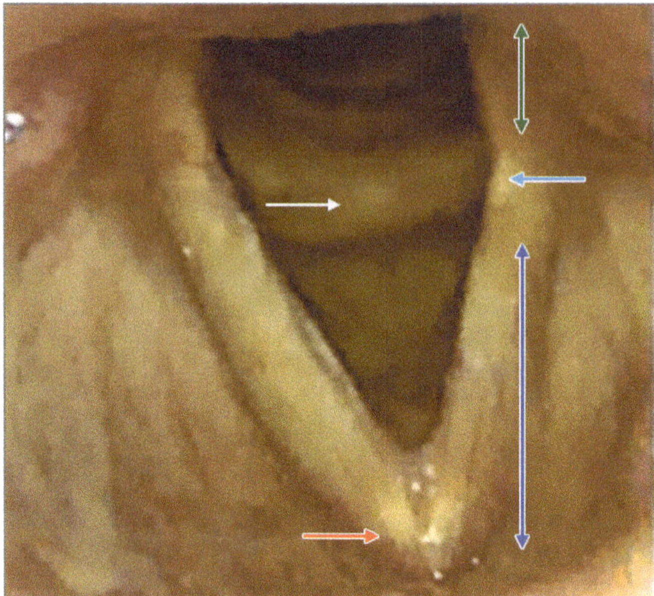

FIG. 1.2: Stroboscopy view with a 70-degree rigid laryngoscope. Red arrow: right macula flava (not to be confused with any lesion); light blue arrow: left vocal process of the arytenoid; dark blue arrow: membranous vocal fold (3/5th length of entire vocal fold); green arrow: cartilaginous vocal fold (2/5th length of entire vocal fold); white arrow: cricoid cartilage indentation in the subglottis

The slit-like space between the true and false vocal fold is the ventricle of the larynx (Morgagni's sinus), which anteriorly leads to a pouch like diverticulum in a vertically upwards direction. This pouch is called the laryngeal saccule or appendix of the laryngeal ventricle or Hiltons pouch and is a mucous membrane lined sac. This sinus lies between the false vocal fold, thyroarytenoid muscle, and the thyroid cartilage. This saccule has a rich cover of mucous glands which when squeezed by the surrounding muscles release mucous to lubricate the vocal folds.

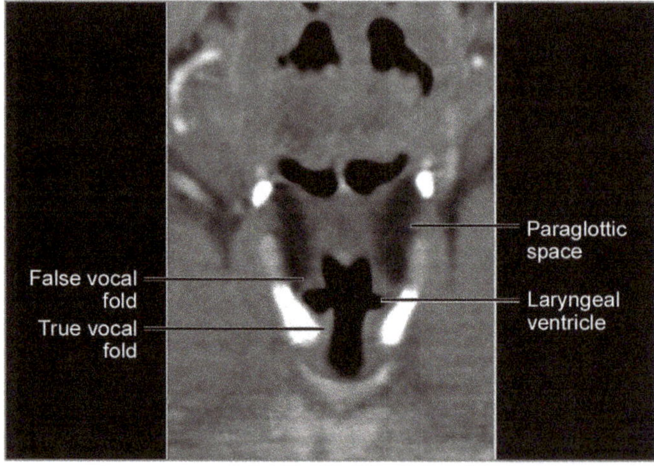

FIG. 1.3: Computed tomography scan coronal image showing the laryngeal ventricle between the false and true vocal folds

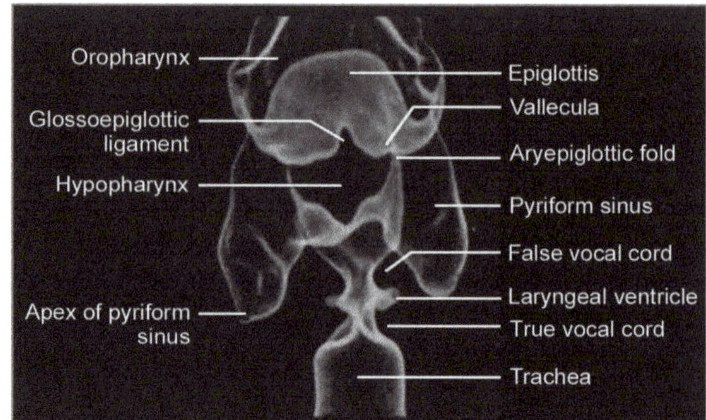

FIG. 1.4: Computed tomography scan 3D reconstruction of a normal larynx

MULTILAYERED ANATOMY OF THE TRUE VOCAL FOLDS

The true vocal folds have a multilayered anatomy, which is the basis of Hirano's cover-body theory of phonation proposed in 1974.[3] Histologically, the vocal folds consists of five layers—squamous epithelium, lamina propria (three layers), and the vocalis muscle. These five anatomical layers work as increasingly stiffer three mechanical layers during vibration. The "cover" is composed of the epithelium and the superficial layer of the lamina propria. The intermediate and deep layers of the lamina propria comprise the "transition" layer and the vocalis muscle act as the "body." As air passes between the vocal folds, the loose "cover" moves in a wave-like motion over the stiffer "body". The cover is pliable and elastic, while the body uses its contractile properties to allow for the adjustment of the stiffness of the vocal fold.

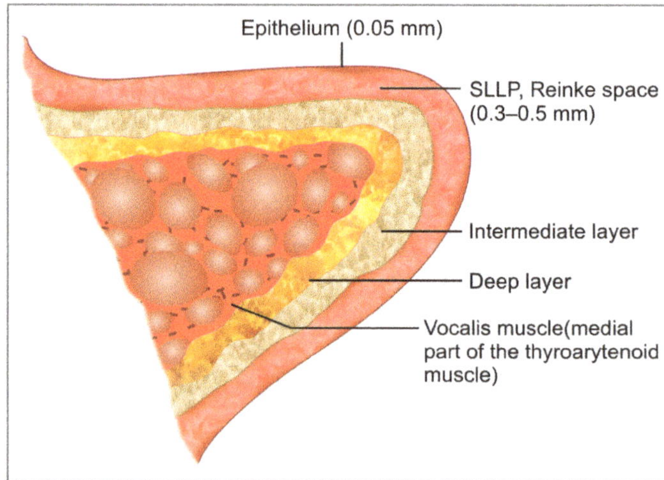

FIG. 1.5: The layered microstructure of the true vocal folds

The epithelium over the membranous vocal folds is only about 5–25 cell thick, the most superficial part containing only 1–3 cells which are lost due to the abrasions produced during phonation. This thin stratified squamous epithelium layer of the mucosa has no mucous glands and this helps to maintain the shape of the vocal folds. The surface cells slough off into the laryngeal lumen as new cells migrate superiorly and medially to replace them. The luminal layer of the mucous blanket is composed of mucin molecules, and ensures adequate moisture and lubrication of the vocal folds. The inner serous layer has high water content and is in direct contact with the squamous cells of the vocal fold epithelium and the cilia of the pseudocolumnar cells of the glottis. This facilitates the mucociliary transport of secretions up from the trachea and through the glottis for expectoration.

The basal lamina or the basement membrane zone provides support to the epithelium, and serves as a transition zone between the epithelium and the Reinke's space. It has two layers: the lamina lucida (low density, clear zone) and lamina densa (higher density of filament).

Anchoring filaments, made of type IV collagen and fibronectin, secure the lamina lucida to the lamina densa. Anchoring fibrils made of type VII collagen loop between the lamina densa and the underlying lamina propria. These anchoring fibrils provide structural integrity to this delicate tissue transition interface, especially in the areas of maximum shear and stress and hence, their density is highest in the midmembranous region which is the area prone to maximum phonotrauma.[4] The number of anchoring fibrils is thought to be genetically determined, which means that there might be a genetic predisposition to developing vocal fold lesions.

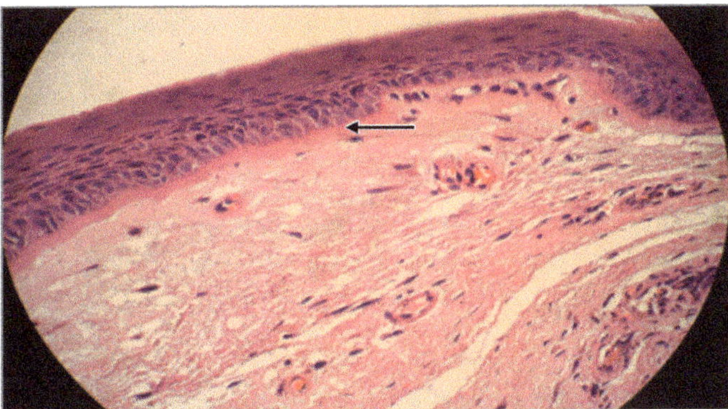

FIG. 1.6: Microscopic image of the epithelium and superficial lamina propria after H&E staining, demonstrating the basement membrane zone of the epithelium (black arrow)

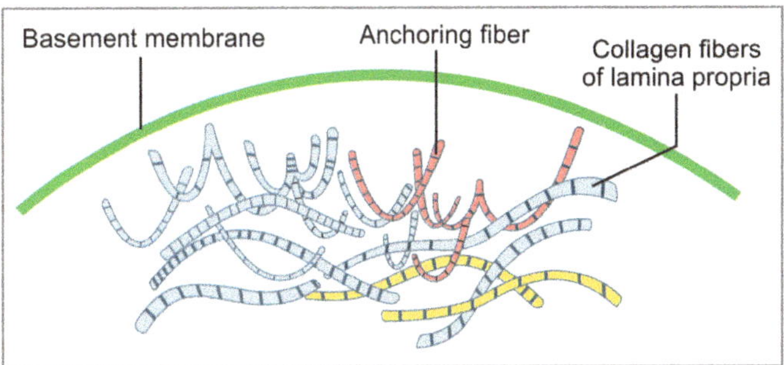

FIG. 1.7: Image of the anchoring fibrils from basal lamina or the basement membrane zone to SLP as described by Dr. Gray in 1994[5]

Beneath the basement membrane is the lamina propria which has three layers: superficial, intermediate, and deep. The superficial lamina propria (SLP), also known as Reinke's space, is acellular and made up of loose fibroareolar tissue and extracellular matrix proteins, water, and loosely arranged fibers of elastin and collagen. The gelatinous nature of the SLP provides it with the visco-elasticity that is needed during vibration and allows the overlying epithelium (cover) to vibrate smoothly and at high speeds over the underlying vocal ligament and muscle (body). This formed the anatomical basis of Hirano's body-cover theory.[3]

The intermediate layer (mostly composed of elastin fibers) and the deep layer (mostly composed of collagen fibers and fibroblasts) together form the vocal ligament. Deep to the vocal ligament lies the thyroarytenoid muscle, medial part of which is referred to as the vocalis.

The vocal folds on either side join anteriorly at the anterior commissure. The tendinous condensation of fibers which joins the vocal folds to the inner perichondrium of the thyroid cartilage is called the Broyles' tendon. The Broyles' tendon contains both lymphatics and blood vessels. It receives the attachments of the ligaments, membranes, and muscles from either sides of the larynx and thus serves as a natural barrier for malignancies of the glottis.[6] Due to this, anterior spread of glottic malignancies is usually supra or infraglottic. Once the Broyles' tendon is breached, the malignancy erodes through to the thyroid cartilage.

The intermediate layer of the lamina propria is thickened at the anterior and posterior ends of membranous vocal folds forming the anterior and posterior macula flava. The macula flavae are located at the anterior and posterior ends of the vocal folds. They have been likened to shock absorbers linking the cartilage at either end of the vocal ligament to the vocal folds. These are elliptical bodies, 1.5 mm × 1.5 mm × 1.0 mm in size, composed of elastic fibers, collagen fibers, fibroblasts, and a ground substance. The macula flava seem to control the synthesis of fibrous components in the vocal ligaments and are responsible for the metabolism of the extracellular matrices which provides viscoelasticity to the lamina propria.[7] They can, therefore, be regarded as the progenitors of the lamina propria.

The posterior glottis or the interarytenoid region is an illdefined area at the junction of the posterior ends of both vocal folds and postcricoid region. It constitutes 35–45% of the entire glottis length and 50–65% of the entire glottis area.[16] Consequently, most of the air passage happens through this region of the glottis. Many authors believe that it is more intimately related to the subglottis rather than the glottis and should be regarded as a part of it as such.[8] The thickening of the interarytenoid region is seen quite often in laryngopharyngeal reflux which is referred to as interarytenoid pachydermia, drawing similarity with the skin of an elephant (pachyderm).

AGE- AND GENDER-RELATED DIFFERENCES IN VOCAL FOLD STRUCTURE

The infant vocal folds are 6–8 mm in length while the adult vocal folds are around 16 mm. The infant lamina propria is only one cell thick and there is no vocal ligament. By the age of 4 years, the vocal ligament begins to appear. The lamina propria becomes two layered by age 6–12 and by adolescence, the layered microstructure is completely established. In females during puberty, the thyroarytenoid becomes thicker but remains narrow and supple. Under the influence of progesterone, there is a diuretic effect which decreases capillary permeability and traps extracellular fluids out of the capillaries causing tissue congestion. This explains why some women experience a subtle change in their voice quality during the menstrual cycle. In men, the testosterone spurt during puberty causes the thyroid prominence to appear (Adam's apple) and the vocal folds to become longer and more rounded. Females have less hyaluronic acid in the Reinke's space than males, which implies lesser protection from vibratory trauma and overuse; and this may explain why women are more prone to vocal lesions than men.[4] As age advances, there is a steady increase in the elastin content of the lamina propria. The vocalis muscle atrophies in both men and women, but in women, the SLP becomes edematous and the epithelium thickens. In men the deep layers of lamina propria show thickening due to increased deposition of collagen.

REFERENCES

1. Neil Weir, Anatomy of the Larynx. In: Milind Kirtane, Chris de Souza, Abir Bhattacharyya, Nupur Nerurkar, editors. Otorhinolaryngology-Head and Neck Surgery Series, Thieme; 2014. pp. 21-37.
2. Antoine Ferrein (1693–1759). Available from: https://en.wikipedia.org/wiki/Antoine_Ferrein.
3. Hirano M. Morphological structure of the vocal cord as a vibrator and its variations. Folia Phoniatr (Basel). 1974;26(2):89-94.
4. Colton R, Casper JK, Leonard R. Morphology of vocal fold mucosa: histology to genomics. In: Colton R, Casper JK, Leonard R, editors. Understanding voice problems: A physiological perspective for diagnosis and treatment, 4th ed. Philadelphia: Lippincott Williams & Wilkins; 2011. pp. 6475.
5. Gray SD, Pignatari SN, Harding P. Morphologic ultrastructure of anchoring fibers in the normal vocal fold basement membrane zone. J Voice. l994;8:48-52.
6. Desloge RB, Zeitels SM. Endolaryngeal microsurgery at the anterior glottal commissure: controversies and observations. Ann Otol Rhinol Laryngol. 2000;109:385-92.
7. Sato K, Hirano M. Histological investigation of the macula flava of the human vocal fold. Ann Otol Rhinol Laryngol. 1995;104(2):138-43.
8. Mcllwain JC. The posterior glottis. J Otolaryngol. 1991;20(Suppl 2):124.

CHAPTER 2

Principles of Phonomicrosurgery

INTRODUCTION

Phonomicrosurgery refers to surgeries performed on the vocal folds at high magnification, which are concerned with improvement or restoration of voice quality through restoration of vocal fold function or more specifically vocal fold vibration.[1]

Prior to any phonomicrosurgical procedure, the patient must receive adequate voice therapy and conservative medical management. Functional and systemic disorders responsible for the voice change should be ruled out. Having exhausted these as treatment modalities, one may move in the direction of surgical intervention. Absence of any guarantee of vocal improvement after surgery with a detailed informed consent (discussed in chapter 3) is essential.

A stroboscopic evaluation or a series of stroboscopies prior to and following surgery is equally essential. Not only does this guide our diagnosis, decision-making and progress of treatment, it gives us an idea of the nonfunctional areas of the vocal fold prior to surgical intervention. Like a computed tomography (CT) scan is needed prior to endoscopic sinus surgery and an audiogram is needed prior to ear surgery, a stroboscopy is essential prior to phonomicrosurgery.

The principles of phonomicrosurgery are based on the cover-body theory of Hirano,[2] which explains the vocal fold vibration, based on the layered microanatomy of the vocal folds as studied under the electron microscope.

The convergence of physiological principles of phonation, i.e., mucosal wave oscillation to microsurgery is phonomicrosurgery. The mantra of phonomicrosurgery is not to remove any excess normal tissue, especially in the superficial lamina propria (SLP), to stay close to the lesion being dissected in benign lesions, to preserve the epithelium in subepithelial lesions, and to respect the anterior commissure.

Since the SLP has a poor propensity towards regeneration, it should be maximally preserved. The epithelium does regenerate slowly, however having an epithelial cover, especially near the anterior commissure, prevents synechiae and web formation.

HISTORICAL ASPECTS

In 1963, Von Leden and Arnold defined the term "phonosurgery."[3] Traditionally, a benign lesion of the vocal fold was excised by holding it and cutting it at its base. This led to the loss of a variable amount of SLP and occasionally the vocal ligament. Often the epithelium was held and torn off in what was referred to as a "mucosal stripping technique"[4] by special instruments made for this purpose, as it was felt at that time that this would help in removal of unhealthy tissue and promote healthy epithelial regeneration.

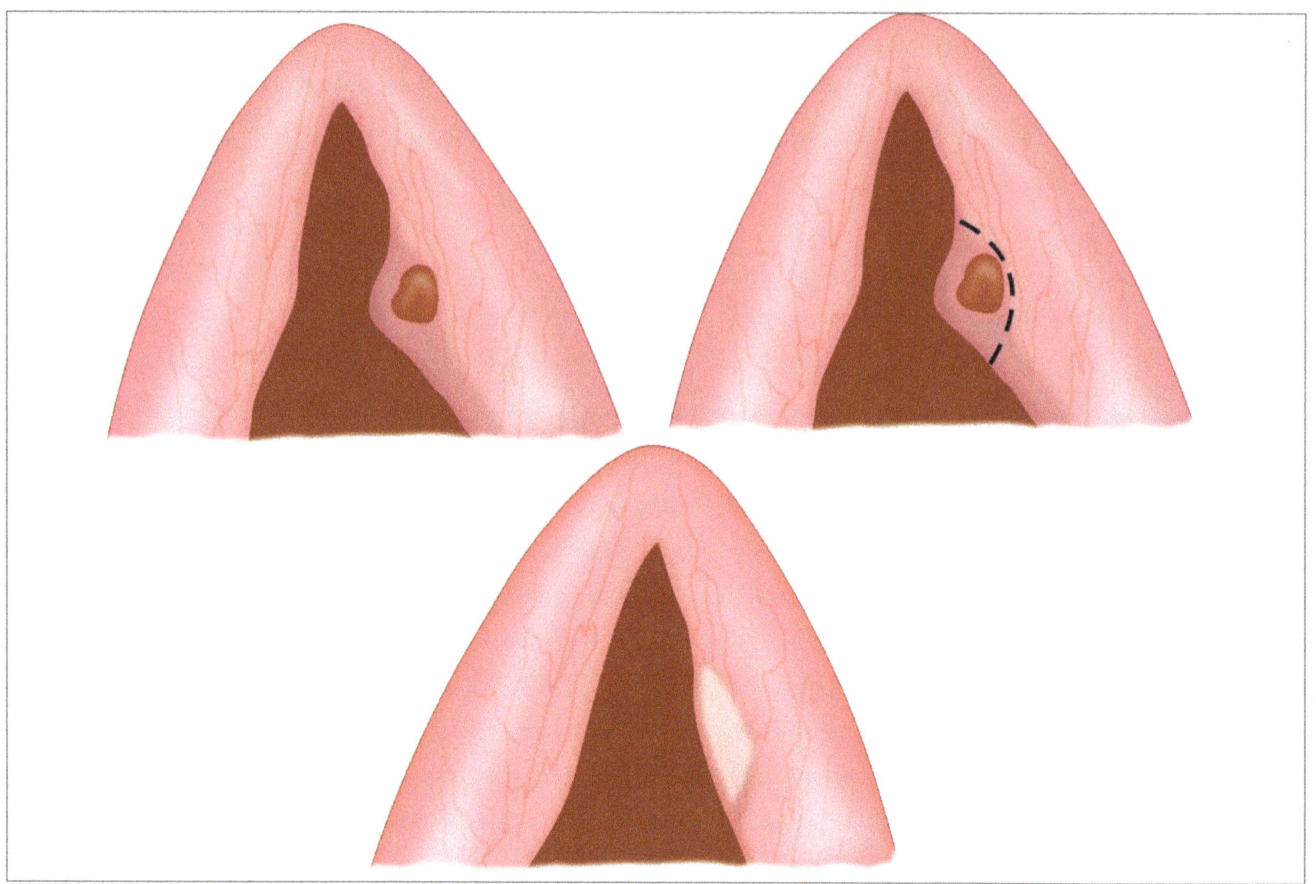

FIG. 2.1: Diagrammatic representation of a right hemorrhagic cyst cut at its base with the exposed vocal ligament seen in white

Once the microanatomy and importance of the microlayered structure of the vocal folds towards vibration was understood, the principles of phonomicrosurgery started developing. The development and routine use of stroboscopy made it easier to understand the correlation between microlayered anatomy preservation for a good mucosal wave formation. Absolutely straight postoperative vocal folds following stripping would be seen to have a poorer vibration than those in whom the dissection had stayed superficial and respected the microlayered anatomy.

Courey et al. proposed the lateral[5] and medial microflap[6] surgery. The principle of the lateral microflap surgery is to take an incision on the epithelium quite lateral to the pathological lesion. The epithelial elevation at this point is easier in deep lesions as identification of the various layers is easier in the absence of pathology. The epithelium is elevated in a medial direction and the subepithelial pathology is dissected, staying close to it, in order to preserve maximum SLP. The epithelial flap is then reposited back into place.

The medial microflap surgery is different from the lateral microflap in that the incision is taken nearer the lesion, but again lateral to it. This is for lesions which are more superficial and where the surgical planes immediately around the lesion are well identifiable.

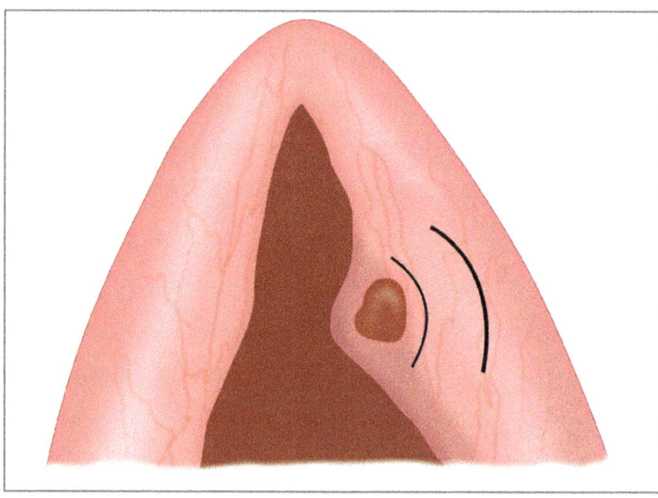

FIG. 2.2: Thicker lateral microflap incision and thinner medial microflap incision in a diagrammatic representation of a right hemorrhagic cyst excision

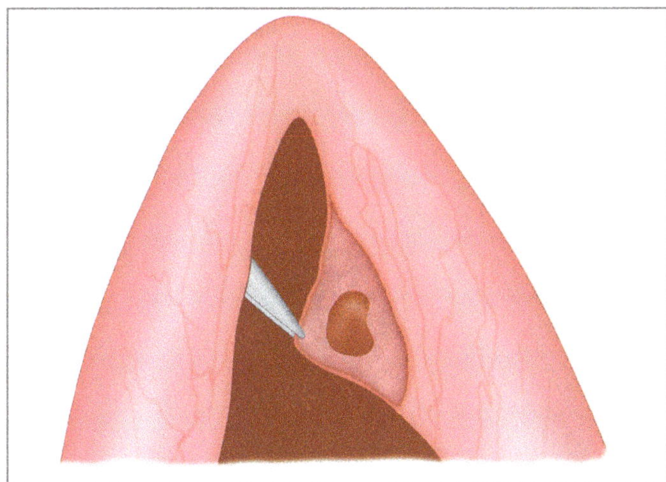

FIG. 2.3: Elevation of the epithelial flap as an inferiorly based one, with dissection around the lesion, staying as close to it as possible

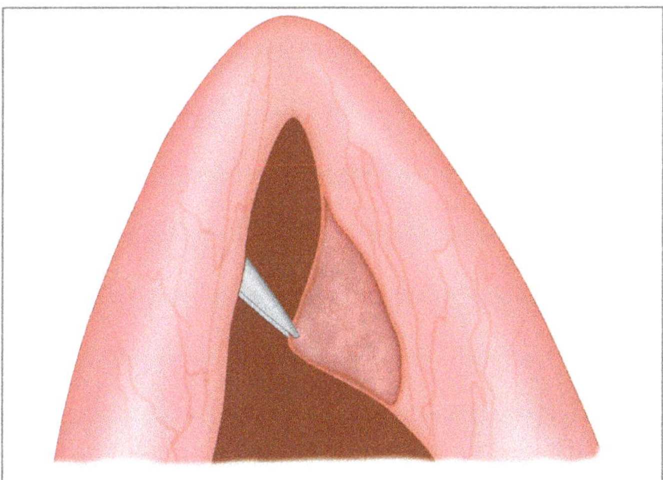

FIG. 2.4: Removal of the cyst with maximum preservation of the superficial lamina propria and the overlying epithelium

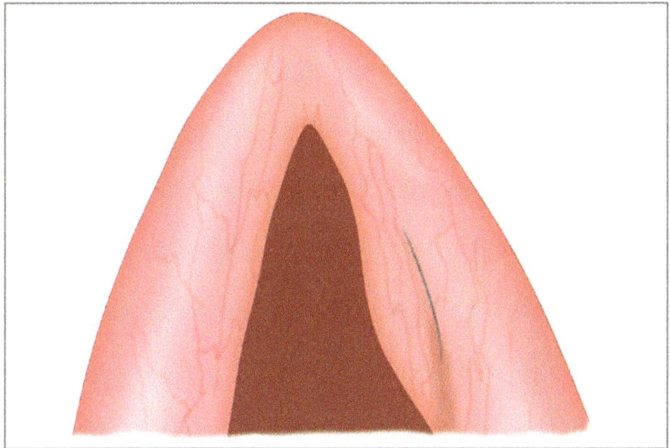

FIG. 2.5: The epithelial flap is now reposited back in position

Gray in 1991[7] demonstrated a complex basement membrane structure between the epithelium and superficial layer of the lamina propria. His studies revealed that the basement membrane is attached to the superficial layer of the lamina propria through an intricate series of type VII collagen loops. These loops emanate from and return to basement membrane cells. Collagen fibers of the superficial layer of the lamina propria pass through them (*see* Chapter 1, Fig. 1.7). This highly sophisticated architectural arrangement is probably variable from person to person and perhaps from family to family.

Thus, the technique of microflap surgery changed with emphasis now placed on minimal epithelial elevation with consequently minimal disturbance to the anchoring loops architecture. The term "mini-microflap" was introduced by Sataloff in 1995,[8] where the epithelial cordotomy is taken directly on the lesion and a very small epithelial flap is elevated or the small epithelial cover over the lesion is sacrificed.

However, the philosophy of minimal elevation of epithelium, preserving maximum SLP, and attempting an epithelial cover remains.

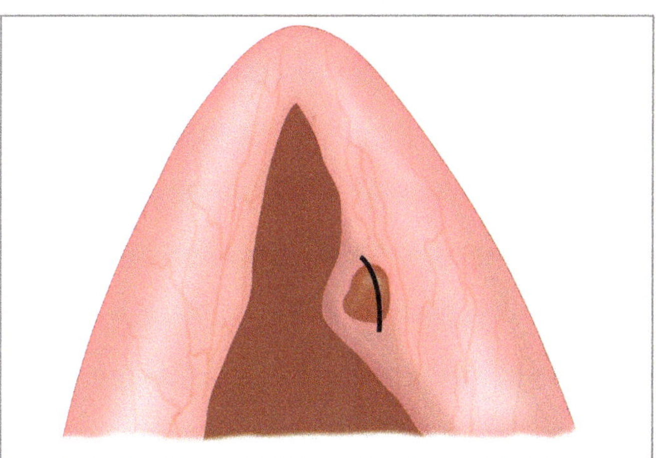

FIG. 2.6: Mini-microflap incision made on the lesion, with minimal overlying epithelium excised with the lesion if needed

What most surgeons propose today is making an incision extremely close to the lesion, minimum elevation of uninvolved epithelium, and staying close to the lesion during dissection to preserve maximum SLP. The most useful epithelium that provides cover of the medial vibrating edge at the completion of surgery is the infraglottic epithelium seen as the dark black area in 2.7

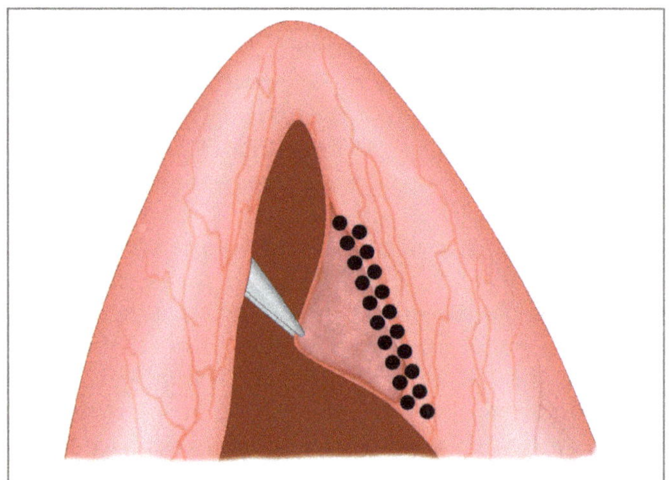

FIG. 2.7: Preservation of the infraglottic epithelium (black dotted area) helps to cover the medial vibrating edge of the operated vocal fold

SUBEPITHELIAL INFILTRATION TECHNIQUE

The concept of laryngeal infusion was introduced in the 1890s for the purpose of anatomic studies.[9,10] The technique has been used for a variety of purposes, including infusion of steroids to disrupt adhesions in vocal fold scar, placement of collagen along the vibratory margin, and separating benign and malignant lesions from underlying structures. The technique has become more popular among clinicians since the 1990s.[11,12]

Many studies highlight the improved vocal outcomes and early return of mucosal wave following SEIT.[13,14] Subepithelial infiltration technique is performed using a 27 gauge needle with 1-2 cc of 1:10,000 saline adrenaline.

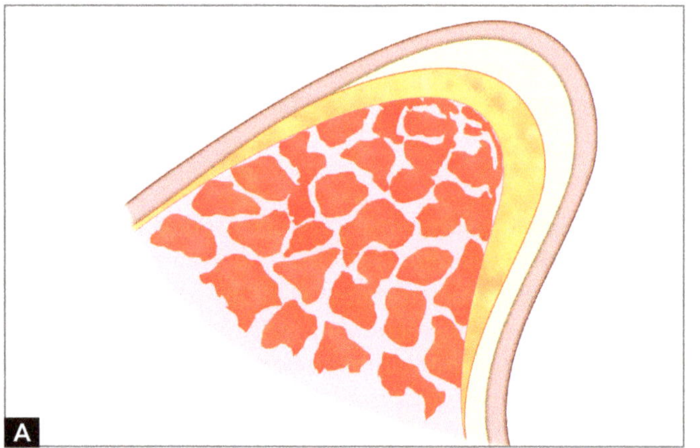

Continued

Continued

B

FIG. 2.8: Diagramatic representation of the ballooning up of the superficial lamina propria after subepithelial infiltration technique. The 27 gauge needle is just below the epithelium

BOX 2.1	Advantages of sub-epithelial infiltration

- Hemostasis
- Clearer demarcation of margins of the lesion
- Depth penetration estimation
- Hydrostatic distention of superficial lamina propria temporarily which allows preservation of layered microstructure
- Hydrodissection
- Acts as heat sink in case laser is being used

Subepithelial infiltration technique may be counter-productive in small cysts as they may be difficult to identify following the infiltration and in Reinke's edema where there already is excess SLP.

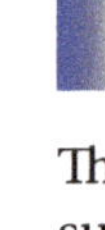

INSTRUMENTATION FOR PHONOMICROSURGERY

The equipment required in order to perform phonomicrosurgery includes:

- High end microscope with a 400 mm lens
- A variety of microlaryngoscopes of different sizes
- Suspension system
- Mayos trolley attached to the operation theater table for fulcrum suspension system
- Telescopes (0, 30, 70 degrees)
- Tooth protection guards
- Microlaryngoscopy chair with arm rest
- Cold steel instruments
- Laser with scanning system (if laser phonomicrosurgery being performed)
- Microdebrider with laryngeal blades.

COLD STEEL INSTRUMENTS IN PHONOMICROSURGERY

Conventional phonomicrosurgery instruments have a tip of 3-4 mm and what is needed for mini-microflap surgery are instrument tips that are 1-2 mm.

Besides a 27 gauge infiltration needle, sharp sickle knife, sharp scissors (right, left, straight, and up-cutting), crocodile (straight, right, and left), microflap suction, the microflap elevators (sharp, blunt—30, 70 degree) and Bouchayer forceps (upward, straight, right, and left) are critical for precise microflap surgery. The Bouchayer forceps allows tissue to be held atraumatically because of the fenestrae present.

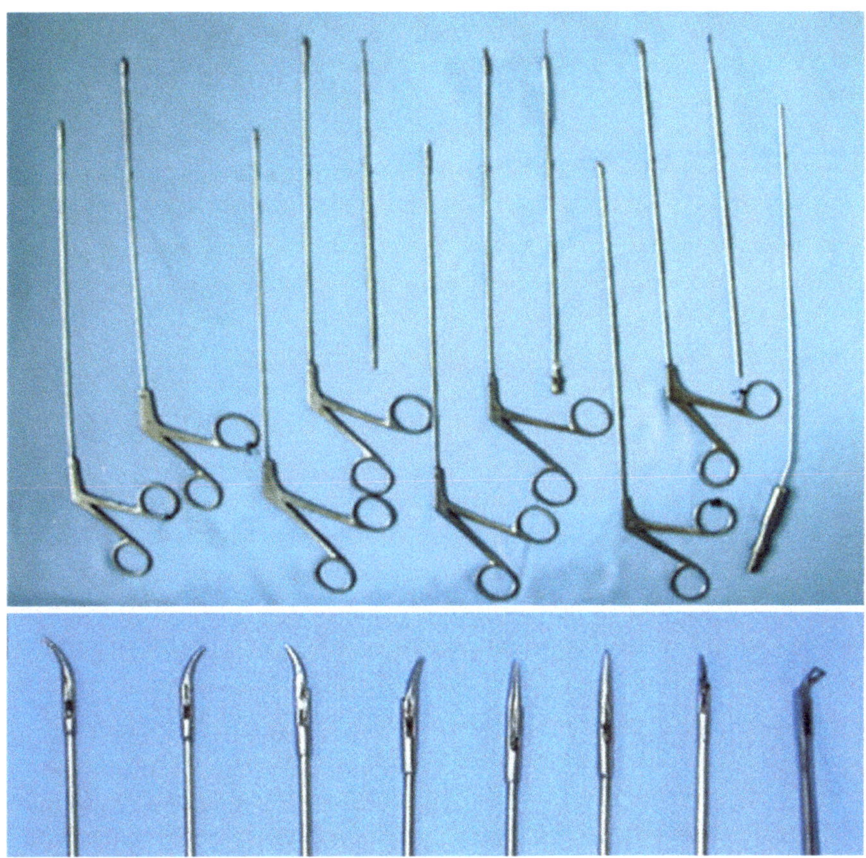

FIG. 2.9: Phonomicrosurgery instruments including crocodile forceps, scissors, and Bouchayer forceps

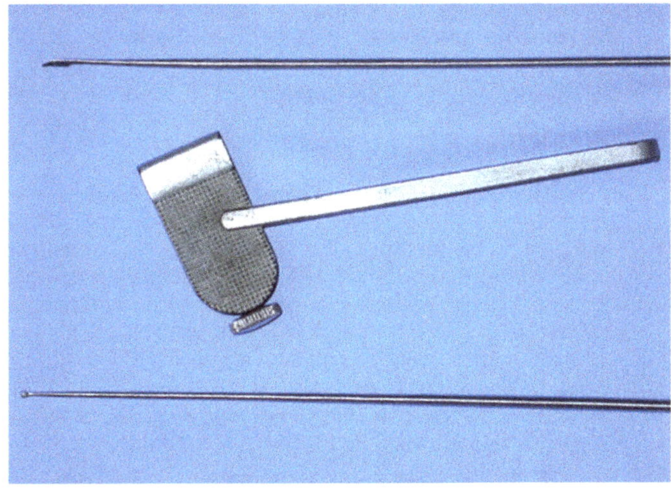

FIG. 2.10: Microflap sickle, universal handle, and microflap elevator

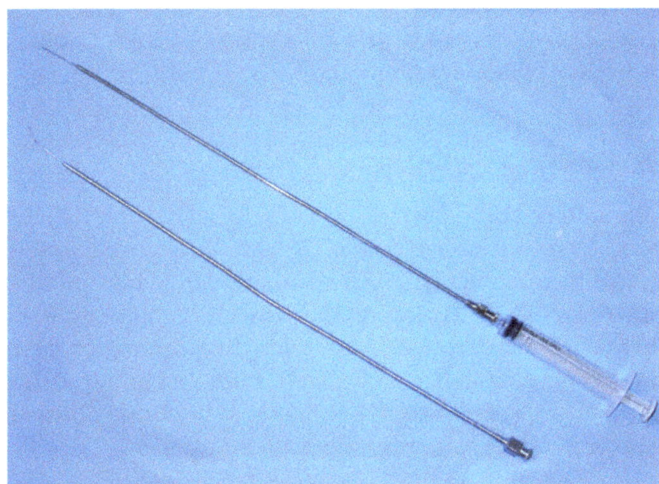

FIG. 2.11: 27 gauge infiltration needle

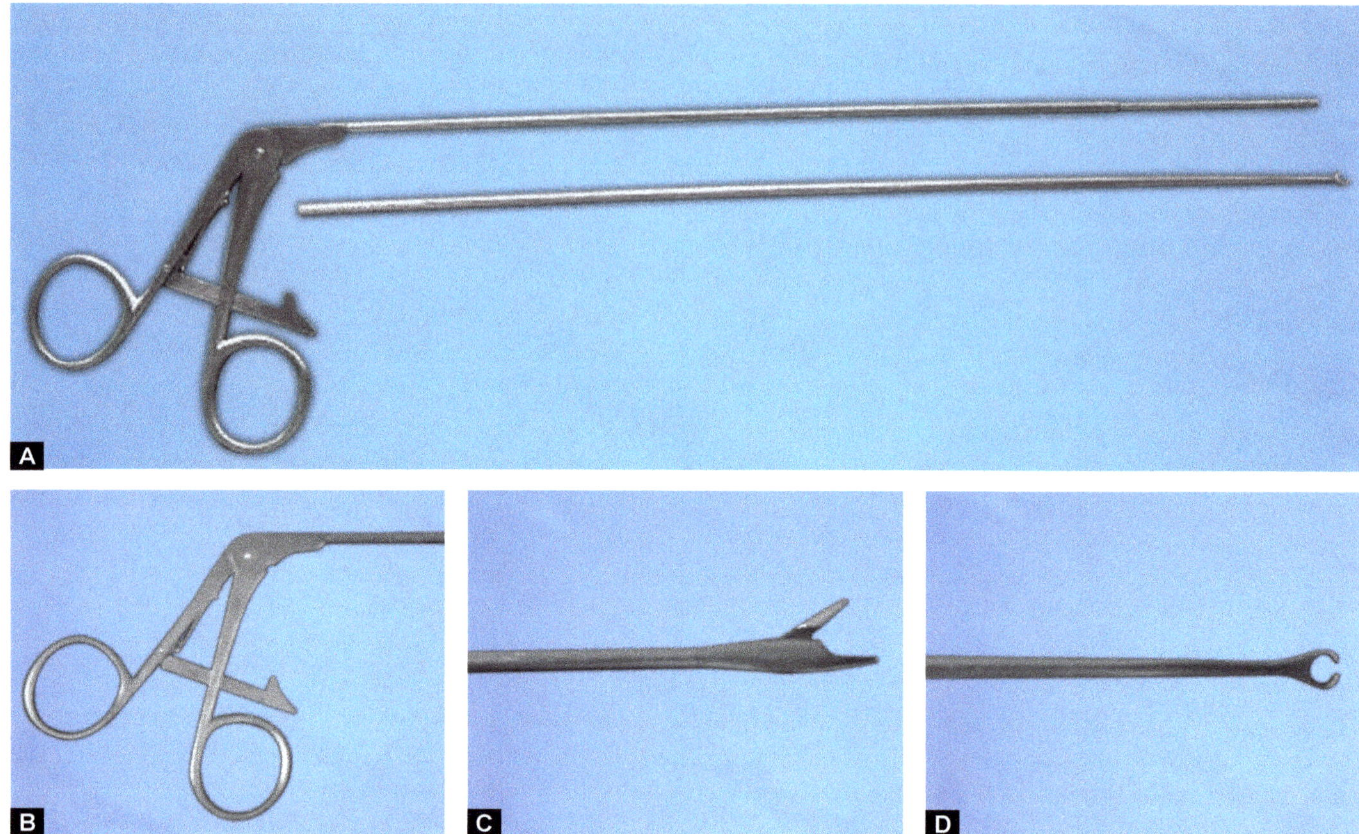

FIG. 2.12: Two instruments needed for suturing in the larynx. A needle holder with a lock and ratchet system and a claw shaped knot slider

POWERED INSTRUMENTS IN PHONOMICROSURGERY

The laryngeal microdebrider is extremely useful in bulky papillomas for which a 3.5 mm Tricut laryngeal blade is used at 1,400–2,000 rpm.

The skimmer laryngeal blade is used for carpet like papillomas over the vocal fold. Typically a 2.9 mm blade is used at 800–1,000 rpm.

LASERS

The commonest laser to be used in laryngology is the CO_2 laser. However, the KTP and pulsed dye lasers (both haemoangiolytic) are also popular. When phonomicrosurgery is being performed, it is advisable to use extremely precise lasers with the scanning system available which have negligible heat dissipation. If such a laser is not available, it is preferable to perform cold steel surgery in benign glottic lesions.

The author uses the CO_2 AcuBlade routinely for phonomicrosurgery. The typical settings are scanner mode, 10 W, superpulse repeat mode with a depth of 2 (500 microns) and a length of the AcuBlade as 1–2 mm. These settings may vary occasionally depending on the case.

Laser safety precautions (discussed in chapter 3) are always maintained.

The motto in phonomicrosurgery should be "to do no harm".

REFERENCES

1. Peter CB, Mark SC. Principles and essentials of phonomicrosurgery. In: Nupur KN, Roychoudhury A, editors. Textbook of laryngology: Official publication of the Association of Phonosurgeons of India. New Delhi: Jaypee Brothers Medical Publishers (P) Ltd.; 2017. pp 139-46.
2. Hirano M. Structure and vibratory behavior of the vocal fold. In: Sawashima M, Cooper FS, editors. Dynamic aspects of speech production. Tokyo, Japan; University of Tokyo Press: 1977. pp. 13-30.
3. Zeitels S. The history and development of phonosurgery. In: Satalo RT, editor. Profes-sional voice: the science and art of clinical care. 3rd ed. San Diego (CA): Plural Publishing, Inc.; 2006. p. 1115-36.

4. Lore JM. Stripping of the vocal chords. Laryngoscope. 1934:44(10):803-16.
5. Courey MS, Gardner GM, Stone RE, et al. Endoscopic vocal fold microflap: A three year experience. Ann Otol Rhinol Laryngol. 1995;104:267-73.
6. Courey MS, Garrett CG, Ossoff RH. Medial microflap for excision of benign vocal fold lesions. Laryngoscope. 1997;107:340-4.
7. Gray S. Basement membrane zone injury in vocal nodules. In: Gauffin J, Hammarberg B, editors. Vocal fold physiology. San Diego (CA): Singular Publishing Group; 1991.p. 21–8.
8. Sataloff RT, Spiegel JR, Heuer RJ, et al. Laryngeal mini-microflap: A new technique and reassessment of the microflap saga. J Voice. 1995;9(2):198–204.
9. Hajek M. Anatomische untersuchungen uber das larynxodem. Arch Klin Chir. 1891;42:46-93.
10. Pressman J, Dowdy A, Libby R, et al. Further studies upon the submucosal compartments and lymphatics of the larynx by the injection of dyes and radioisotope. Ann Otol Rhinol Laryngol. 1956;65:963-80.
11. Welsh LW, Welsh JJ, Rizzo TA Jr. Laryngeal spaces and lymphatics: Current anatomic concepts. Ann Otol Rhinol Laryngol Suppl. 1983;105:19-31.
12. Kass ES, Hillman RE, Zeitels SM. Vocal fold submucosal infusion technique in phonomicrosurgery. Ann Otol Rhinol Laryngol. 1996;105(5): 341-7.
13. Nerurkar N, Narkar N, Joshi A, et al. Vocal outcomes following subepithelial infiltration technique in microflap surgery: A review of 30 cases
14. Hochman II, Zeitels SM. Phonomicrosurgical management of vocal fold polyps: The subepithelial microflap resection technique. J Voice. 2000;14(1):112-8.

CHAPTER 3

Microlaryngoscopy for Phonomicrosurgery

INTRODUCTION

A satisfactory visualization of the larynx, particularly the lesion being operated upon, is a prerequisite for phonomicrosurgery. Handling situations of an anterior larynx, anterior laryngeal lesion, large tongue, edentulous patient, restricted mouth opening, short stiff neck with reduced neck extension, reduced occipitoatlanto extension, and retrognathia are discussed in this chapter.

PREDICTING A DIFFICULT MICROLARYNGOSCOPY

Presently available studies shows thyromandibular angle value >120 degrees in men and 130 degrees in women,[1] body mass index of >25.0 kg/m,[2] thyroid-mental distance of <5.5 cm,[2] neck circumference >40 cm,[3] horizontal thyromental distance <6.05 cm,[3] sternomental distance <13.9 cm,[1] and modified Cormack-Lehane Score[4] as the significant parameters for a difficult laryngeal exposure. A study done by Paul et al. in 2016 concludes that neck girth, atlanto-occipital extension, and the modified Cormack-Lehane Score are significant in predicting difficult laryngeal exposure for microlaryngoscopy (MLS).[5]

Typically, a Pickwickian person[6] (short, fat, short neck) is thought to be a difficult MLS. However, many of these patients are not difficult to intubate or operate upon. However, they can desaturate postextubation repeatedly if they are not completely awake, at the time of extubation, and in an upright position. The Malampati classification is an indicator used by the anesthetists for the ease of intubation. The author finds that if a preoperative 70-degree rigid laryngoscopy reveals a good view of the entire larynx, then the exposure for MLS is usually not a challenge. However, if the larynx is not visible with a rigid laryngoscope, but only visible with a flexible laryngoscope, then the laryngeal exposure during MLS may be difficult. The ease of intubation for the anesthetist immediately serves as a guide to the ease of MLS.

It is advisable to have a difficult intubation cart ready for all cases. This should include a flexible pediatric intubating bronchoscope and small endotracheal tubes with atraumatic but firm stillettes. Once the anesthetist can achieve good ventilation with a bag and mask, the patient can be given a relaxant. The patient is oxygenated for 5–7 minutes and the anesthetist attempts laryngoscopy. If the larynx is difficult to visualize but the posterior opening can be seen, an attempt is made to gently introduce a stillete into the airway, over which the endotracheal tube may be rail-roaded. If this is unsuccessful, an under vision flexible laryngoscopy guided intubation is performed. In order to have a per-oral intubation, the anesthetist holds the Macintosh laryngoscope (without a light) and the flexible laryngoscope with the endotracheal tube railroaded on it is introduced under vision in to the subglottis. Once the tracheal rings are seen, the tube in held in position and the flexible scope is withdrawn. The Macintosh laryngoscope not only provides easy oral access but also prevents the teeth from suddenly biting and damaging the flexible scope.

TECHNIQUE OF MICROLARYNGOSCOPY

Jackson, years ago, advised that the upper airway is seen best when the cervical spine is straight and the chin is thrust forward, and today, when we use the Boyce-Jackson "sniffing position" while performing indirect laryngoscopy, we continue to follow this advice.[7] A flexion of the neck on the chest with an extension of the head on the neck (atlanto-occipital joint) is the Boyce's position. During MLS, this is best achieved with a 15-degree head elevation. Many surgeons use the Boyce-Jackson position for MLS. In most MLS cases, the author prefers no head elevation but a head and neck extension, with head elevation preferred only for difficult cases. Tooth guards are placed, especially for the upper teeth. For edentulous patients, a moist cottonoid covered by the tooth guard or foam may be used. It is important to have various types of microlaryngoscopes to select from. The author routinely uses a Kleinsasser laryngoscope or a Dedo laryngoscope. Occasionally, the Kantor-Berci video laryngoscope system is used when the laser is not needed. There are various techniques to introduce a microlaryngoscope. The aim is to introduce the largest size scope that can fit atraumatically and without infolding of the epiglottis.

For a right handed surgeon, the mouth is opened with the right hand, the scope is held in the left hand and introduced keeping the tongue central. The lips should be under view and not caught between the teeth and the scope. The scope is passed parallel to the tongue till the tongue base is reached, . Once the epiglottis is visualized, the scope is passed underneath it with the endotracheal tube posterior to the scope and directly under vision. The direction of the scope is now anterior and upward till the ventricle is reached. At this point the fulcrum suspension system is fixed with the chest piece fixed onto the microlaryngoscope and over a Mayo's trolley above the patients chest, but not in contact with it. If a Boston University suspension system is being used, it fixes to the side of the operation theater (OT) table.

If however there is inadequate space between the epiglottis and the endotracheal tube, the epiglottis may infold on attempted MLS. In such a situation, another technique of introduction from posterior to the endotracheal tube is useful. The scope is passed along the ventral aspect of the tongue up to the posterior pharyngeal wall with the endotracheal tube anterior to the scope. Once the interarytenoid region is seen, the microlaryngoscope is gently maneuvered anterior to the endotracheal tube, crossing over the right pyriform and right aryepiglottic fold.

In very difficult anatomical situations of the epiglottis, it may be held with a forceps or a suture taken through it while performing MLS.

Endotracheal tubes are typically fixed at the left angle of the mouth. A cloth pocket attached at the surgeons end allows placement of suction for easy access by the surgeon. Whichever type of microlaryngoscope the surgeon is most comfortable with should be first used. It is preferable to always place the chest piece on a chest support rather than on the patient's chest as this prevents undue pressure on the chest, and also provides good extension without any movement of the assembly with the ventilatory movements of the chest.

THE DIFFICULT EXPOSURE

When the exposure of the larynx is becoming a challenge during MLS, various measures can be attempted.

- Anterior commissure pressure
  A sponge is placed on the neck of the patient and a 4 inch mastoid bandage is placed over this sponge at the level of the cricothyroid membrane, anchored on both sides of the OT table, so as to provide constant and steady anterior commissure pressure. With time, the larynx is seen to slowly drop further improving the exposure
  The use of both external counterpressure and internal distention as an adjunct to MLS was most helpful for the surgical management of lesions located near the anterior commissure. Seemingly, the two resultant forces are in opposition to each other, but in fact they are complementary, both to each other and to the orthodox laryngoscopic principle of elevated-vector suspension[8]
- Using one size smaller microlaryngoscope
- Rather than going closer to the vocal folds, withdraw the microlaryngoscope to the level of the false vocal folds. Along with the anterior commissure pressure, this often suffices in adequate exposure
- Anterior commissure laryngoscope
  This is extremely useful in the situation of the anterior larynx. A Dedo laryngoscope has helped us in most of our difficult cases. The Zeitels universal modular glottiscope has been described to be very useful, especially in the difficult larynx
- A flexion-flexion position may be attempted in visualizing the very anterior larynx, extreme anterior flexion of the head on the neck and of the neck on the chest produces the shortest distance between the lips and larynx and results in maximum flaccidity of the soft tissues and the easiest exposure of the glottis. In difficult patients, this may be the only position that permits visualization of the anterior of the glottis. However, it is difficult to perform microscopic surgery with the patient in this position[9]
- A 70-degree telescope may be used to operate off the monitor, along with flexible tip instruments. When a biopsy or polyp excision is planned, the lesion should be detached by downward pressure in the direction of

the subglottis . This decreases the chances of epithelial tears on the vocal fold vibrating edge
- A flexible bronchoscope with a side channel may be used via the microlaryngoscope for taking biopsies.

ANESTHESIA AND LASER SAFETY

Most of the Author's patients are intubated as potential laser cases with all laser safety protocols in place, regardless of whether cold steel or laser work is finally needed.

General anesthesia is administered by orotracheal intubation with a number 5 (adult female) or 5.5 (adult male) laser safe Mallinckrodt's/Medtronic/red rubber tube or by ventilation through a tracheostomy tube. The anesthetist places the endotracheal tube cuff well below the vocal folds, such that extension of the head and neck does not cause a resultant upward movement of the endotracheal tube cuff upto the glottis. Once the patient is in position for MLS, the cuff should be seen 5-6 cm below the vocal folds. The endotracheal tube is fixed to the left angle of the mouth in all cases.

As a part of the laser safety protocol, nitrous oxide as an inhalational anesthetic agent is not used and the oxygen flow in the ventilator is kept below 30%, which is equivalent to atmospheric air. Availability of pressurized atmospheric air is a must while performing laser cases. A large saline soaked cotton pledget is kept in the subglottis, the cuff of the laser safe tube is filled with cold sterile water with methylene blue and the patients eyes and face are covered by moist gauze. Personnels in the OT wear laser safe spectacles and a bucket of water is placed in the operating room (OR). The OR door has a signage stating, "laser in use," and unnecessary movement and people in the OT are avoided.

The anesthetist and nursing staff are trained in laser use, and a trained OT technician is present.

During extubation in MLS cases, it is extremely important to have a completely awake patient who is breathing spontaneously. At the end of the surgery, a 10% lignocaine spray over the vocal folds prevents laryngospasm and pain. A good endotracheal and oral suctioning is vital. Patients who are sleep apnoeic may often desaturate if not widely awake at extubation. They often need a 90 degree propped up position postoperatively and need to be woken up repeatedly if they doze off.

COMPLICATIONS

The patient undergoing a MLS should be informed about the possibility of chipping of teeth; accidental tooth extraction; cuts to the anterior tonsillor pillar, tongue, or lips; short-term change in taste sensation; and very rarely a possibility of hypoglossal paresis.

The possibility of having to abandon the surgery in a difficult exposure or due to anesthetic complications should also be discussed. Pneumothorax, pneumomediastinum and cardiac complications are possible complications.

The very small possibility of a laser fire or need for a tracheostomy is also discussed.

Spending time personally explaining the possibility and types of complications prior to the procedure is essential. In case of a complication, an immediate and frank discussion with the relatives is important and most relatives and patients are very understanding of the physician's efforts.

REFERENCES

1. Hsiung MW, Pai L, Kang BH, et al. Clinical predictors of difficult laryngeal exposure. Laryngoscope. 2004;114(2):358-63.
2. Roh JL, Lee YW. Prediction of difficult laryngeal exposure in patients undergoing microlaryngosurgery. Ann Otol Rhinol Laryngol. 2005;114(8):614-20.
3. Pinar E, Calli C, Oncel S, et al. Preoperative clinical prediction of difficult laryngeal exposure in suspension laryngoscopy. Eur Arch Otorhinolaryngol. 2009;266(5):699-703.
4. Hekiert AM, Mick R, Mirza N. Prediction of difficult laryngoscopy: does obesity play a role? Ann Otol Rhinol Laryngol. 2007;116(11):799-804.
5. RR Paul, AM Varghese, et al. Difficult laryngeal exposure in microlaryngoscopy: Can it be predicted preoperatively? Indian J Otolaryngol Head Neck Surg. 2016;68(1):65-70.
6. Obesity hypoventilation syndrome. Wikipedia. Available from: https://en.wikipedia.org/ wiki/Obesity_hypoventilation_syndrome.
7. Greenland KB. A proposed model for direct laryngoscopy and tracheal intubation. Anaesthesia. 2008;63:156-61.
8. Zeitels SM, Vaughan M. "External counterpressure" and "internal distention" for optimal laryngoscopic exposure of the anterior glottal commissure volume. 1994;103(9):669-75.
9. Vaughan GW. Vocal fold exposure for glottic surgery via a rigid scope. Available from: www.bumc.bu.edu/orl/.

CHAPTER 4

Vocal Fold Polyp

DEFINITION

Vocal fold polyps are generally acellular, with thickened epithelium over superficial lamina propria (SLP) and increased vascularity in an abundant delicate fibrin stromal matrix.[1]

They are typically found on the striking zone of the vocal fold (mid membranous vocal fold) and unlike vocal fold nodules are usually unilateral.

CASE 1

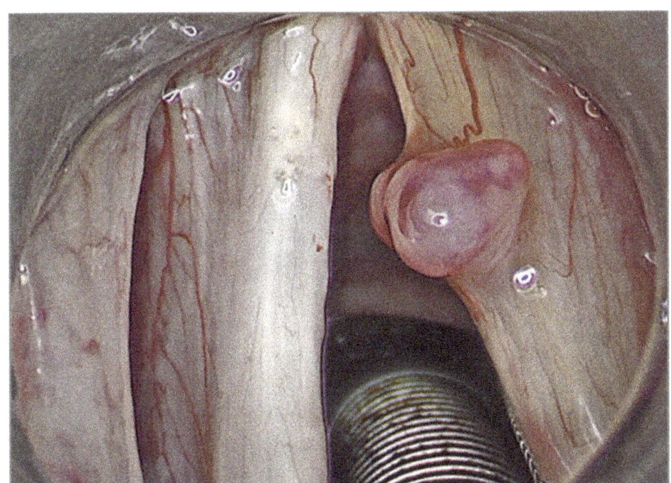

FIG. 4.1: A hemorrhagic polyp with a feeding vessel seen on the striking zone of the right vocal fold. A yellow tinge of the right vocal fold is suggestive of hemosiderin pigment of resolving subepithelial hemorrhage. A 5.5 Mallinckrodt laser tube is seen *in situ* in the posterior larynx. (E-CC).

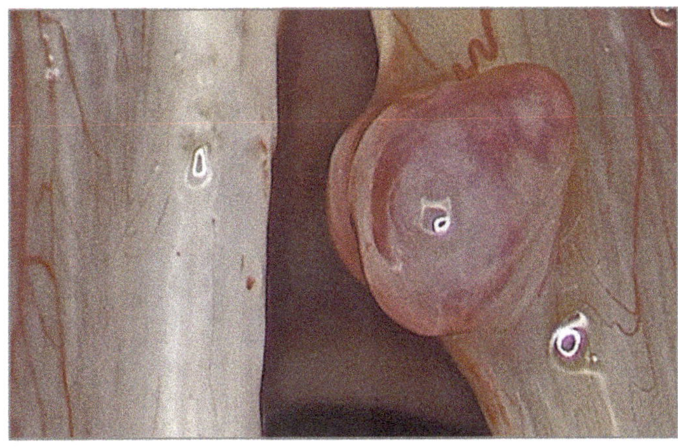

FIG. 4.2: Note the bilobed appearance of the same polyp (4.1) due to constant phonation indentation by the opposite vocal fold. (E-CC)

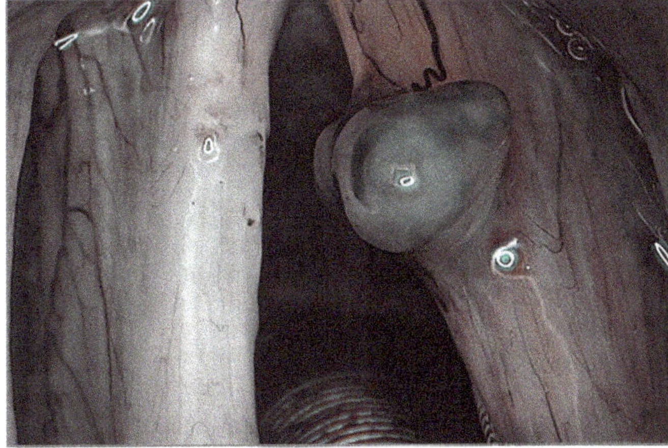

FIG. 4.3: Same polyp (4.1) seen in SA mode revealing a type 1 Ni pattern of vasculature[2] on both vocal folds. (E-SA)

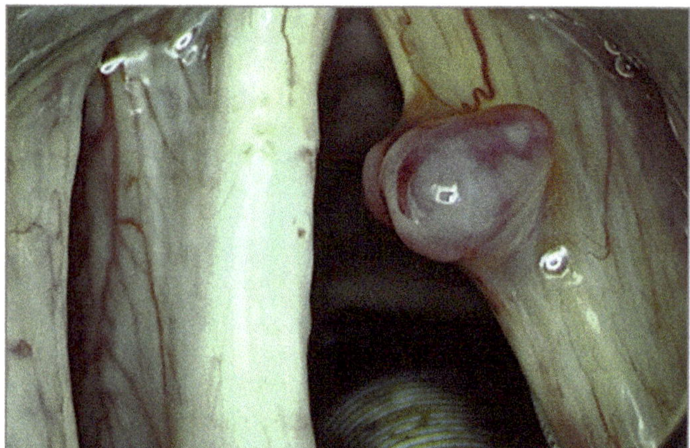

FIG. 4.4: Same polyp (4.1) seen in SB mode. (E-SB)

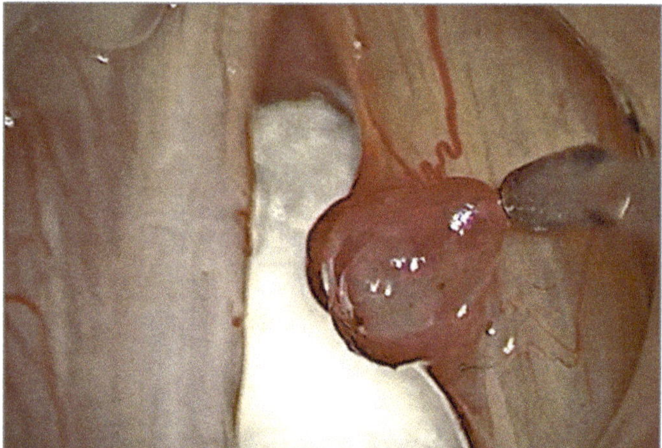

FIG. 4.5: Palpation of the attachment of the polyp with a blunt microflap elevator. A laser plume suction is seen in the left upper corner of the image. Prior to starting work with the laser, a moist cotton pledget is placed in the subglottis, protecting the cuff of the Laser tube. (M-CC)

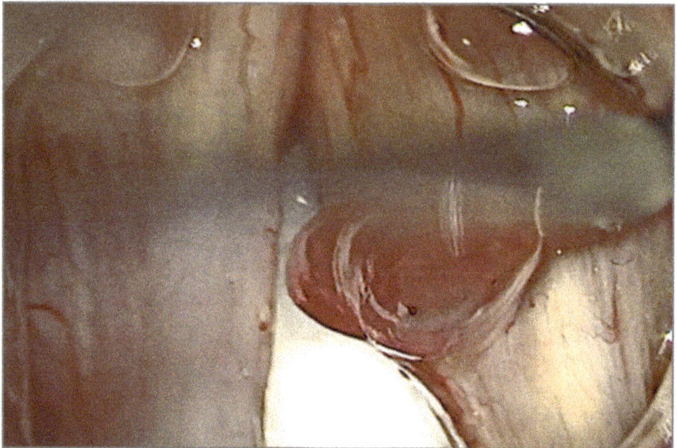

FIG. 4.6: Subepithelial infiltration of 1-2 cc of 1:10,000 saline adrenaline being performed in the Reinke's space of the right vocal fold. This infiltration helps with hemostasis, medialization of the lesion, depth penetration estimation of the lesion, and temporary bulking up of the Reinke's space which works as a good buffer zone when working with the CO_2 laser.[3] (M-CC).

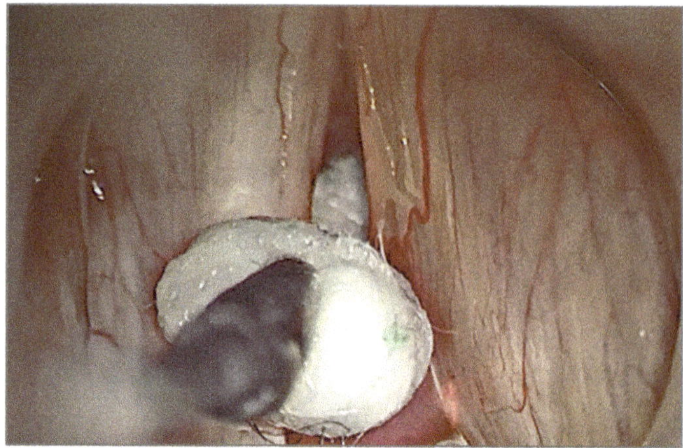

FIG. 4.7: A cotton ball is being used to mediatize the polyp so as to reveal the pedicle of the polyp. The AcuBlade (red line) is directed just at the edge of the pedicle of the polyp posteriorly. (M-CC)

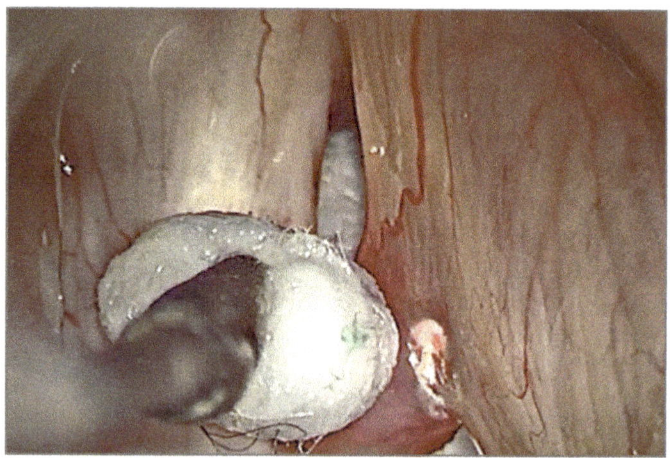

FIG. 4.8: An epithelial cordotomy being performed by the AcuBlade CO_2 laser. The laser is being used in scanner super-pulse mode. The grey unfocussed area on the left upper corner is the laser plume suction.(M-CC)

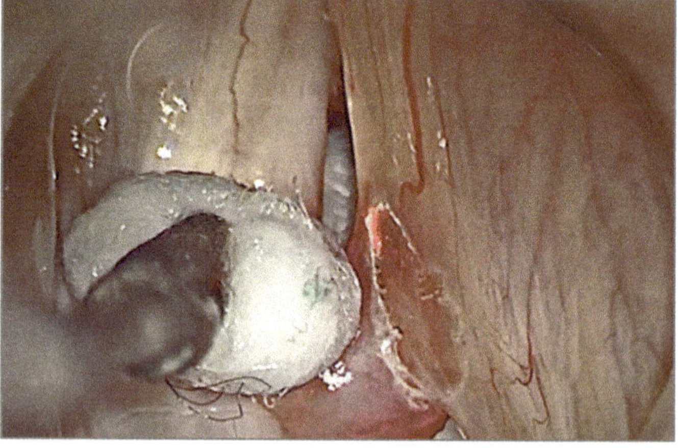

FIG. 4.9: Completion of the epithelial cordotomy with laserisation of the entry point of the feeding blood vessel. (M-CC)

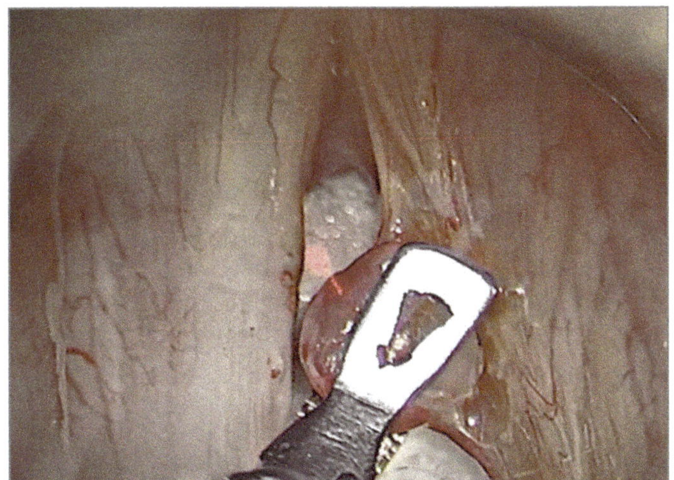

FIG. 4.10: An upward Bouchayer forceps holds the polyp and provides gentle traction. (M-CC)

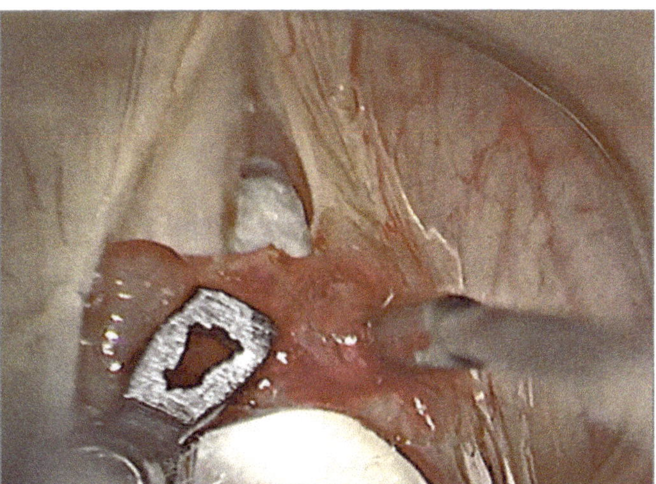

FIG. 4.13: Dissection of the polyp from the infraglottic epithelium with a blunt microflap elevator. (M-CC)

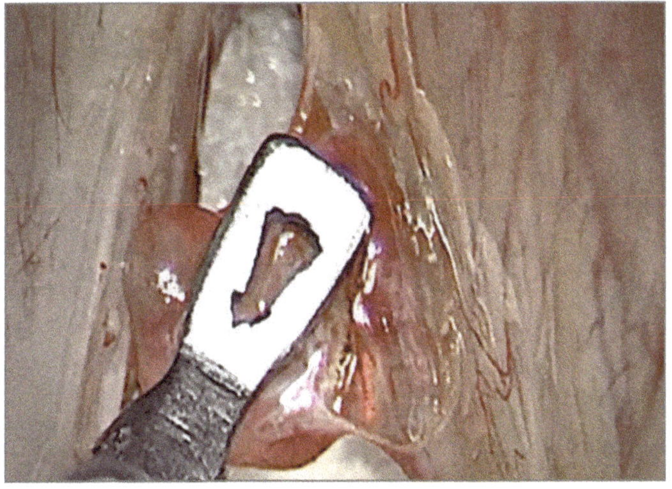

FIG. 4.11: The AcuBlade is used to excise the epithelium near the polyp such that maximum infraglottic epithelium may be preserved. (M-CC)

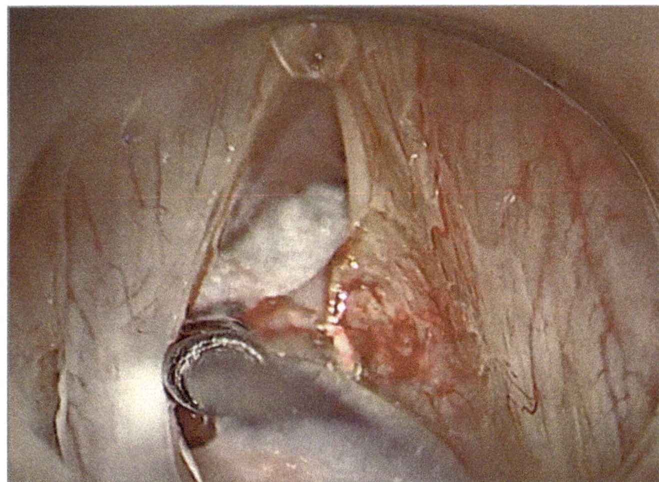

FIG. 4.14: Dissection of the polyp from the infraglottic epithelium with the AcuBlade. (M-CC)

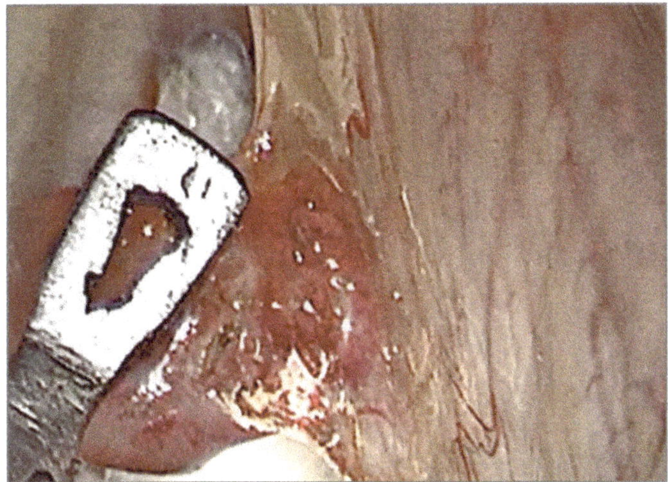

FIG. 4.12: Dissection of the polyp from the infraglottic epithelium with the AcuBlade. (M-CC)

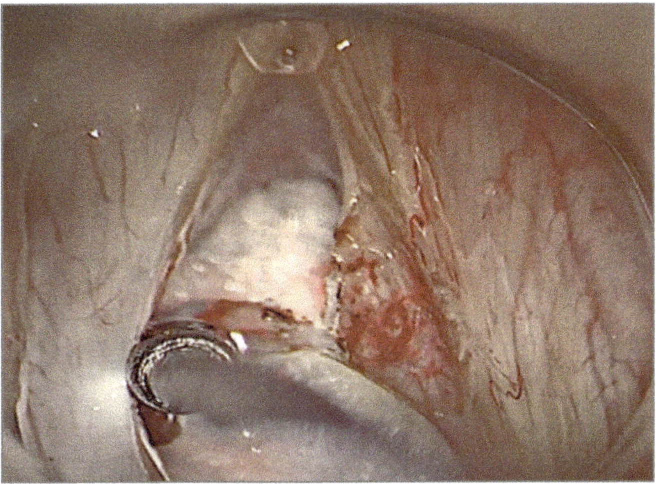

FIG. 4.15: Final dissection of the polyp from the infraglottic epithelium with the AcuBlade. (M-CC)

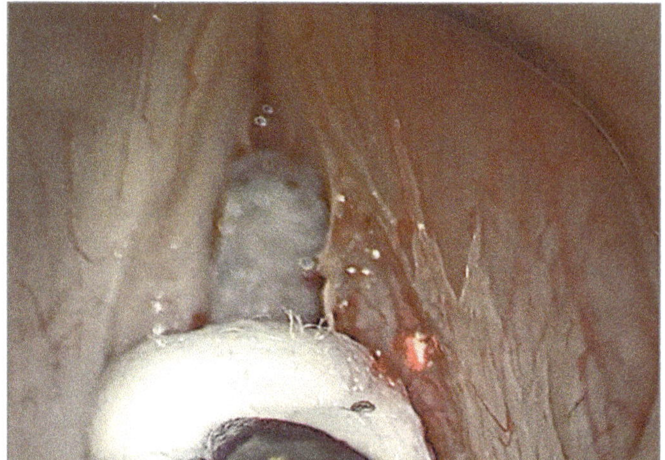

FIG. 4.16: Laser coagulation of the varices of the infraglottic epithelium. (M-CC)

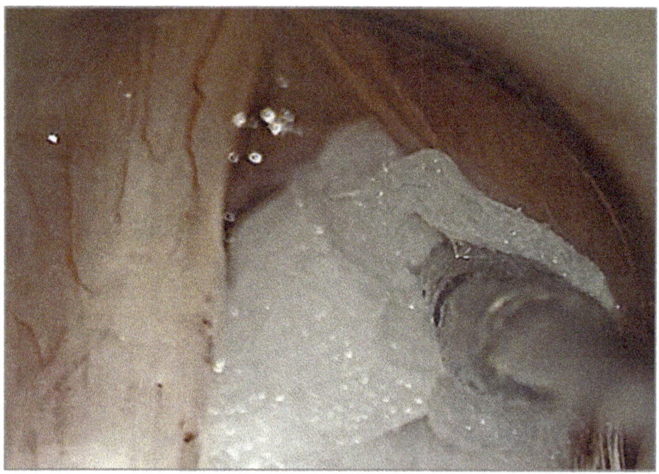

FIG. 4.17: A moist cotton pledget being used to redrape the medial vibrating edge of the right vocal fold with the infra glottic epithelium. (M-CC)

FIG. 4.18: Laser coagulation of the feeding blood vessel as ascertained by the direction of the red blood corpuscles. (M-CC)

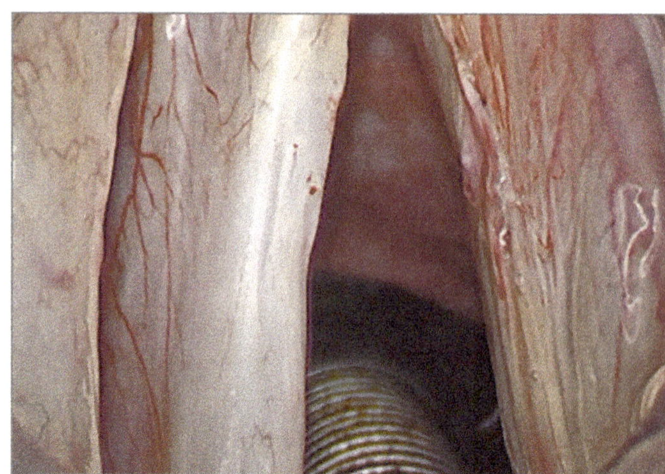

FIG. 4.19: Postoperative endoscopic view revealing a good edge-to-edge approximation at the incision site.(E-CC)

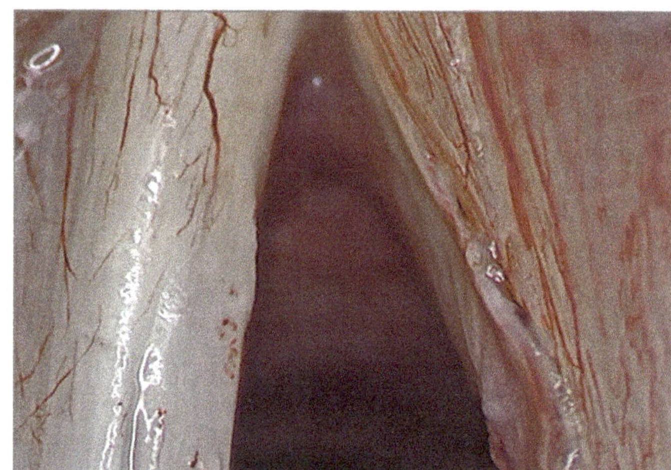

FIG. 4.20: Magnified view of 4.19 (E-CC)

CASE 2

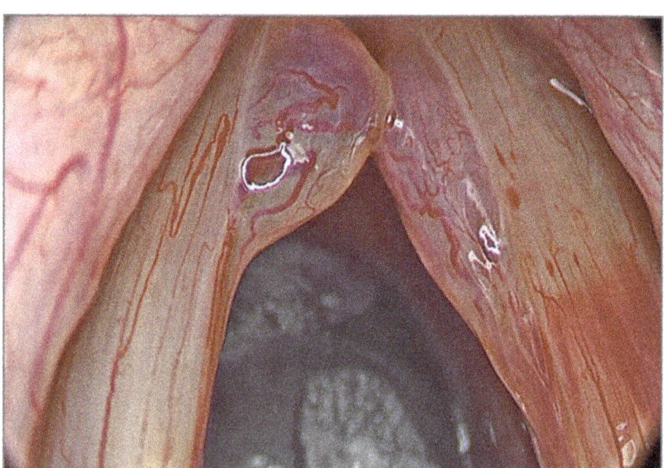

FIG. 4.21: Bilateral hemorrhagic polyps with right vocal fold SEH observed posteriorly. This was following a steroid course given for right severe SEH. (E-CC)

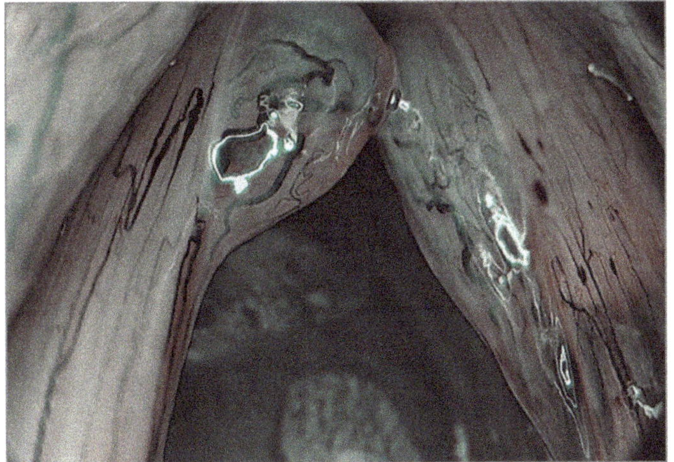

FIG. 4.22: SA mode revealing cyan (blue) subepithelial vessels within the polyps, and within the area of the SEH (right vocal fold posterior). (E-SA)

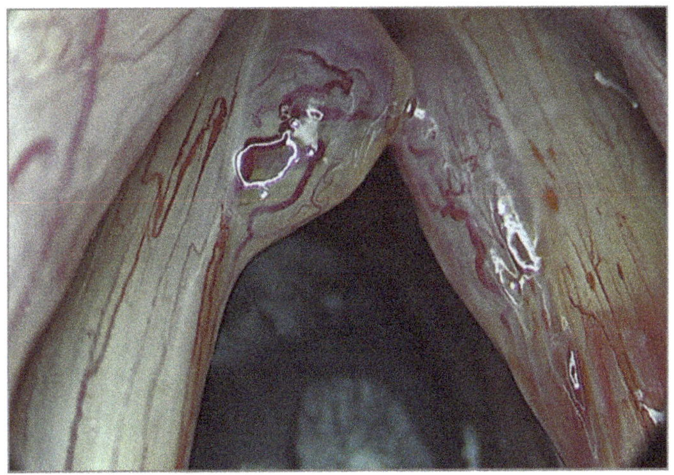

FIG. 4.23: SB mode revealing a better delineation of the subepithelial vessels (red) from surrounding SEH (right vocal fold posterior) due to a sharper contrast with the surrounding tissue. (E-SB)

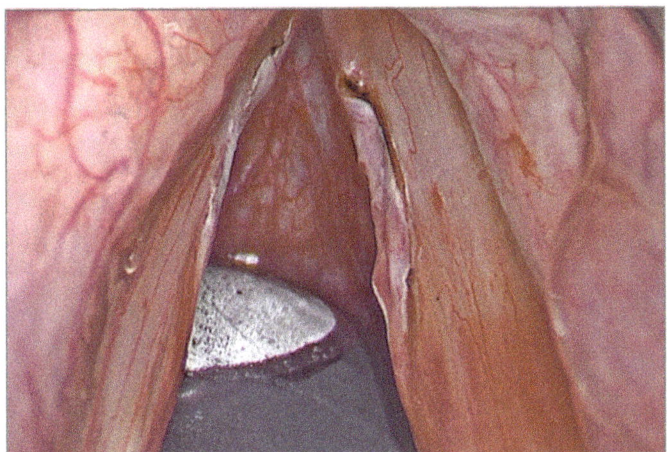

FIG. 4.24: Postoperative picture revealing epithelial cover of both vocal folds at the surgical site. The cuff of the laser safe Xomed tube is seen filled with methylene blue and saline (CC). The SEH seen posteriorly on the right vocal fold is surgically untouched and resolution with voice rest and anti-inflammatory medication is planned for the patient

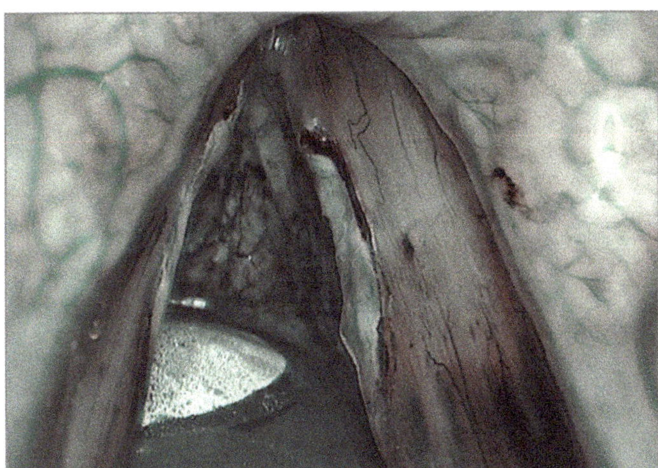

FIG. 4.25: SA image of 4.24. (E-SA)

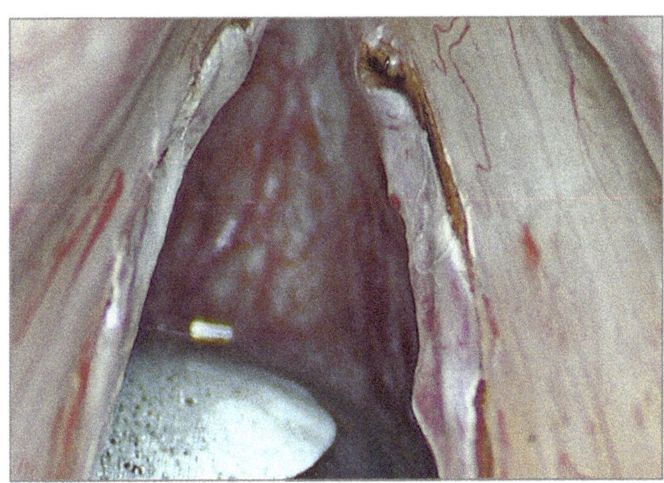

FIG. 4.26: SB image of 4.24 (E-SB)

CASE 3

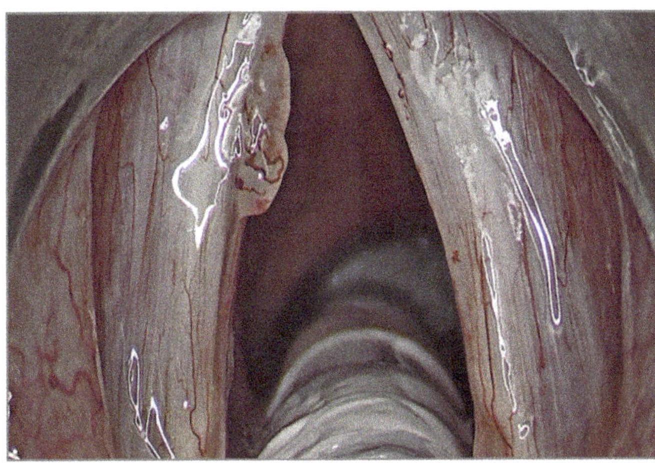

FIG. 4.27: A myxomatous polyp on the striking zone of the left vocal fold with varices within the polyp (E-CC)

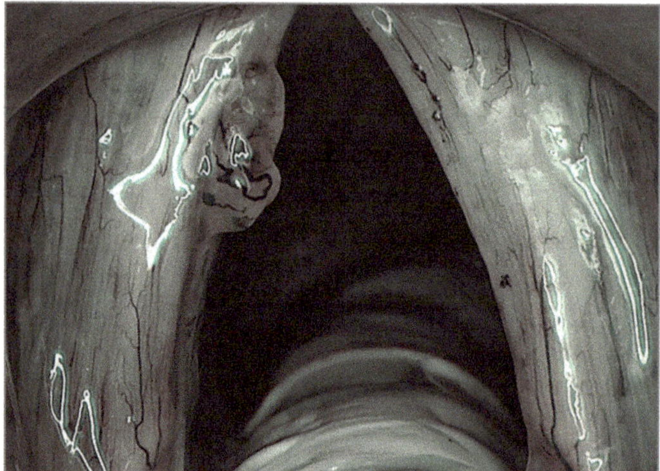

FIG. 4.28: SA image of 4.27. (E-SA)

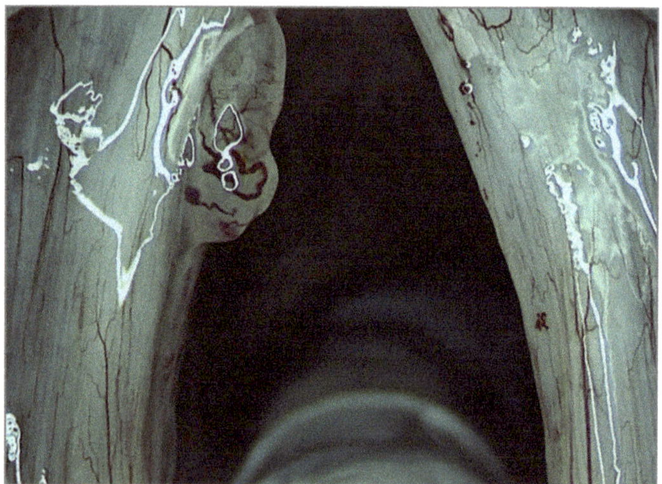

FIG. 4.29: SB image of 4.27. (E-SB)

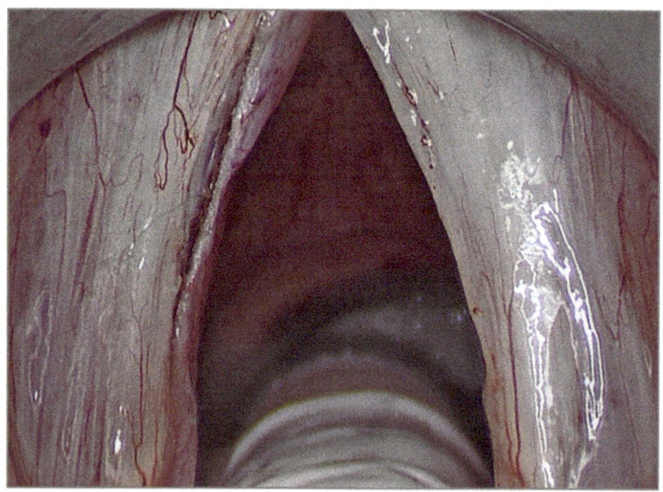

FIG. 4.30: Postoperative image of the patient revealing a slit epithelial loss on the superior surface of the left vocal fold, at the incision site. (E-CC)

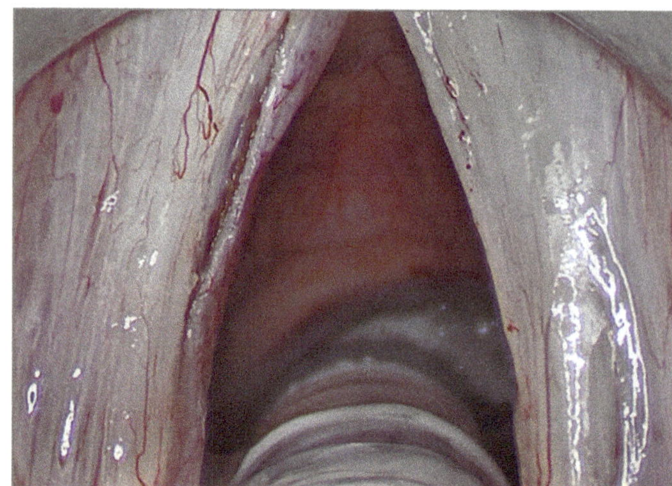

FIG. 4.31: Magnified image of the epithelial slit gap seen in 4.30. Epithelial regeneration bridges such gaps effectively, however, large epithelial gaps take longer to heal. Once epithelium is elevated from the underlying SLP, it does not retain the architecture of the intertwining anchoring and collagen fibers between the basement membrane and the SLP even if reposited in place. [4] (E-CC)

CASE 4

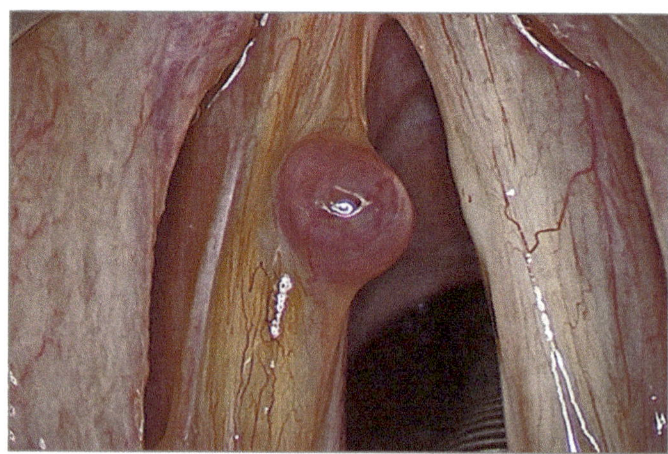

FIG. 4.32: Left hemorrhagic polyp with left resolving SEH (yellow hue). (E-CC)

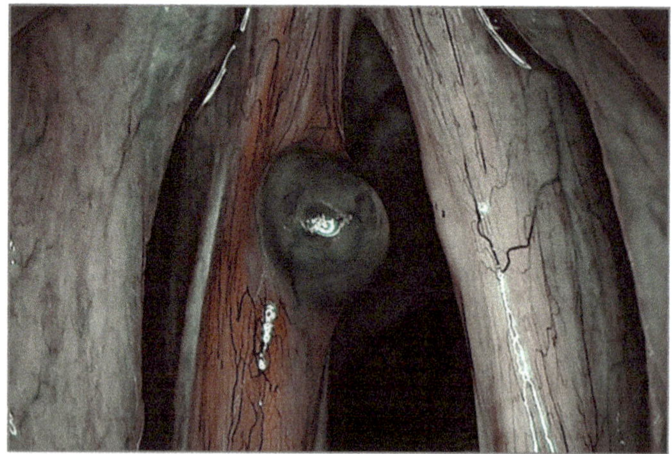

FIG. 4.33: SA image of 4.32 revealing cyan subepithelial veins and pink SEH (resolving). (E-SA)

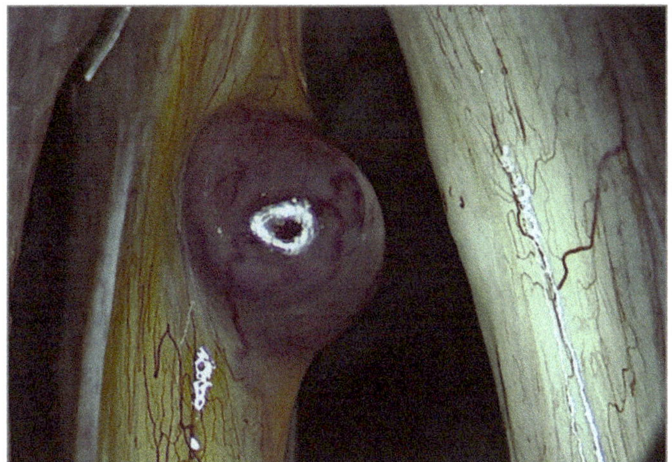

FIG. 4.34: SB image of 4.32 revealing red subepithelial veins and yellow SEH (resolving). (E-SB)

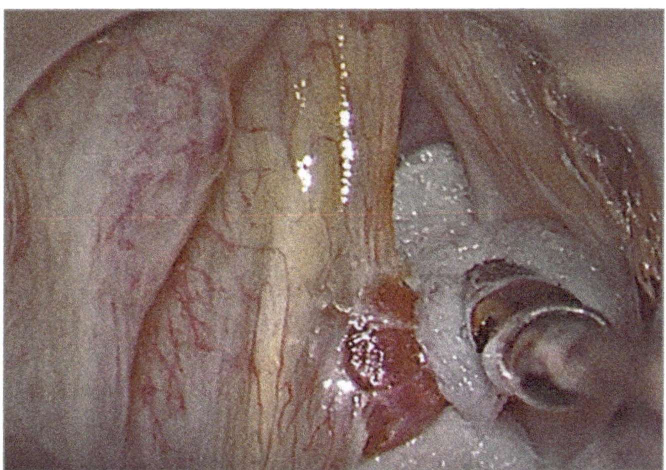

FIG. 4.35: A cotton ball is being used to palpate and medialize the lesion. The white vocal ligament can be clearly appreciated through the translucent epithelium and SLP. (M-CC)

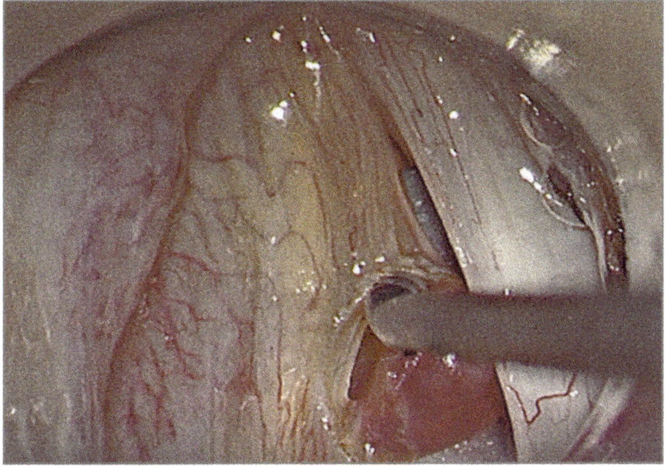

FIG. 4.36: A sickle knife is being used to perform an epithelial cordotomy. This is performed on the immediate lateral edge of the lesion (mini-microflap surgery). SEIT has been performed prior to this incision. (M-CC)

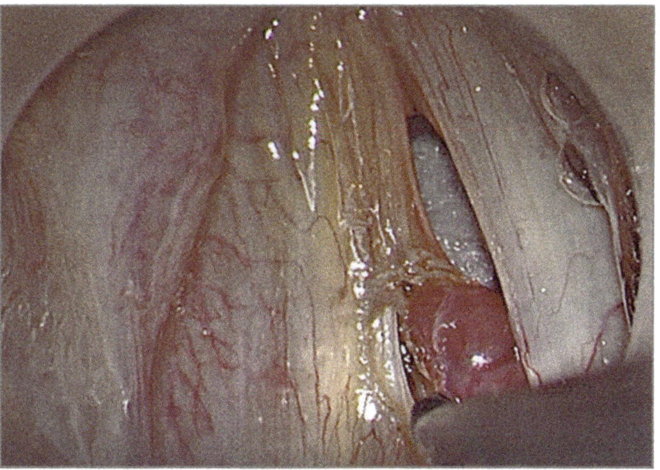

FIG. 4.37: Blunt dissection of the polyp from the underlying SLP. (M-CC)

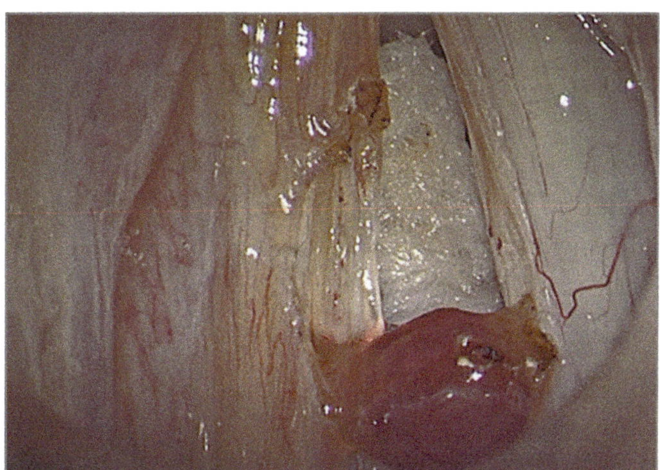

FIG. 4.38: Decision made to excise the overlying epithelium along with the polyp using a CO_2 AcuBlade system. (M-CC)

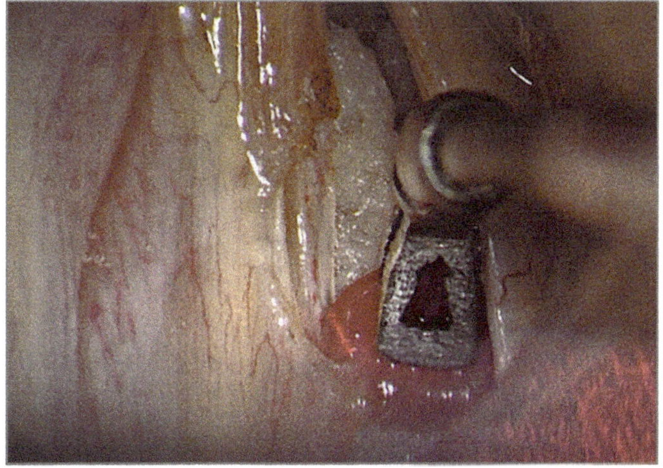

FIG. 4.39: Bouchayer forceps being held in a downward direction for a better grip on the polyp, while excising the posterior attachment with the AcuBlade. (M-CC)

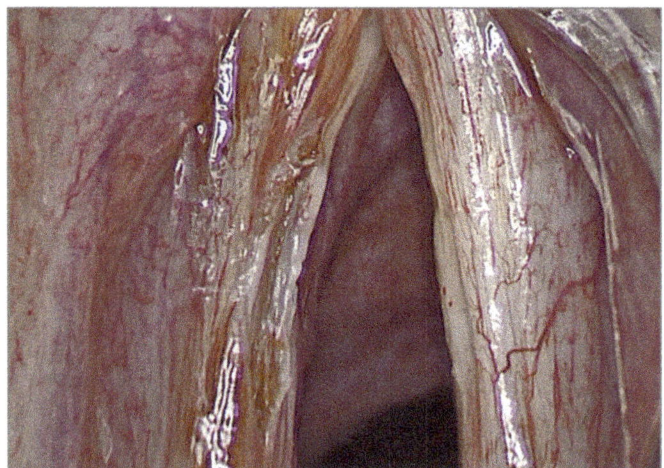

FIG. 4.40: Postoperative image, revealing slight loss of epithelium at the left medial vibrating edge. (M-CC)

CASE 5

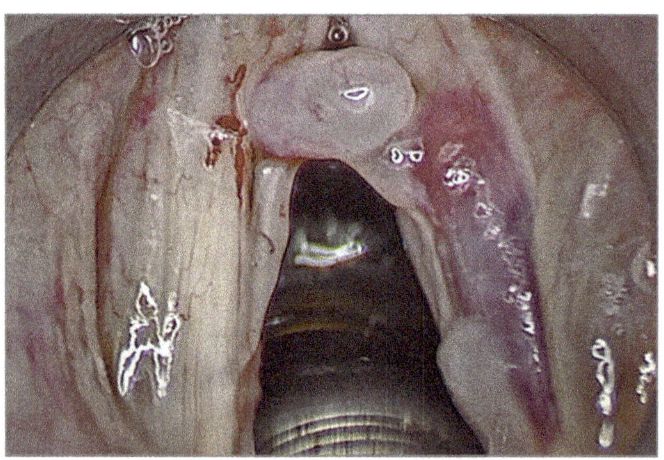

FIG. 4.41: A left polyp originating within a sulcus, also seen is a right hemorrhagic cyst. Varices are observed lateral to the polyp on the left vocal fold. A Mallinckrodt laser safe tube is seen in the posterior larynx. (M-CC)

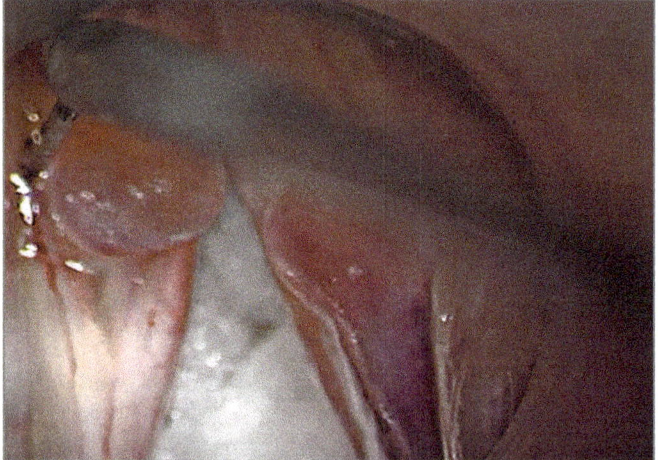

FIG. 4.42: Left subepithelial infiltration being performed. A cotton pledget is placed in the subglottis, protecting the cuff of the endotracheal tube during laser surgery. (M-CC)

FIG. 4.43: A Bouchayer forceps holding and providing gentle medial traction on the polyp. The CO_2 AcuBlade is aimed at the immediate lateral margin of the polyp. (M-CC)

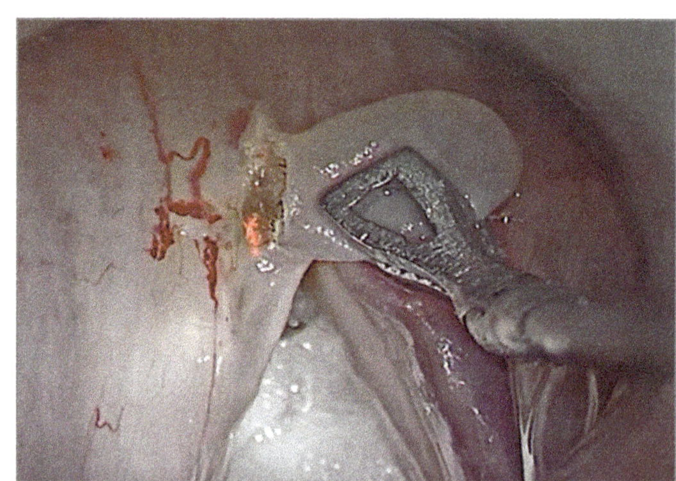

FIG. 4.44: Laser epithelial cordotomy performed. (M-CC)

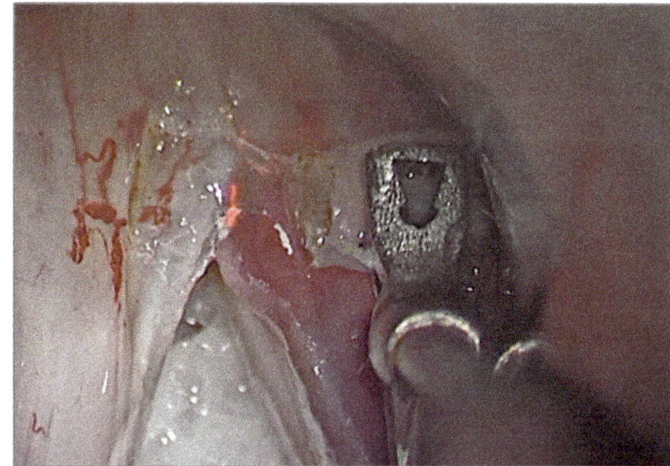

FIG. 4.45: Laser excision of the polyp being performed while retaining maximally the infraglottic epithelium and existent SLP. The gelatinous material seen at the base of the polyp suggests that the sulcus is superficial and not extending to the ligament.(M-CC)

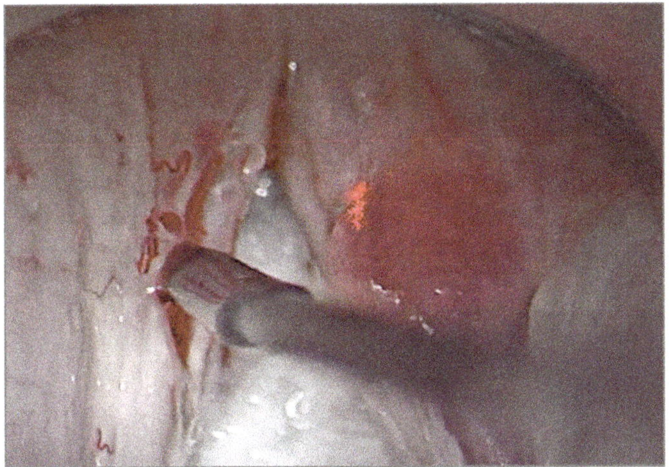

FIG. 4.46: Infraglottic epithelium covering the medial vibrating edge. A decision not to operate on the left sulcus at this time was taken, keeping in mind its superficial nature. (M-CC)

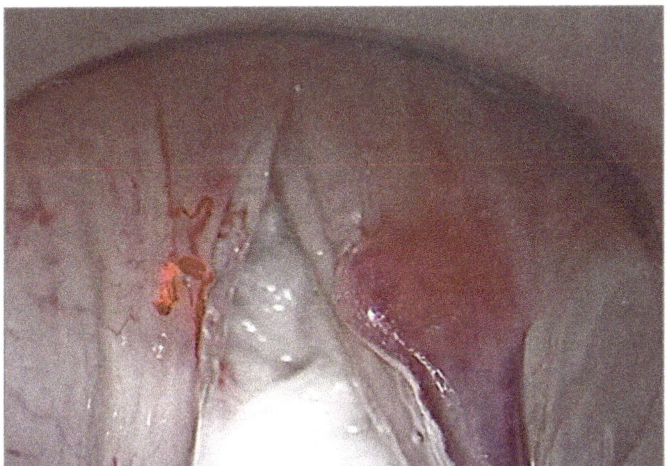

FIG. 4.47: Laser coagulation of the varices of the left vocal fold. A good edge-to-edge approximation of the epithelium can be observed at the incision site. (M-CC)

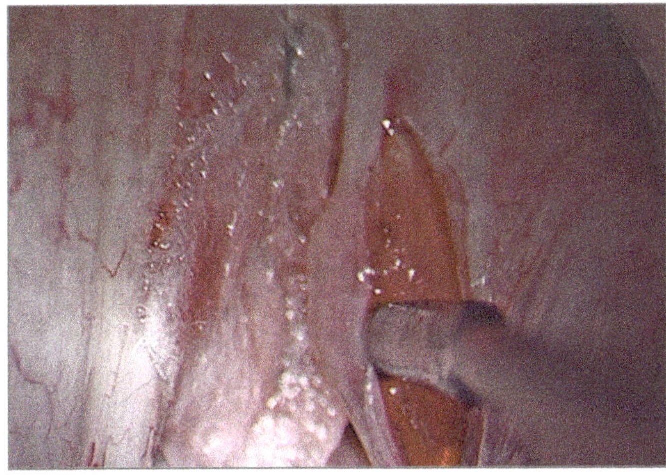

FIG. 4.48: A laser epithelial Cordotomy has been performed just lateral to the right hemorrhagic cyst. (M-CC)

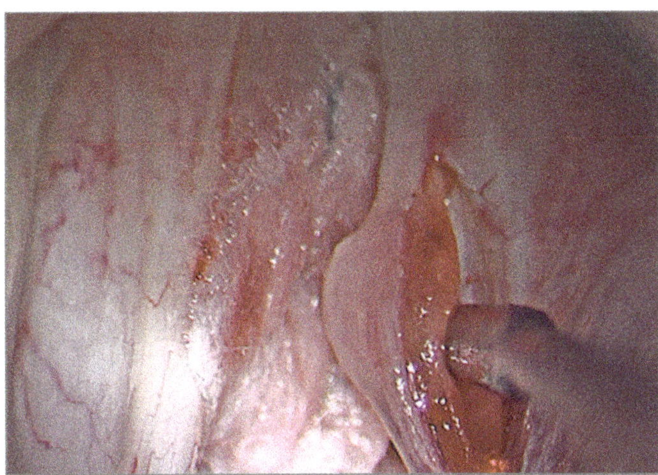

FIG. 4.49: Cold steel dissection of the cyst from the underlying SLP using a blunt microflap elevator is being performed. (M-CC)

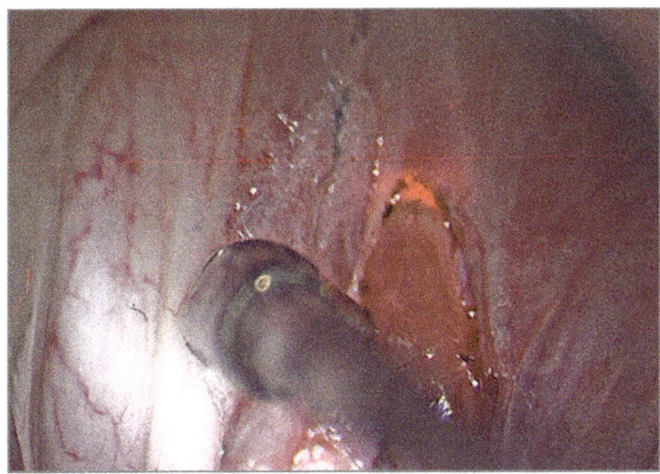

FIG. 4.50: CO_2 laser excision of the anterior fibrotic band tethering the cyst.[5] (M-CC)

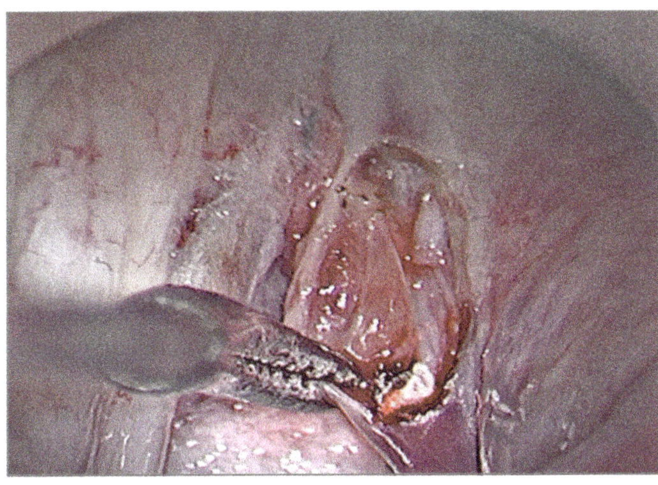

FIG. 4.51: CO_2 laser excision of the posterior fibrotic band tethering the cyst. (M-CC)

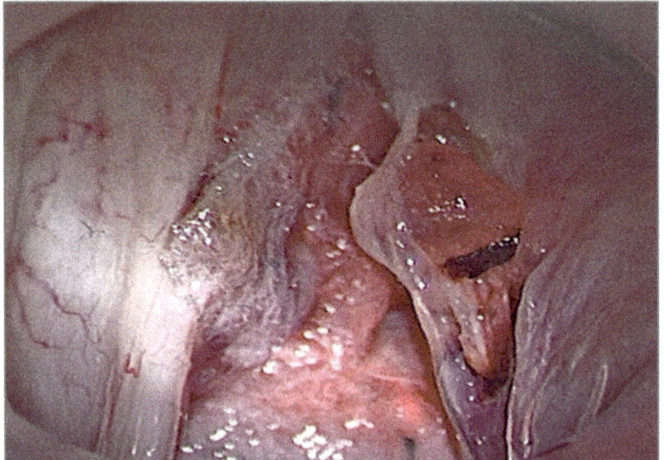

FIG. 4.52: Cyst lying attached to overlying epithelium and a small portion of its bed. (M-CC)

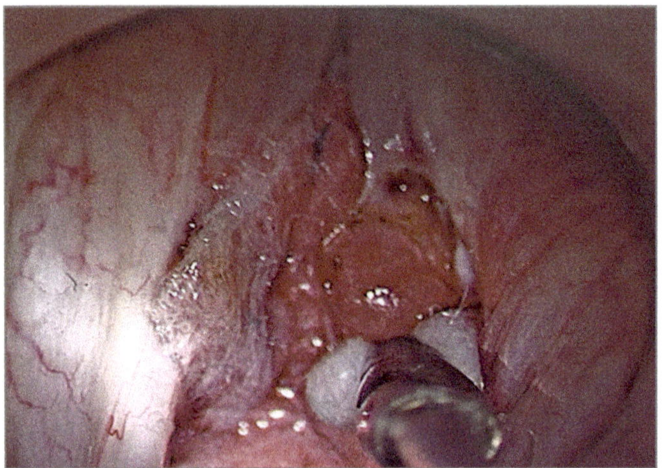

FIG. 4.53: A cotton pledget is being used to complete the dissection. (M-CC)

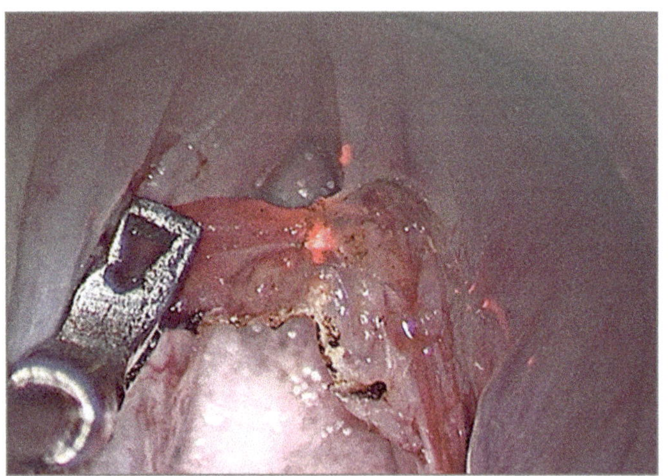

FIG. 4.54: Final anterior excision using a CO_2 laser. (M-CC)

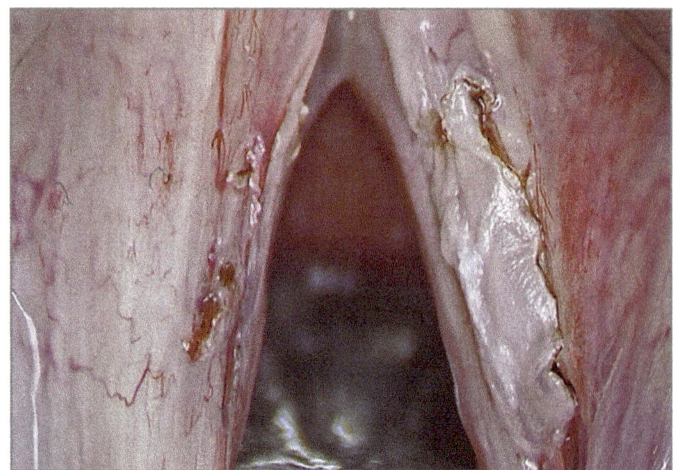

FIG. 4.55: Final postoperative endoscopic view revealing a good epithelial cover bilaterally. (E-CC)

CASE 6

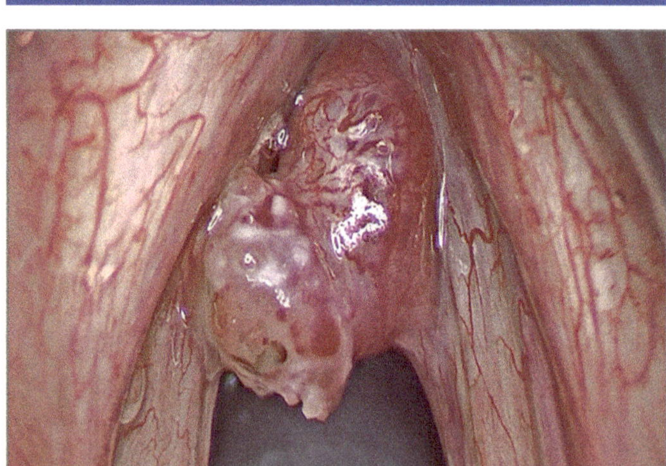

FIG. 4.56: A right bilobed hemorrhagic polyp. (E-CC)

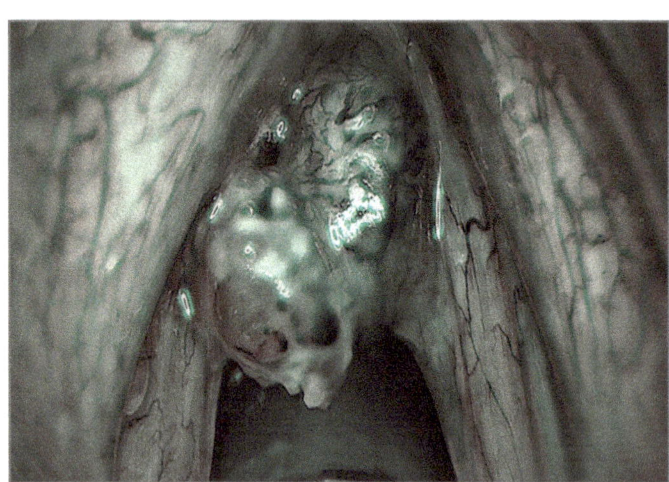

FIG. 4.57: SA image of 4.56. (E-SA)

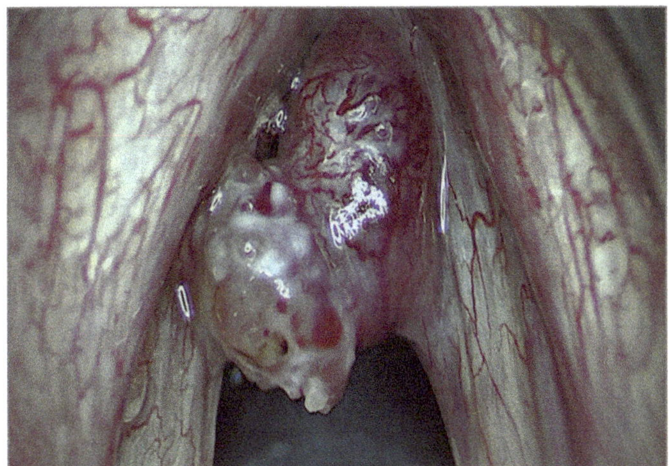

FIG. 4.58: SB image of 4.56. (E-SB)

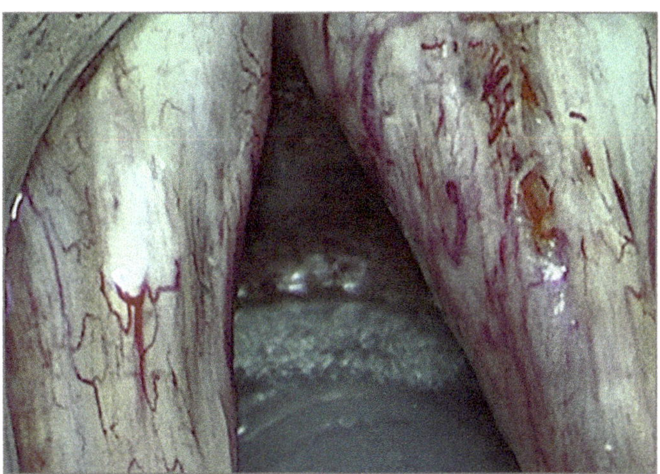

FIG. 4.61: SB image of 4.59. (E-SB)

FIG. 4.59: Good epithelial cover following excision (E-CC)

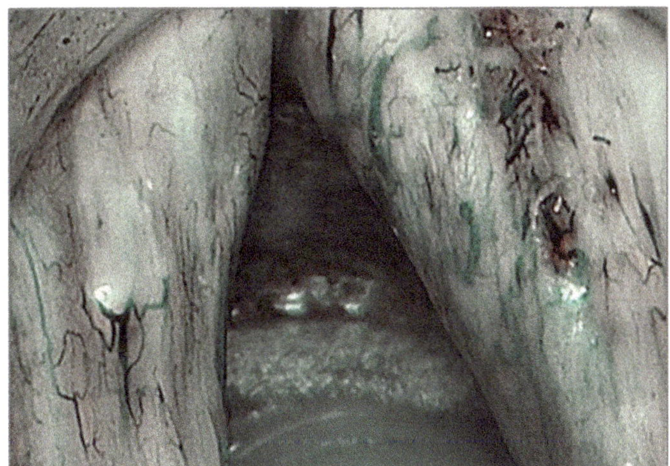

FIG. 4.60: SA image of 4.59. (E-SA)

CASE 7

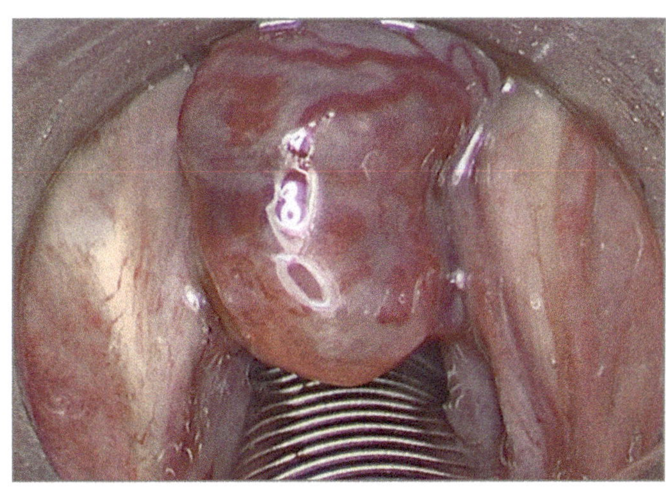

FIG. 4.62: A large right hemorrhagic polyp with dilated subepithelial vessels. A contact lesion of the left vocal fold is hidden from view by this large polyp. (E-CC)

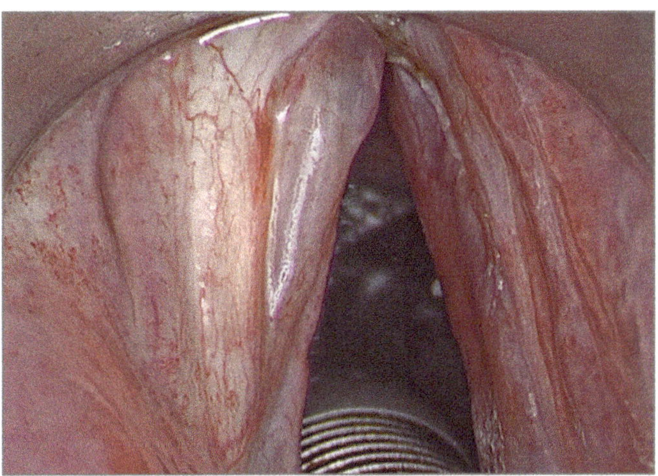

FIG. 4.63: Postoperative view showing good epithelial cover on both sides. (E-CC)

CASE 8

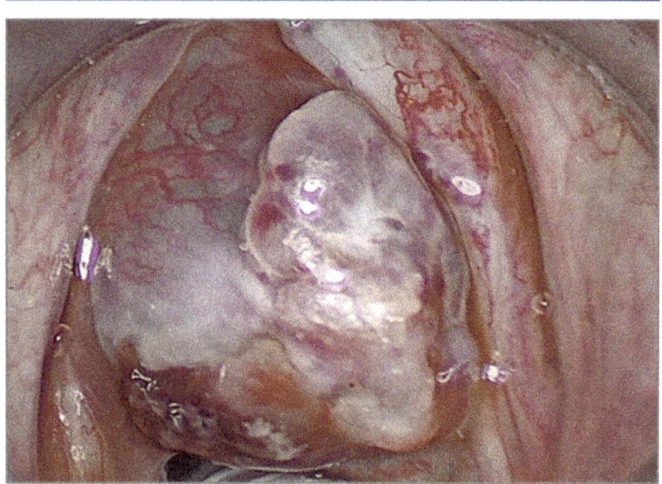

FIG. 4.64: An extremely large left hemorrhagic polyp with multiple blood vessels (E-CC)

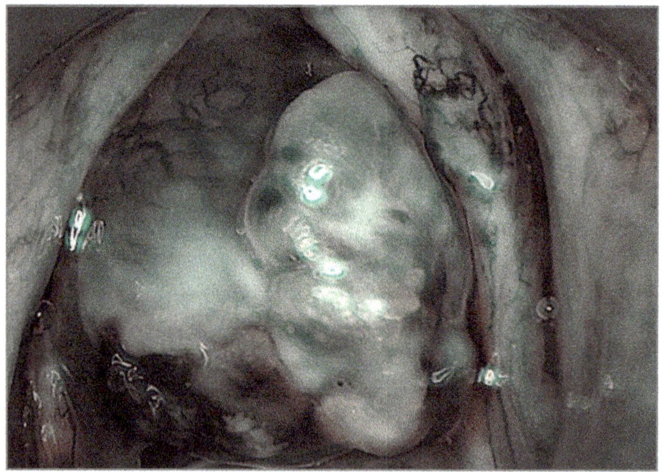

FIG. 4.65: SA image of 4.64 revealing cyan subepithelial veins of the polyp and of contralateral (right) vocal fold. Also seen is posterior hemorrhage within the polyp. (E-SA)

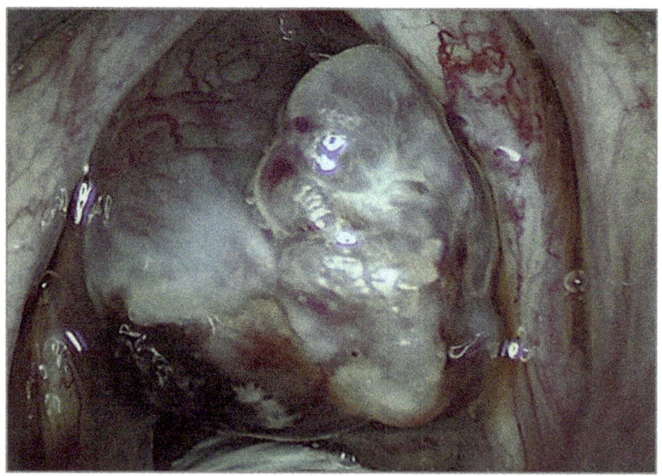

FIG. 4.66: SB image of 4.64. (E-SB)

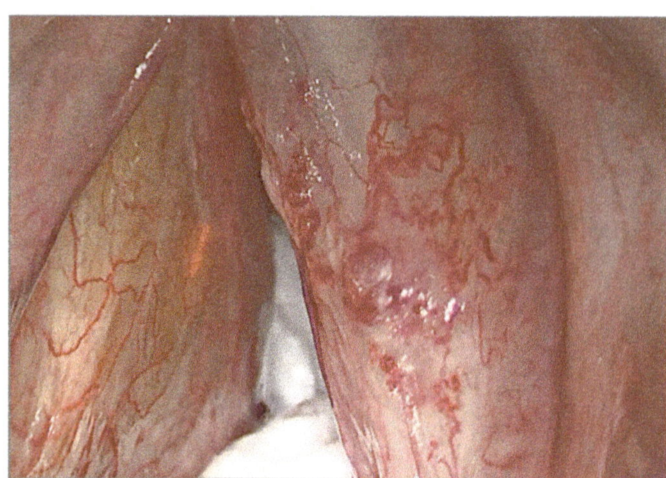

FIG. 4.67: Huge polyps, such as this one, are best medialized into the laryngeal introitus, so as to clearly visualize the edge of the pedicle. The CO_2 laser AcuBlade can be seen directed towards this pedicle edge. (M-CC)

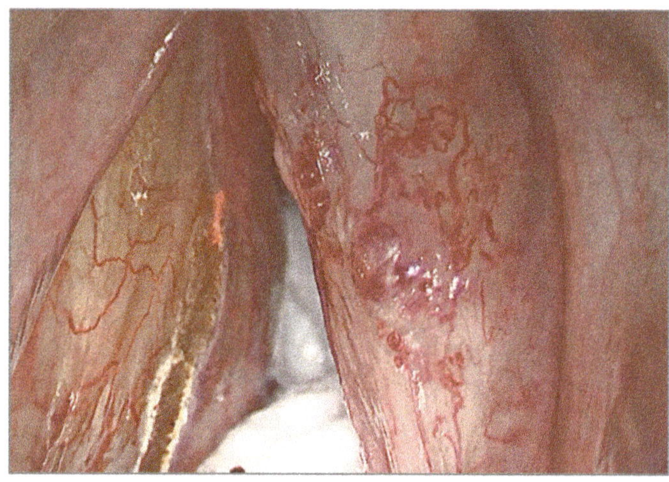

FIG. 4.68: Laser epithelial cordotomy being performed just at the lateral edge of the left polyp. (M-CC)

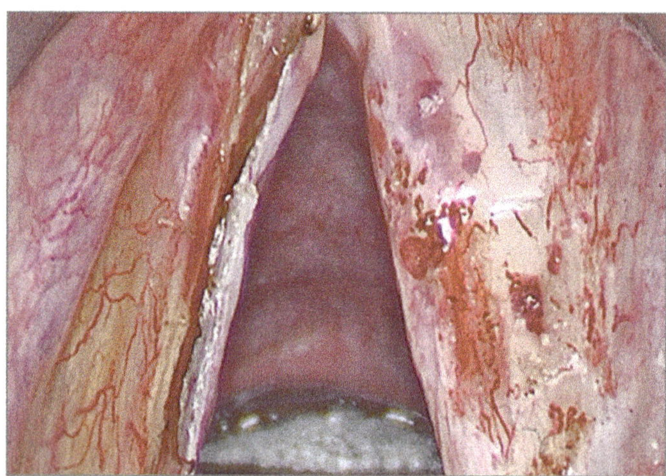

FIG. 4.69: Postoperative endoscopic view revealing a good epithelial cover (E-CC)

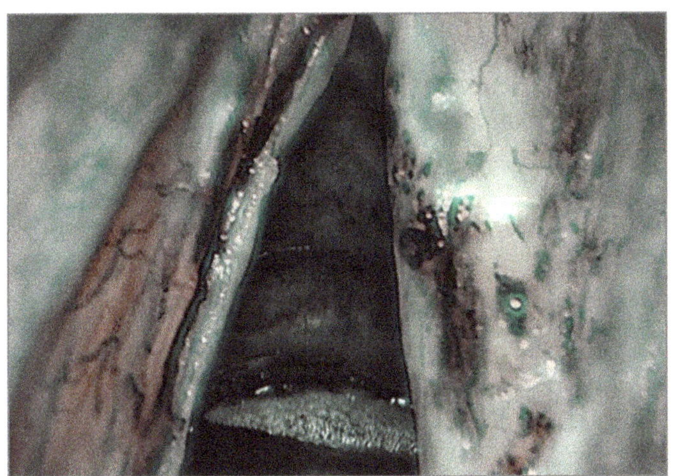

FIG. 4.70: SA image of 4.69. (E-SA)

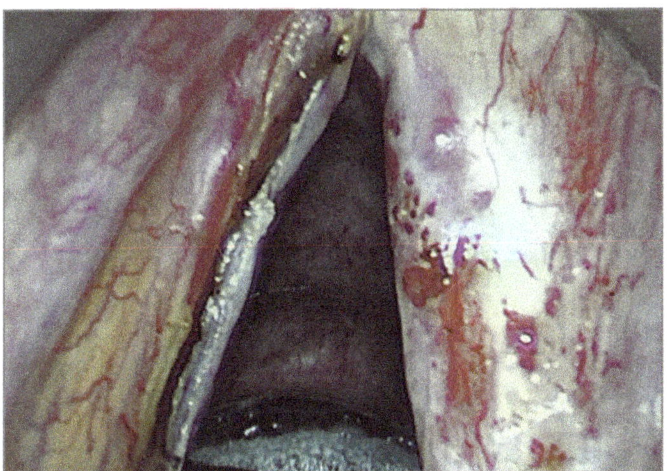

FIG. 4.71: SB image of 4.69. (E-SB)

CASE 9

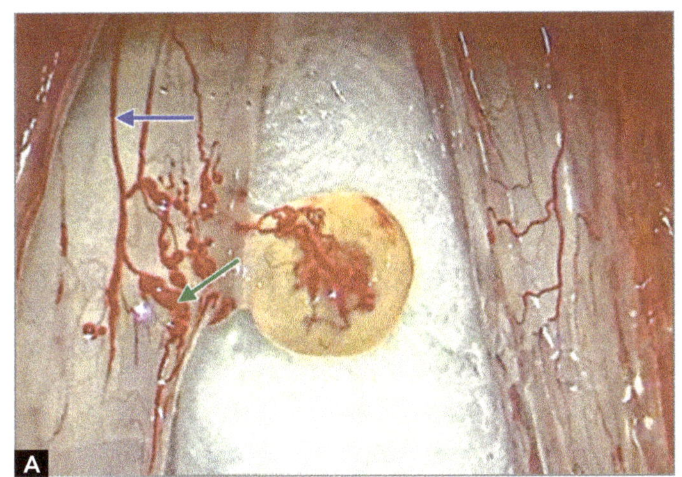

Continued

Continued

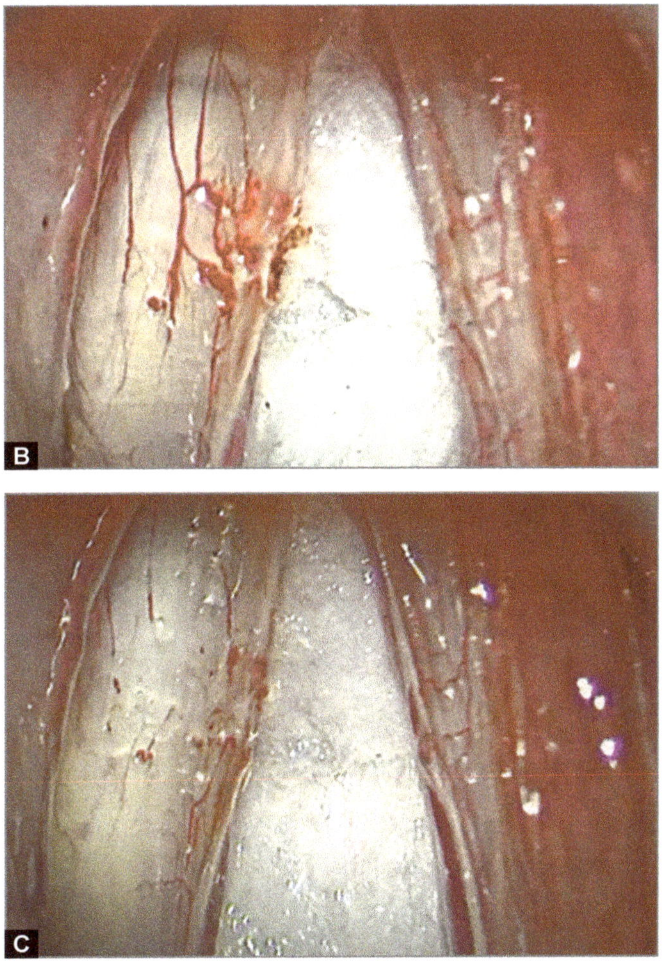

B

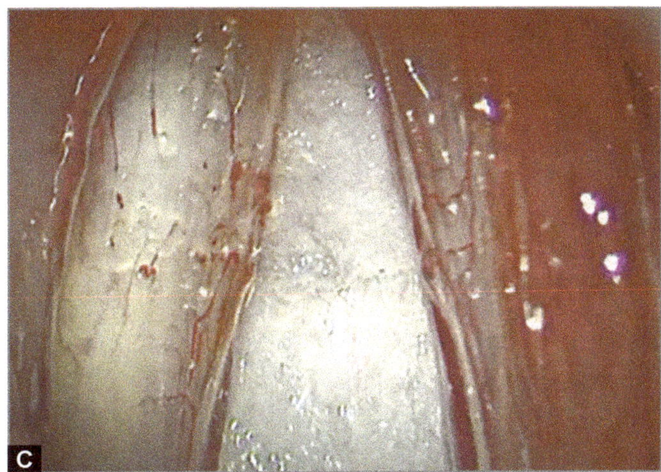

FIG. 4.72: A, Left vocal fold vascular lesions with an associated polyp, Blue arrow—varix, green arrow—ectasia; **B,** Polyp excised using CO_2 laser; **C,** Laser ablation of the varices

REFERENCES

1. Kotby MN, Nassar AM, Seif EL, El et al. Ultrastructural features of nodules and polyps, Acta Otolaryngol. 1998;105(5-6):477-82.
2. Ni XG, He S, Xu ZG, et al. Endoscopic diagnosis of laryngeal cancer and precancerous lesions by narrow band imaging. J Laryngol Otol. 2011;125(3):288-96.
3. Nerurkar N, Narkar N, Joshi A, et al. Vocal outcomes following subepithelial infiltration technique in microflap surgery: a review of 30 cases. J Laryngol Otol. 2007;121(8):768-71.
4. Gray SD, Pignatari SS, Harding P. Morphologic ultrastructure of anchoring fibers in normal vocal fold basement membrane zone. J Voice. 1994;8(1):48-52.
5. Nupur N, Sunita C. Subepithelial vocal fold cyst-pearl on a string? Int J Phonosurg Laryngol. 2012;2(2):53-6.

CHAPTER 5

Vocal Fold Cyst

DEFINITION

A cyst is a benign well-encapsulated collection of fluid of varying consistency. In the vocal fold, a cyst is typically found lying free in the superficial lamina propria (SLP) underneath the epithelial layer and is thus referred to as a sub-epithelial cyst.[1]

Occasionally, this cyst may be adherent to the overlying epithelium, or it may open into the laryngeal lumen (open cyst) or it may extend into the vocal ligament. This lesion (vocal fold cyst-ligament) does not respond to voice rest or voice therapy, and the prognosis for prompt recovery of the voice after surgical excision is less compared with a vocal fold polyp or subepithelial cyst. [2]

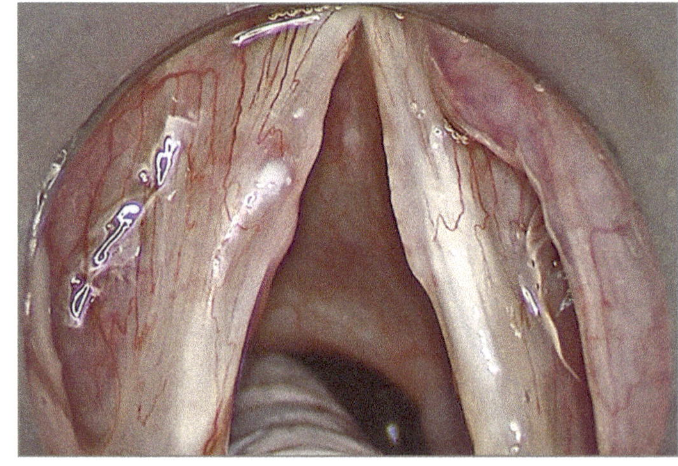

FIG. 5.2: Open cyst of the left vocal fold. (E-CC)

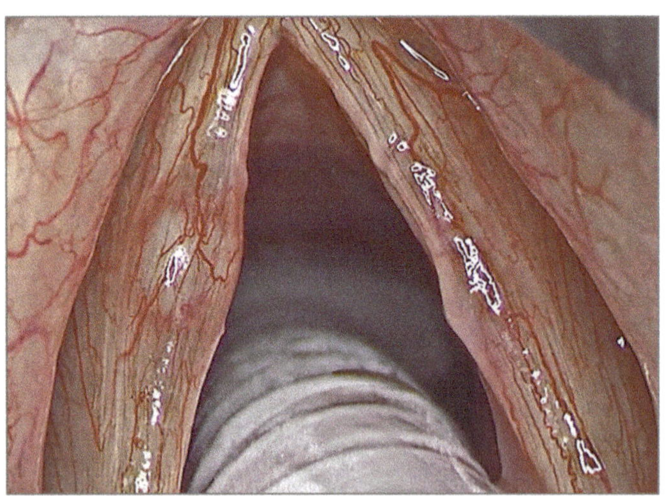

FIG. 5.1: Left subepithelial cyst. (E-CC)

Glottic subepithelial cysts may be mucous retention cysts or epidermoid cysts. Though these cysts differ histologically from one another, the treatment for symptomatic patients remains surgical in both cases.

TYPES OF SUBEPITHELIAL CYST

Histopathologically, a subepithelial cyst of the vocal fold may be epidermoid with a thick capsule wall of squamous epithelium and cheesy material, typically found on the medial vibrating edge or mucous retention with a thin capsule wall of respiratory epithelium, clear fluid within, and typically on the superior surface of the vocal fold.

Though surgery is recommended for all symptomatic cysts, it is usually easier to excise epidermoid cysts due to the thicker capsule wall, which makes its identification easier even in the event of a rupture.

Diagrammatic Representation

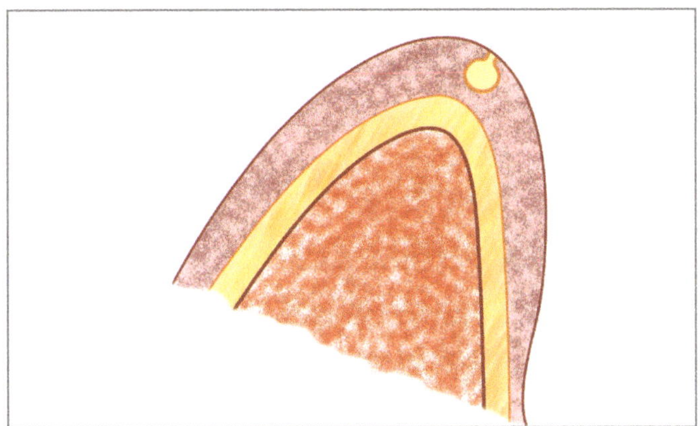

FIG. 5.3: Open epidermoid cyst

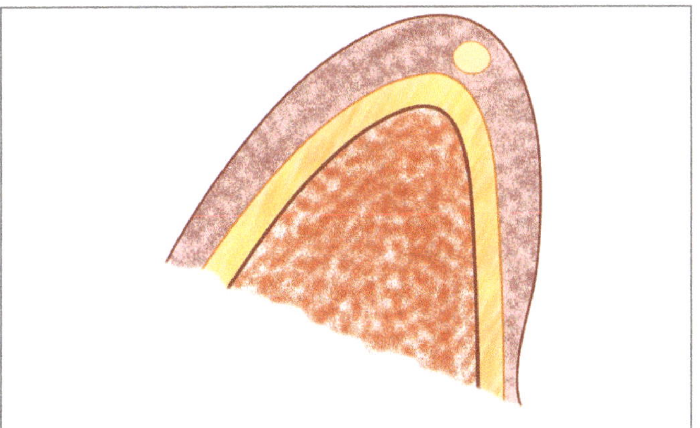

FIG. 5.4: Subepithelial mucous retention cyst

H&E Stained Sections Demonstrating Histopathology

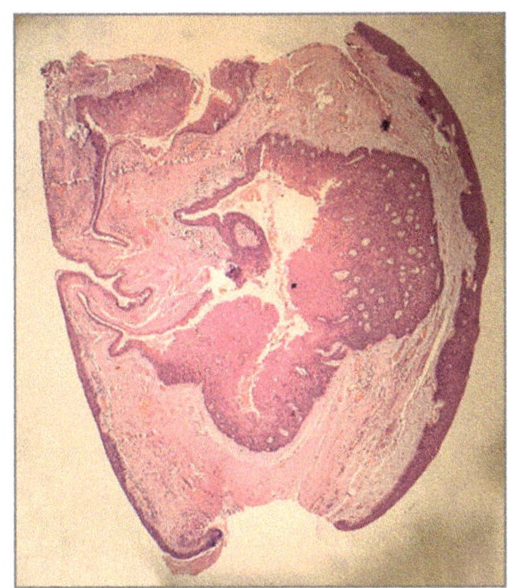

FIG. 5.5: Epidermoid cyst

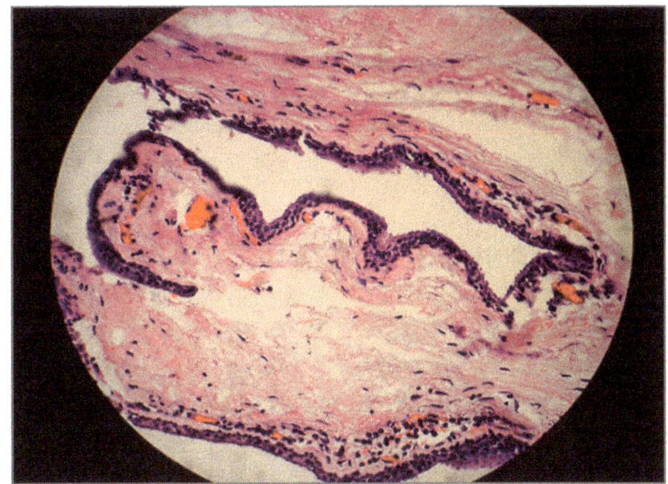

FIG. 5.6: Mucous retention cyst

Postsurgical Specimens

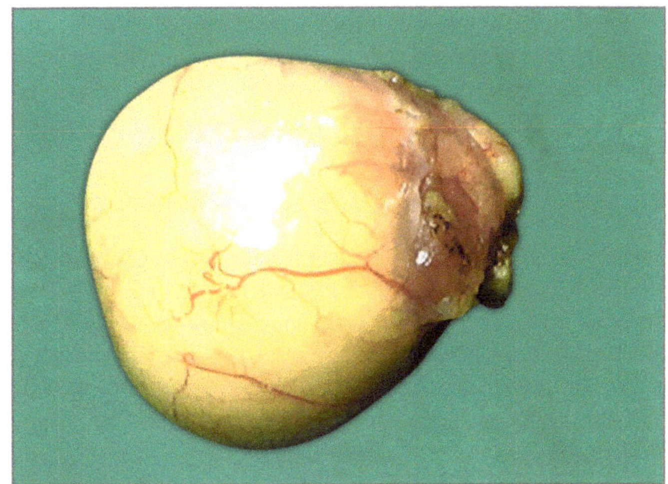

FIG. 5.7: Epidermoid cyst

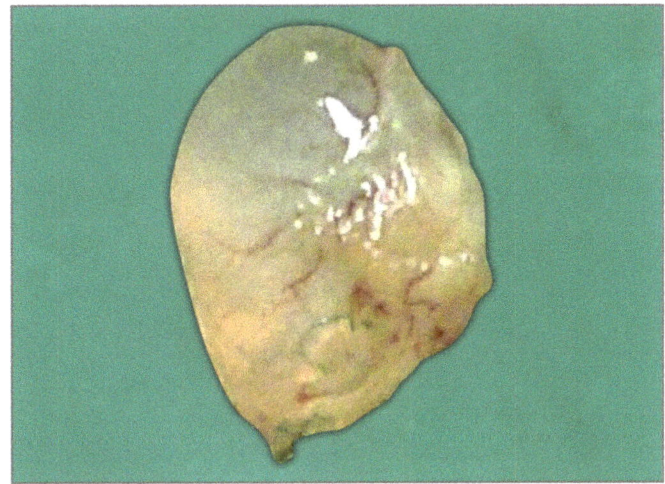

FIG. 5.8: Mucous retention cyst

Epidermoid	Mucous retention
Cyst lining stratified squamous epithelium	Cyst lining columnar epithelium
Cyst content keratin so cheesy, pultaceous	Cyst content liquid and so transparent
Congenital, ? Phonotrauma	Aquired
Cell rests in SLP of remnants of 4th and 6th branchial arch	Blockage of duct of mucous gland
Constant in size	May wax and wane in size
Easier to excise	Tend to rupture easily during excision

FIG. 5.9: Differences between epidermoid and mucous retention cysts

Palpation
↓
Subepithelial infiltration technique
↓
Incision, laser, or cold steel
↓
Blunt dissection
↓
Sharp dissection of anterior and posterior fibrotic bands, using laser or scissors
↓
Complete removal of cyst wall
↓
Preservation of overlying epithelium

FIG. 5.11: Surgical steps

SURGICAL STEPS

The main challenge during surgical excision of symptomatic cysts is rupture during excision with part of the cyst wall being left behind resulting in recurrence. The second concern is postoperative healing, which often depends on the depth of penetration of the cyst.

As a rule in phonomicrosurgery, maximum SLP should be preserved, thus staying close to the cyst during dissection is ideal.

It has been the authors experience that cysts tend to have anterior and posterior fibrotic bands tethering it, giving the appearance of a pearl (cyst) on a string (the bands).[3]

Identifying and cutting these bands or laserising them allows for an easier cyst excision with less chances of rupture. Blunt dissection of these bands is not usually successful and to be avoided.

CASE 1

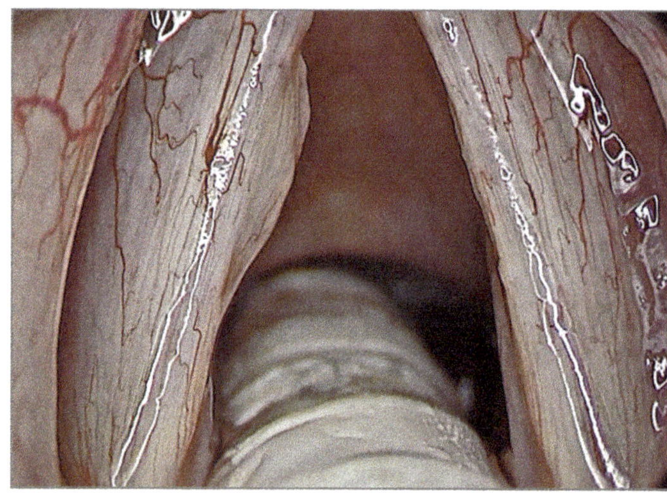

FIG. 5.12: A subepithelial cyst seen on the medial vibrating edge of the left vocal fold. Also seen is a Medtronic laser safe tube *in situ*. (E-CC)

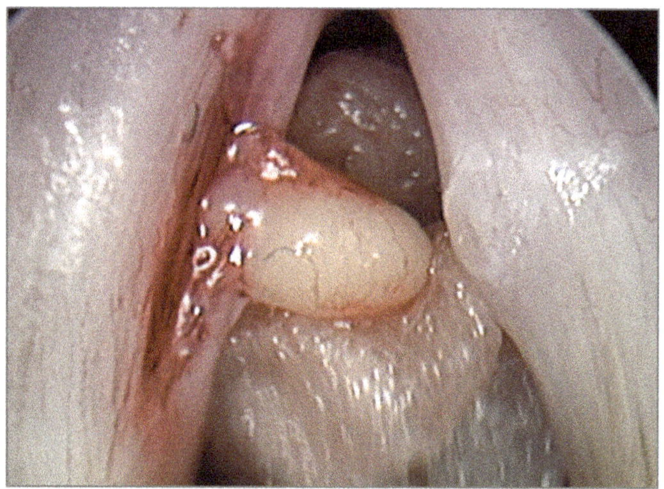

FIG. 5.10: An epidermoid cyst of the left vocal fold demonstrating the anterior and posterior fibrotic bands.

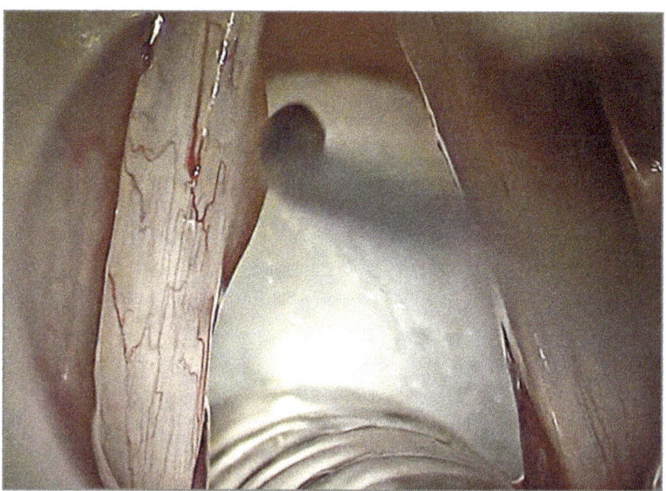

FIG. 5.13: Palpation of the cyst by a blunt microflap elevator to ascertain its firmness and to palpate its lateral extent. (M-CC)

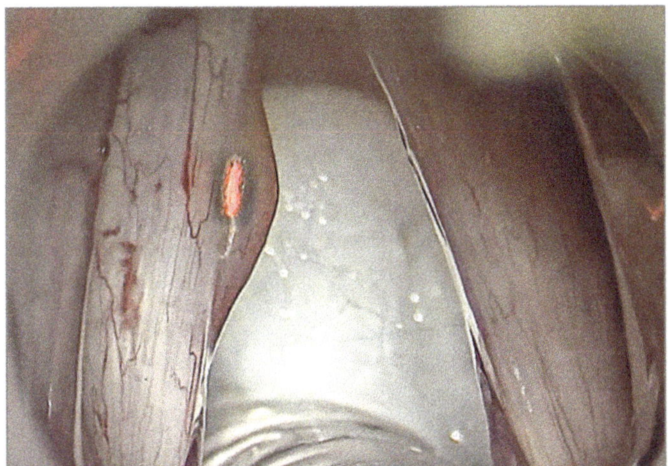

FIG. 5.14: An epithelial cordotomy being made at the immediate lateral edge of the cyst using a CO_2 laser AcuBlade. A wet cotton pledget is protecting the cuff of the laser endotracheal tube. The blurred image on the right upper corner is the laser plume suction. The SEIT has been used prior to this incision. (M-CC)

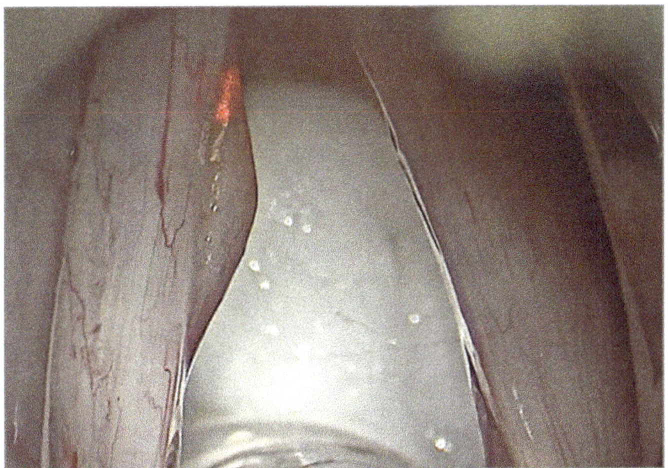

FIG. 5.15: Anterior extension of the epithelial cordotomy. (M-CC)

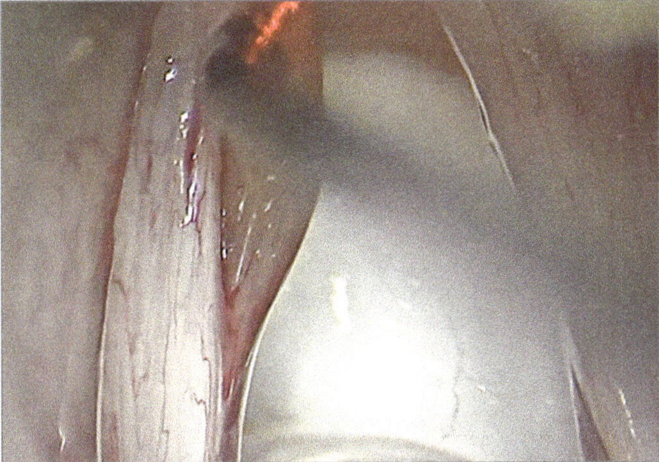

FIG. 5.16: Making a laser cut on the epithelium over the anterior most extent of the cyst while a microflap elevator is placed under this epithelium to protect inadvertent opening up of the cyst by the laser beam. This step reveals the underlying anterior fibrotic band. (M-CC)

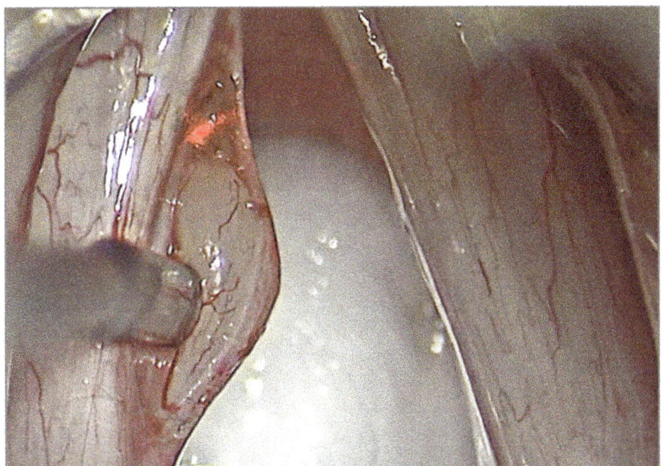

FIG. 5.17: The anterior fibrotic band tethering the cyst is now excised with the AcuBlade. This step is best performed by sharp dissection, either using a laser or a scissors. (M-CC)

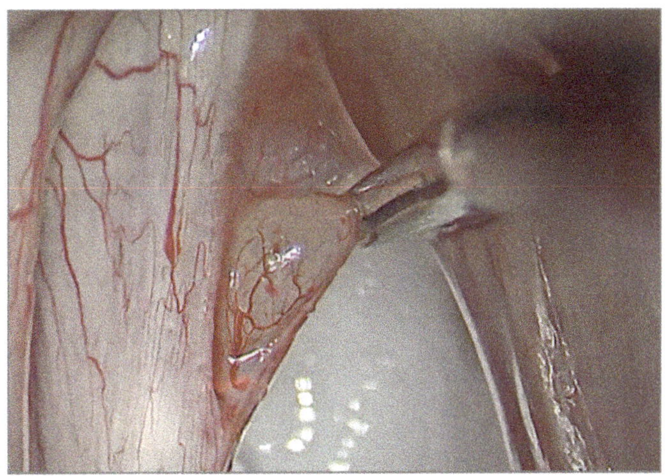

FIG. 5.18: Once the anterior fibrotic band has been excised, the cyst retracts posteriorly. It is safe to hold the epithelial edge or any connective tissue on the cyst; however, the cyst if held directly has a high propensity towards rupture. (M-CC)

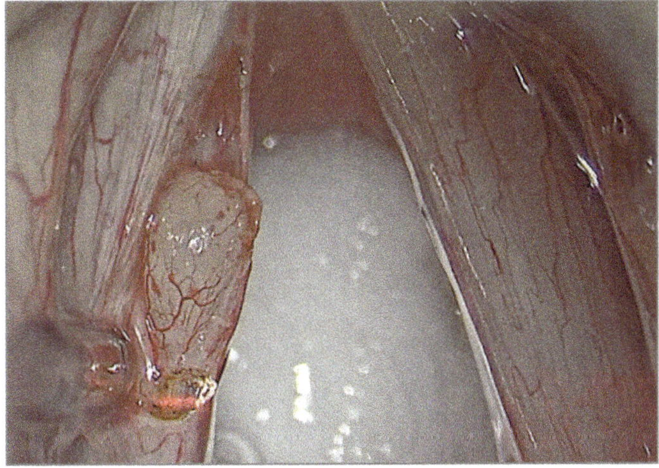

FIG. 5.19: The posterior fibrotic band is now being excised by the AcuBlade. These anterior and posterior fibrotic bands tethering the cyst are a common observation and have been referred to as a " pearl on a string" by the author.[3](M-CC)

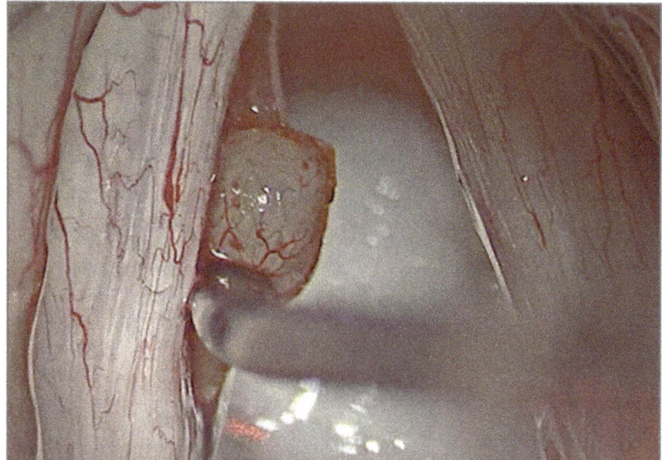

FIG. 5.20: There is now an anterior retraction of the cyst. The excision of the remaining attachments of the cyst from its bed is performed using a blunt microflap elevator. (M-CC)

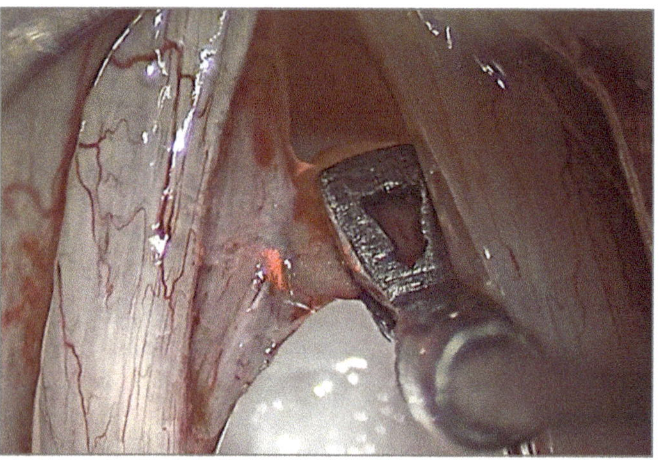

FIG. 5.21: The final laser excision of the epithelial attachment of the cyst is being performed. The cyst is being lightly held with a Bouchayer forceps. The fenestrae of this forceps allow the cyst to fill the space within the fenestra such that the cyst is held in an atraumatic fashion. Rupture of the cyst at this point is not worrisome, as almost all the attachments have been released. (M-CC)

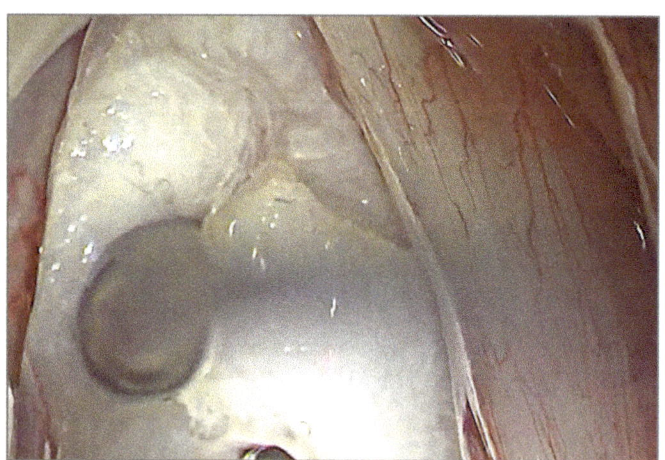

FIG. 5.22: A cotton pledget is being used to apply pressure on the infraglottic epithelium to stick onto the vibrating edge of the vocal fold. (M-CC)

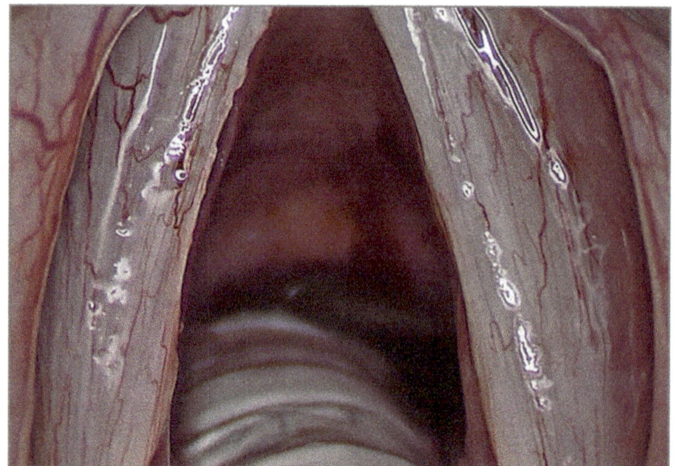

FIG. 5.23: The postoperative view of the vocal folds. (E-CC)

CASE 2

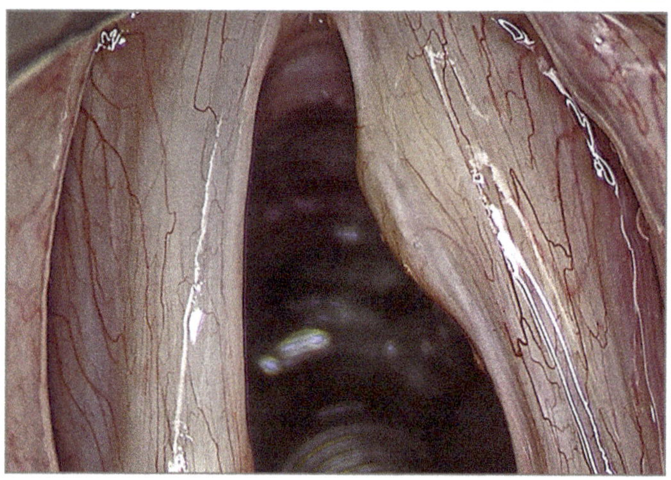

FIG. 5.24: A subepithelial cyst seen on the medial vibrating edge of the right vocal fold extending to the lower lip. (E-CC)

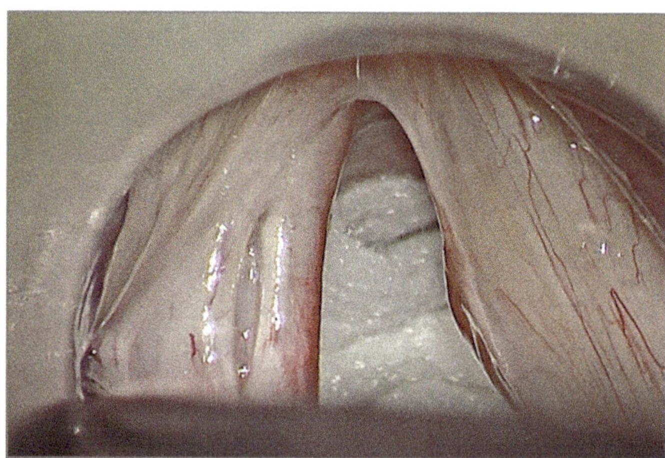

FIG. 5.25: Eversion of the left vocal fold reveals a sulcus vergeture on the lower lip of the left vocal fold. This finding had not been picked up on preoperative stroboscopy. A moist cotton pledget is protecting the cuff of the laser tube. (M-CC)

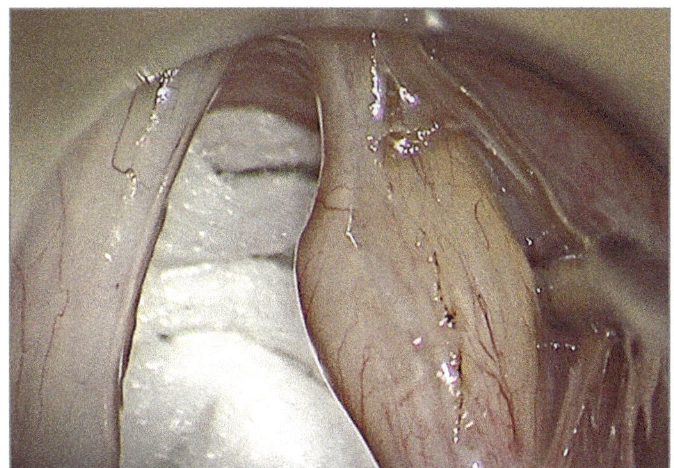

FIG. 5.26: An epithelial cordotomy has been performed on the lateral edge of the cyst. A blunt microflap elevator is seen separating the cyst from the underlying SLP. (M-CC)

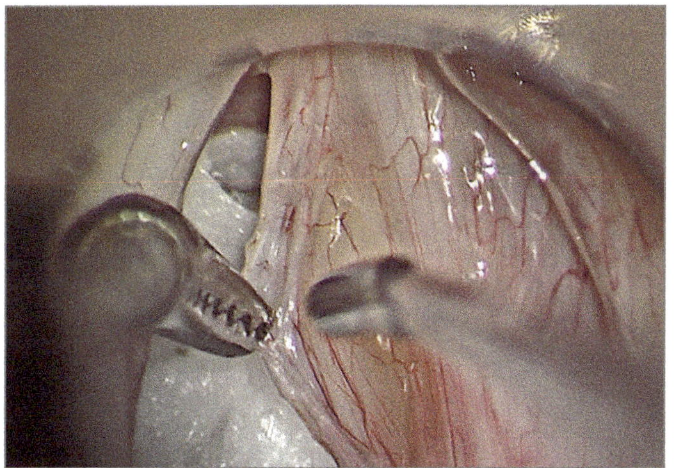

FIG. 5.27: A blunt microflap elevator being used to dissect the cyst from the overlying epithelium

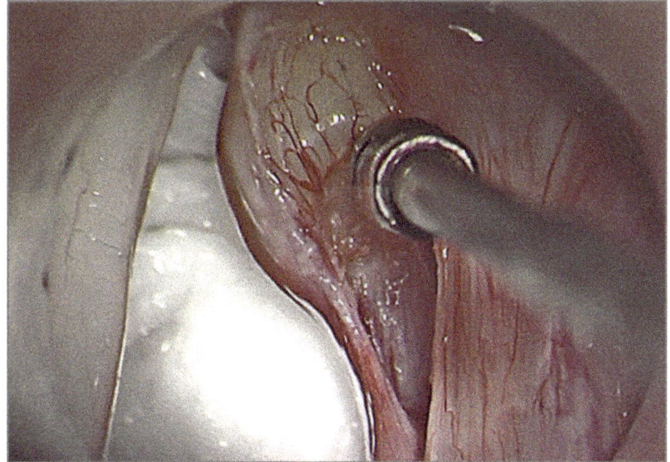

FIG. 5.28: Release of the posterior fibrotic band allows the posterior dissection of the cyst. (M-CC)

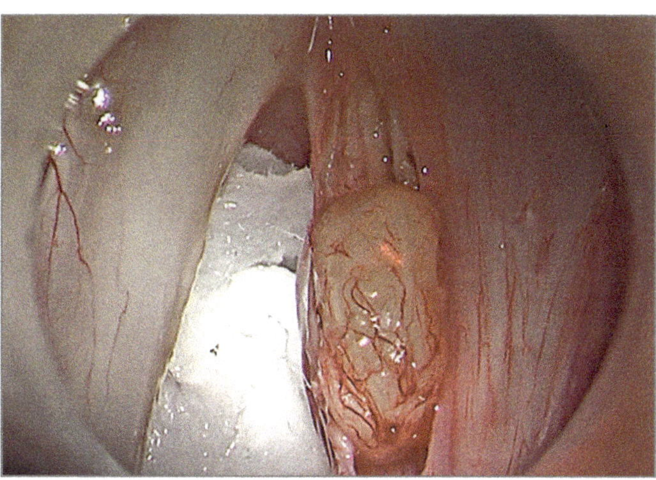

FIG. 5.29: The cyst has been separated from both the anterior and posterior fibrotic bands. (M-CC)

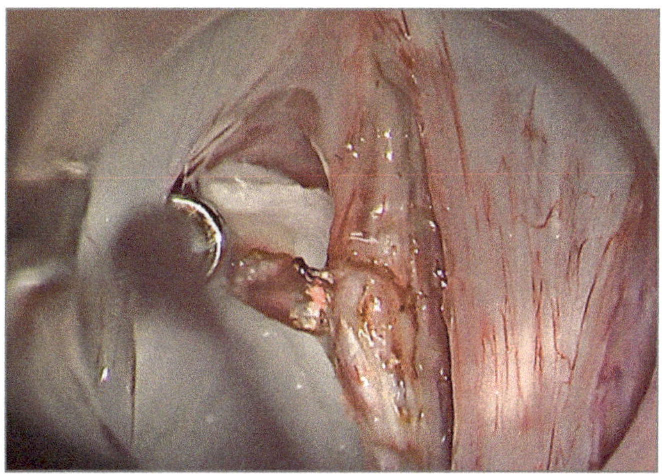

FIG. 5.30: Laser excision of the final epithelial attachment of the cyst. (M-CC)

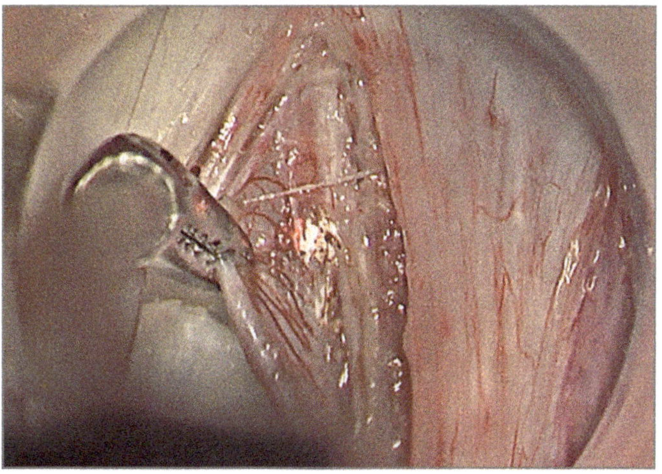

FIG. 5.31: Laser coagulation of the epithelial varices and laser thinning of the epithelial flap so as to achieve a good inversion and reposition of it on the medial vibrating edge of the vocal fold. (M-CC)

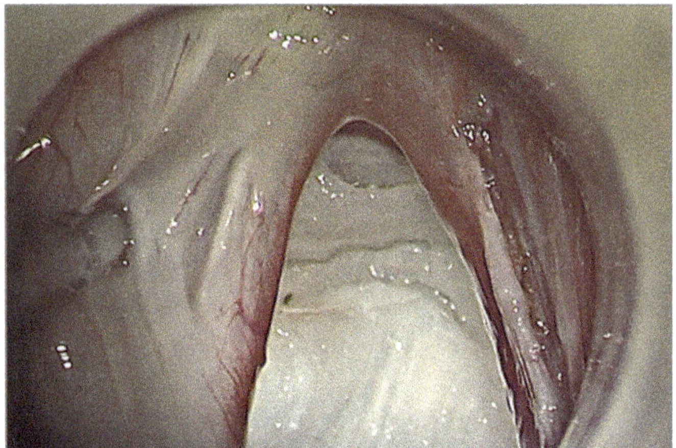

FIG. 5.32: Epithelial flap reposited back to cover the medial vibrating edge of the right vocal fold. A blunt microflap elevator is laterally retracting the left vocal fold to reveal the sulcus vergeture on the infraglottic edge of the vocal fold. (M-CC)

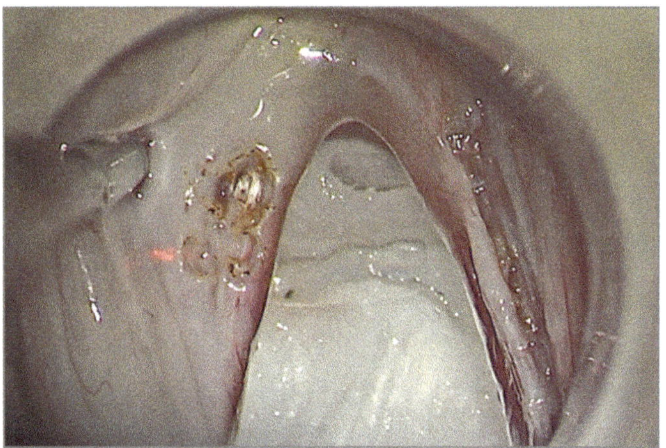

FIG. 5.33: Small release incisions are being taken, using the AcuBlade, perpendicular to and at the edges of the sulcus. This allows for gradual reepithelialization of the raw area interspersed with the epithelial areas and is used by the author for sulci that dip upto the ligament. It is based on the Pontes method but does not cut through the ligament and is used for sulci that reach up to but do not involve the ligament. (M-CC)

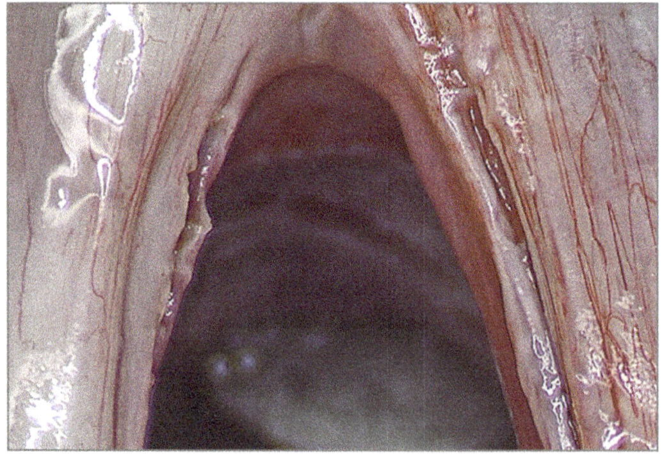

FIG. 5.34: Final postoperative view of the vocal folds. (E-CC)

CASE 3

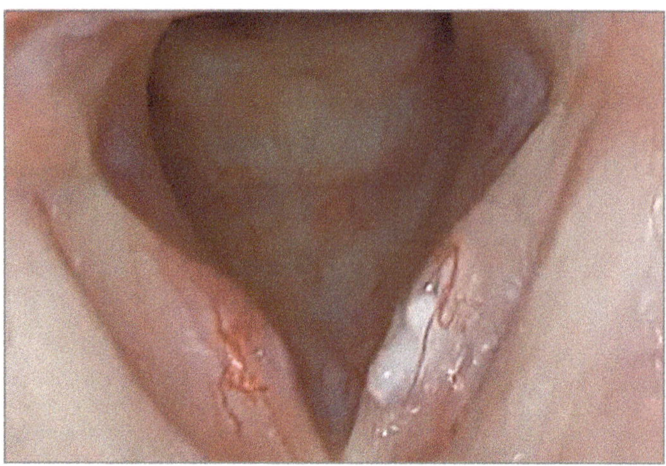

FIG. 5.35: White light 70-degree laryngoscopy revealing an open cyst of the left vocal fold with varices. Also seen are varices on the right vocal fold and a suspicious cyst on the superior surface of the right vocal fold

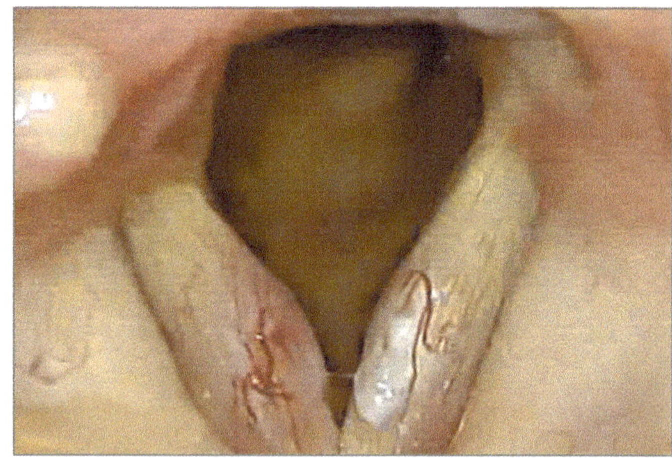

FIG. 5.36: Stroboscopy of case 3 using the Olympus system revealing a possible sulcus of the left vocal fold in addition to the open cyst contained within it

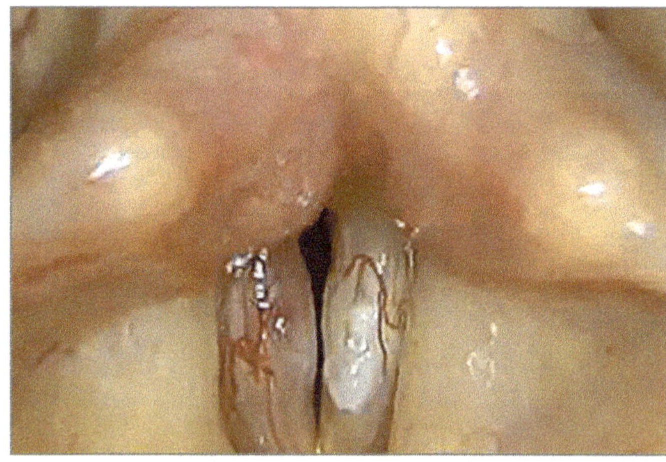

FIG. 5.37: Stroboscopy of case 3 with the vocal folds in adduction with an hourglass pattern of phonatory gap. The right vocal fold seems to have a subepithelial lesion also.

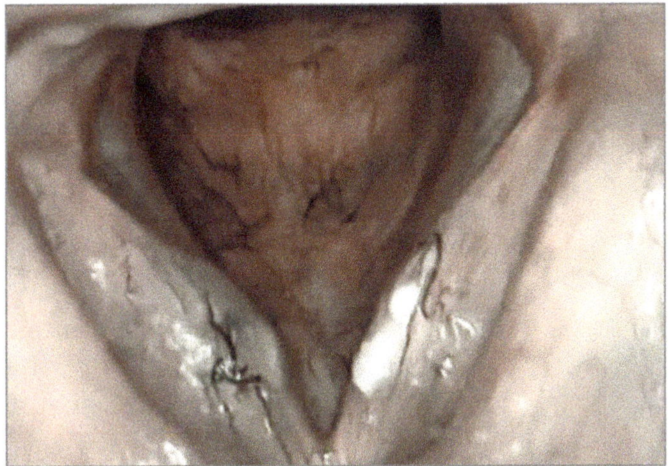

FIG. 5.38: Narrow band imaging of case 3 highlighting the white open cyst from the surrounding mucosa and the cyan subepithelial veins.

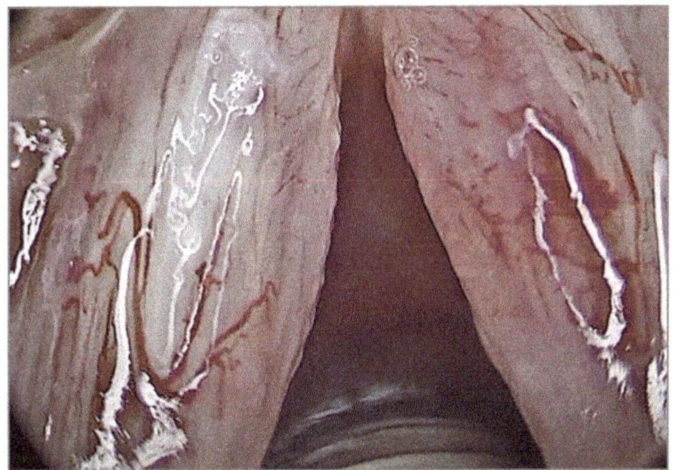

FIG. 5.39: An open epidermoid cyst is confirmed to lie within a sulcus vocalis of the left vocal fold with varices at its posterior margin on direct endoscopic evaluation with a 0 degree 10 mm telescope. The right vocal fold also reveals varices and ectasias on the superior surface. (E-CC)

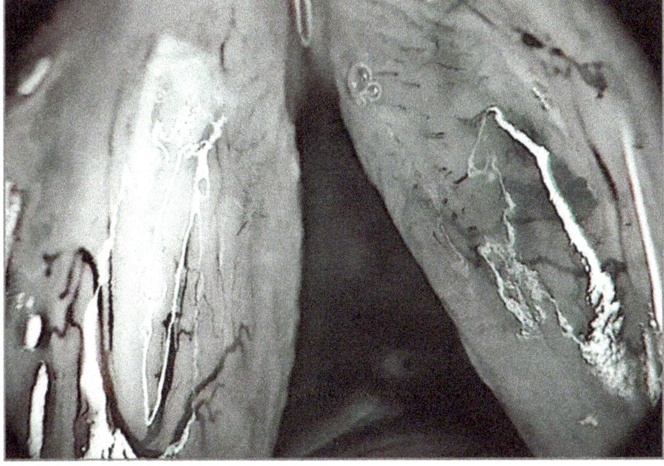

FIG. 5.40: The SA image of case 3 revealing brown surface capillaries and cyan subepithelial veins. (E-SA)

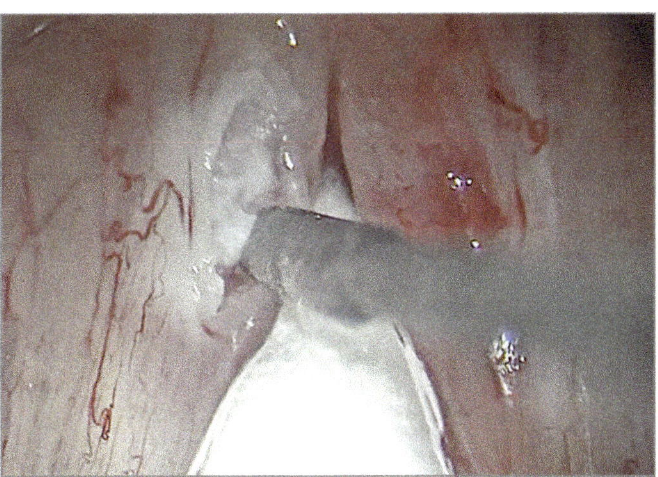

FIG. 5.41: A blunt microflap elevator retracting the medial lip of the left vocal fold sulcus. (M-CC)

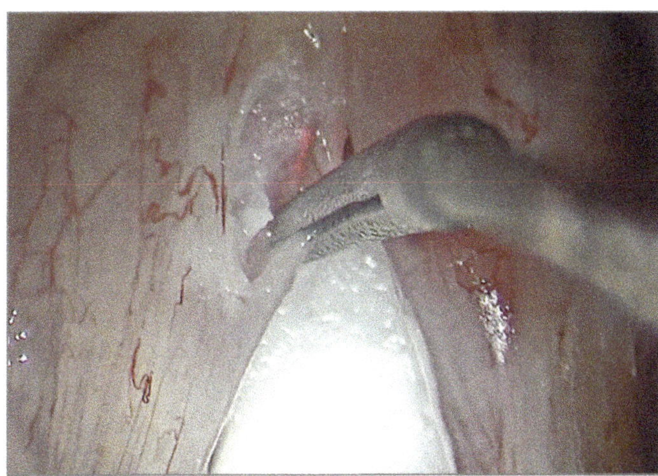

FIG. 5.42: A left crocodile forceps holding the medial lip of the sulcus while the AcuBlade is used to excise the open epidermoid cyst. (M-CC)

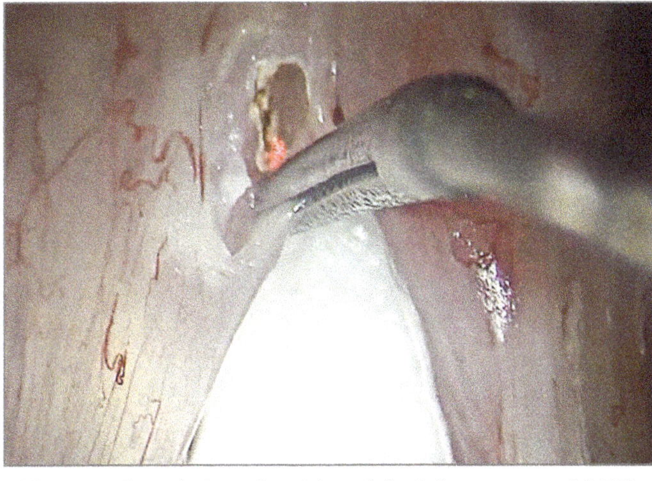

FIG. 5.43: Completion of excision of the left open cyst. (M-CC)

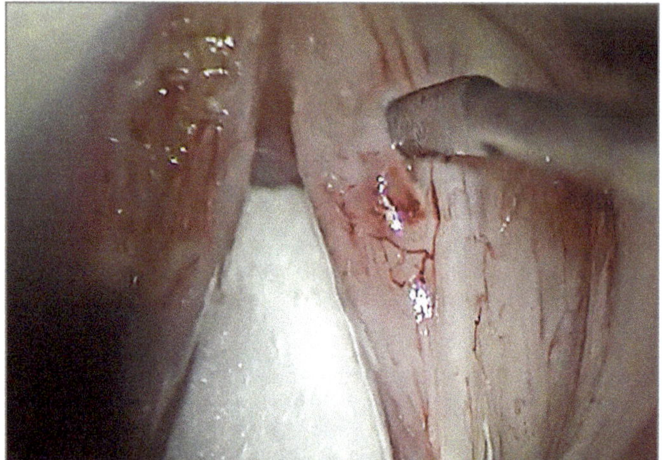

FIG. 5.44: Palpation of the right vocal fold with a blunt microflap elevator reveals a slit like focal pit, giving the impression of an incomplete mucosal bridge. (M-CC)

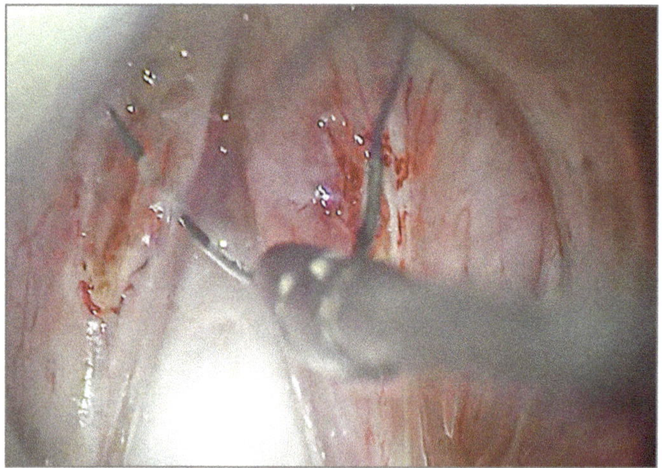

FIG. 5.45: 5-0 vicryl being used to suture the edges of the left vocal fold sulcus after completely excising (with laser) the epidermoid cyst contained within. The needle is seen passing through the medial epithelial edge. (M-CC)

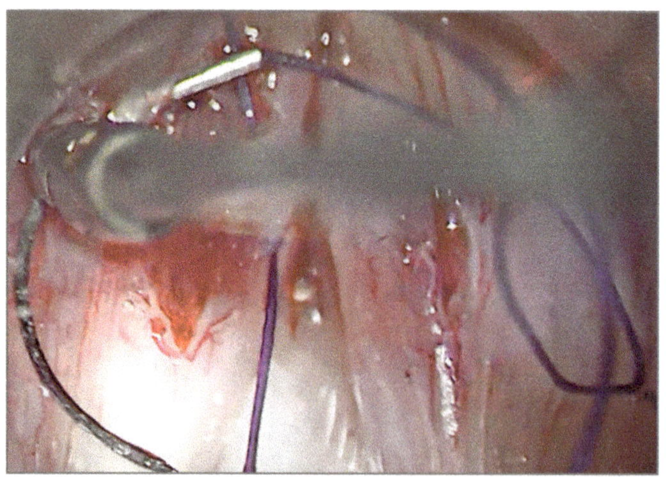

FIG. 5.46: The needle is now passed through the lateral epithelial edge. (M-CC)

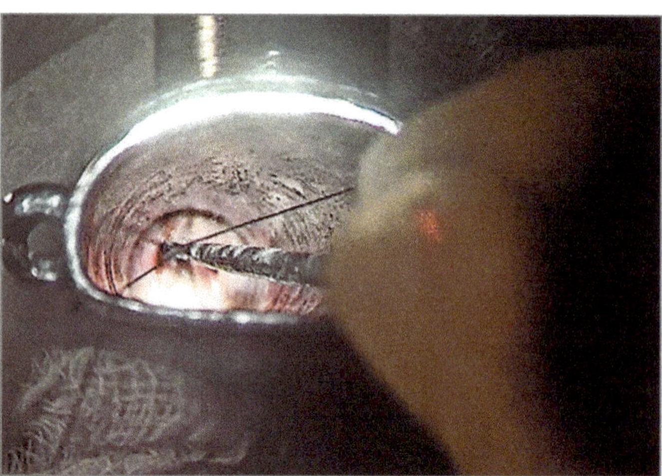

FIG. 5.47: Both the needle and non-needle end of the vicryl are brought out of the microlaryngoscope where a knot is made and then slid down to the vocal fold level with the help of a claw-like knot slider

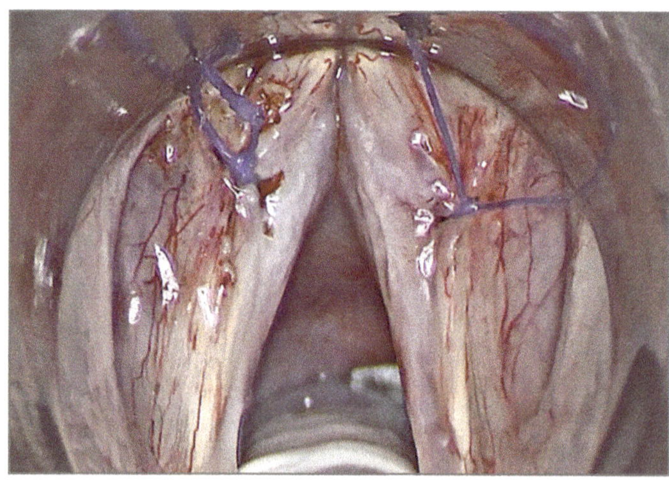

FIG. 5.48: Final postoperative image taken after the sulcus of both the sides has been freshened and edges sutured to one another. (E-CC)

CASE 4

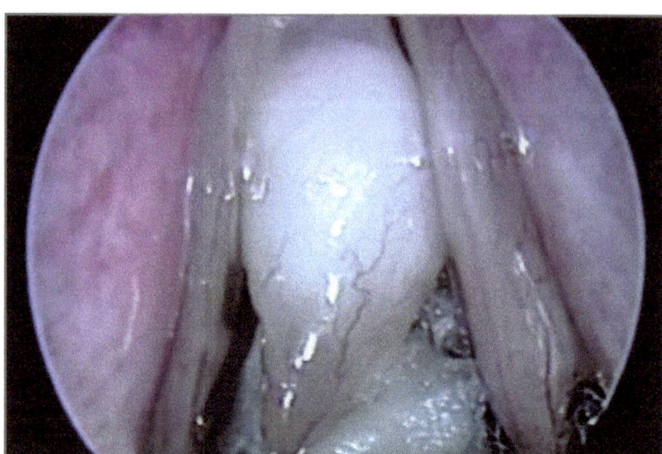

FIG. 5.49: A blunt microflap elevator is being used to palpate the lateral extent of a large epidermoid subepithelial cyst of the left vocal fold. A moist cotton pledget is seen in the subglottis. (VLS- -3 chip)

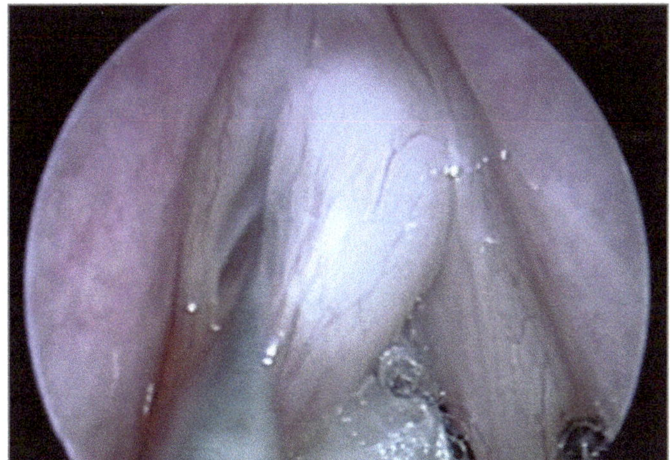

FIG. 5.50: A sickle knife directed upwards being used to make an epithelial cordotomy just lateral to the left subepithelial cyst. (VLS-3 chip)

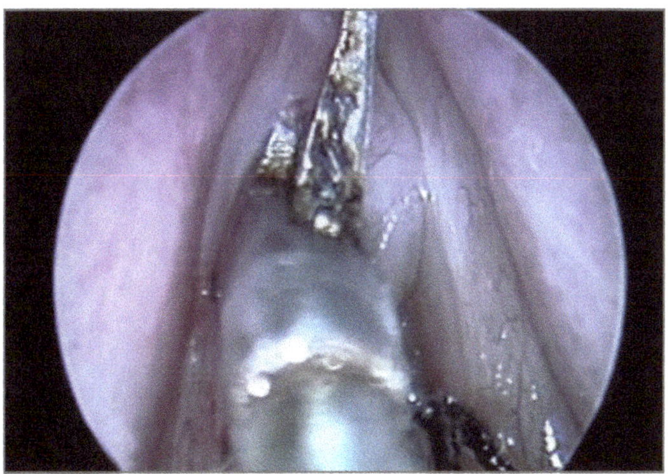

FIG. 5.51: Extension of the epithelial cordotomy anteriorly using an upward directed scissors. (VLS-3 chip)

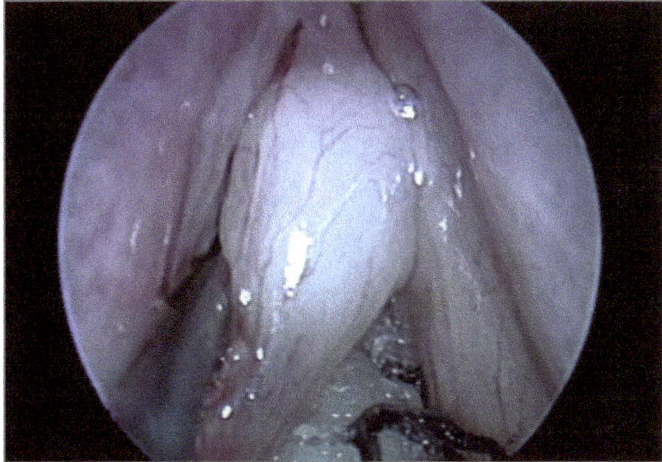

FIG. 5.52: A blunt microflap elevator being used to separate the cyst from the underlying SLP. (VLS-3 chip)

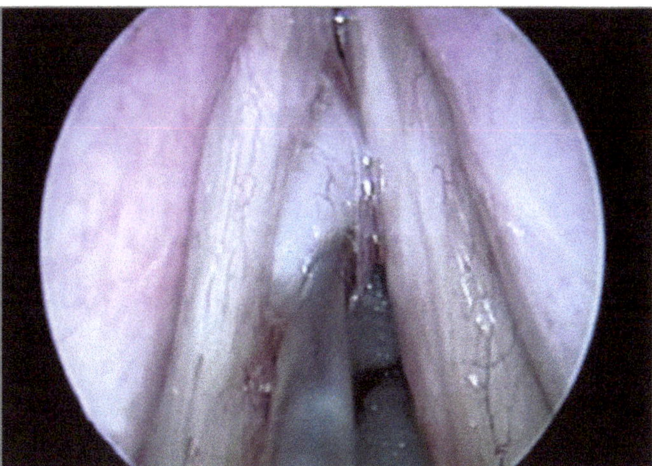

FIG. 5.53: A blunt microflap elevator being used to separate the cyst from the overlying epithelium. (VLS-3 chip)

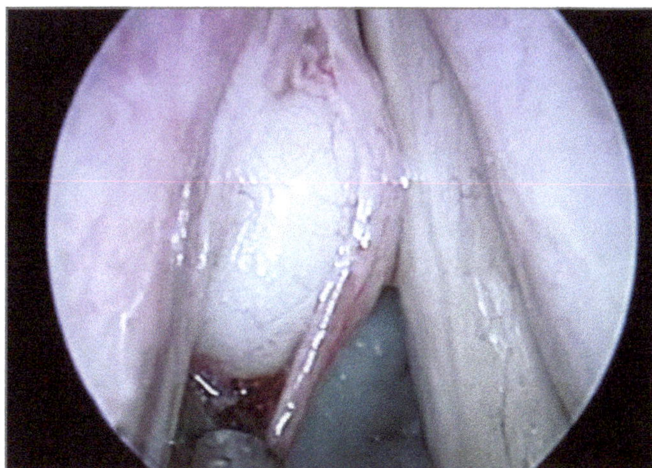

FIG. 5.54: Cutting the posterior fibrotic band with a straight scissors. The anterior fibrotic band has not been cut. Being one of the earlier cases in the author's experience, the importance of excising these anterior and posterior fibrotic bands was not clearly appreciated then. (VLS-3 chip)

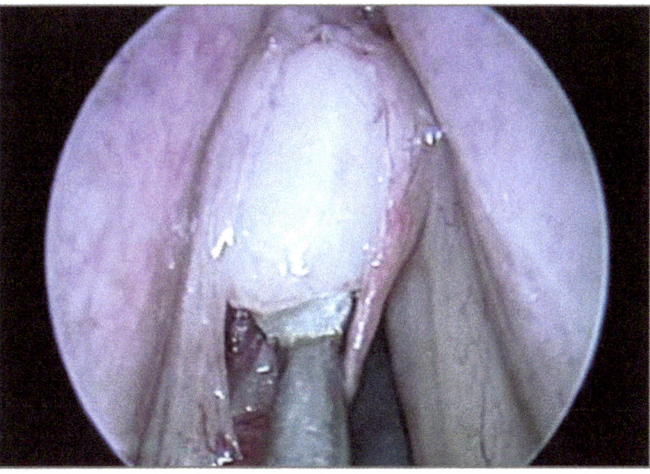

FIG. 5.55: Delivering the cyst from its bed with the help of a 90-degree microflap elevator. (VLS-3 chip)

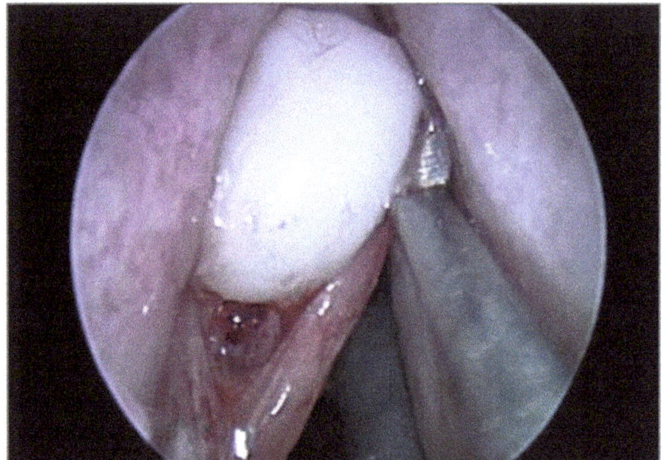

FIG. 5.56: Cyst being delivered out of its bed. (VLS-3 chip)

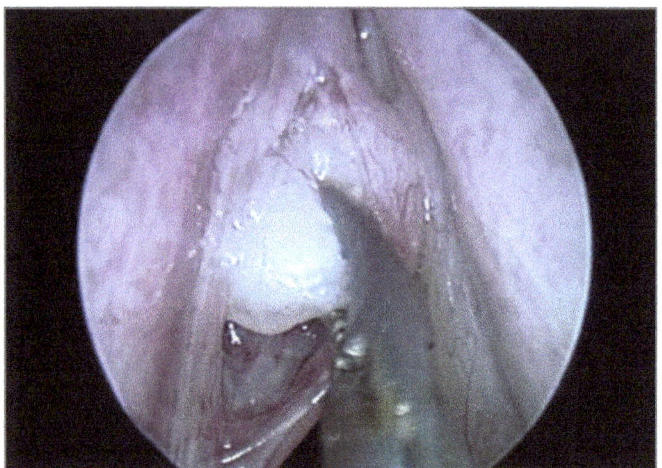

FIG. 5.57: Holding the cyst with a left crocodile to complete the excision. (VLS-3 chip)

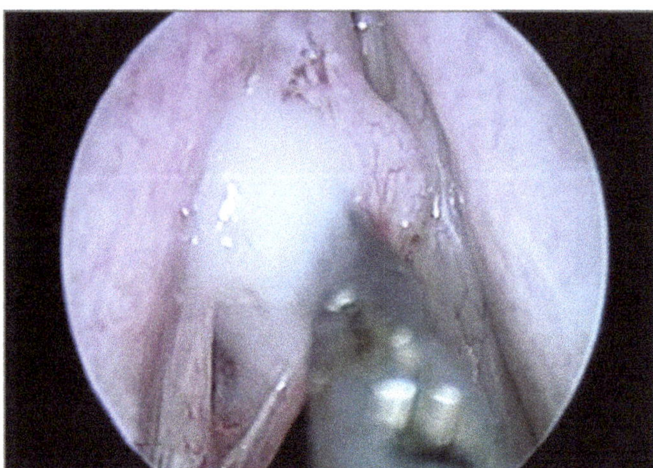

FIG. 5.58: Rupture of the cyst caused by the pressure exerted by the left crocodile forceps. A large Bouchayer held very gently, instead of the crocodile, may have prevented this rupture. Prior cutting of the anterior fibrotic band also may have facilitated complete removal of the cyst without a need to hold it. (VLS-3 chip)

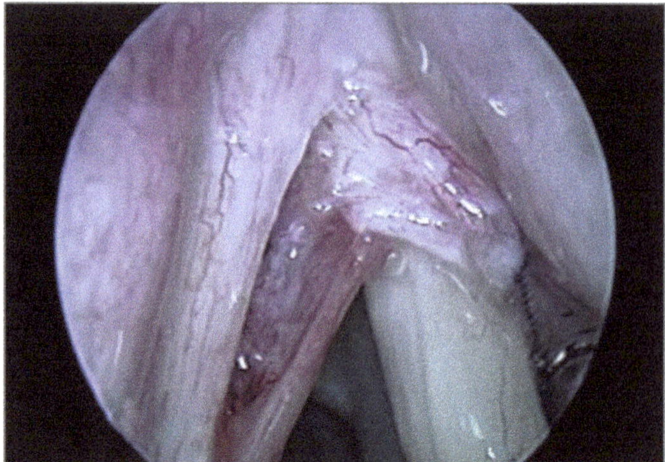

FIG. 5.59: Once a large cyst such as this is ruptured, it is essential to identify the entire cyst capsule and excise it. Holding the cyst capsule with medial traction makes the rest of the surgery easier in this case, however, in cases of thin cyst capsules the identification of the capsule may be tricky. (VLS-3 chip)

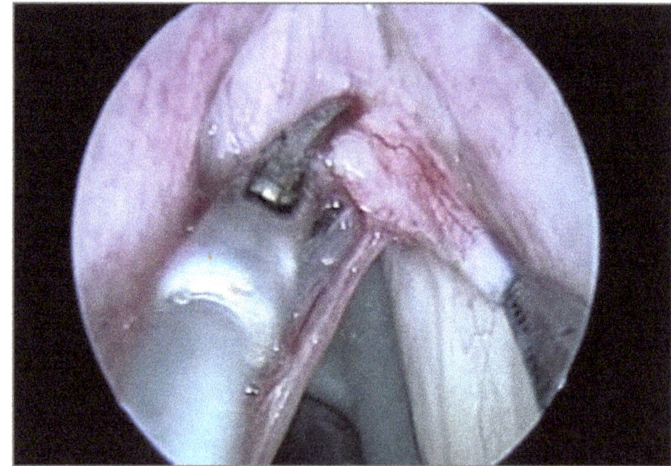

FIG. 5.60: Cutting the anterior fibrotic attachment with a scissors. Prior dissection of this band may have prevented cyst rupture. (VLS-3 chip)

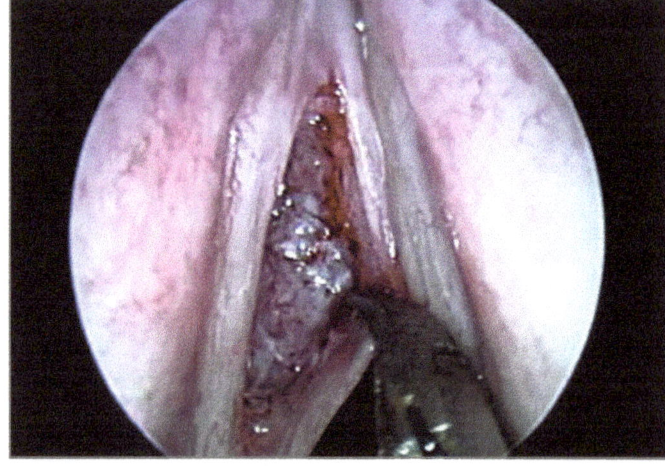

FIG. 5.61: Inspection of the cyst bed to confirm absence of any remnant cyst wall. (VLS-3 chip)

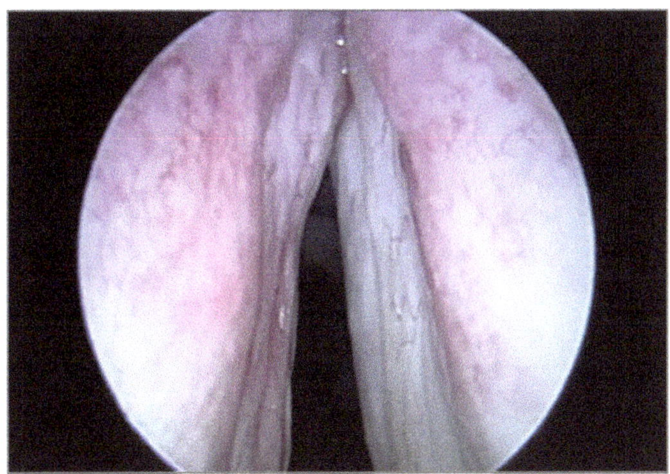

FIG. 5.62: Reposition of the overlying epithelium with a good edge to edge approximation at the site of epithelial cordotomy. (VLS-3 chip)

CASE 5

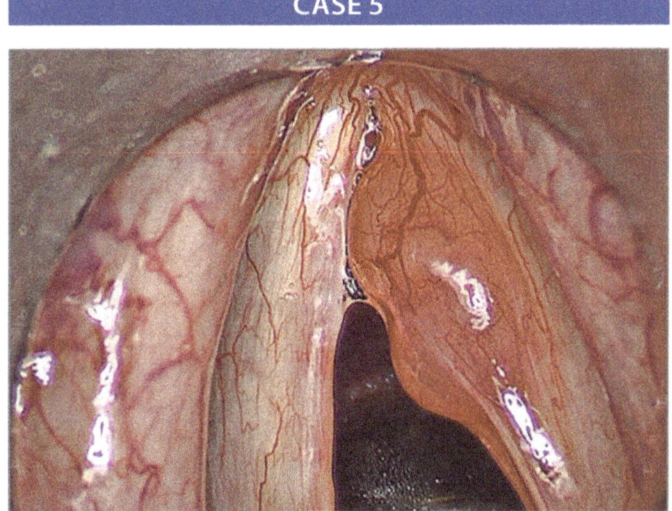

FIG. 5.63: Right bilobed cyst with anterior feeding vessels. (E-CC)

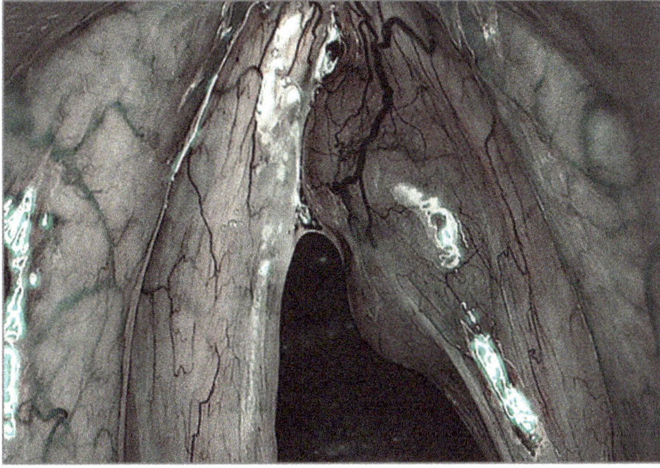

FIG. 5.64: Spectra A image of case 5, the subepithelial cyan vessel is clearly seen

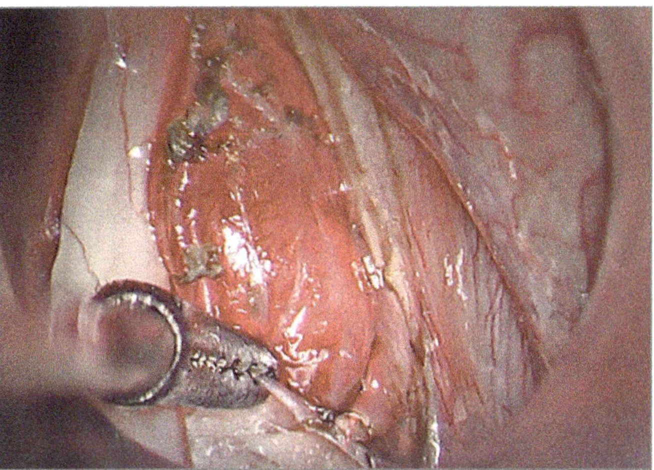

FIG. 5.65: Following an epithelial cordotomy just lateral to the cyst, it is dissected away from the underlying SLP. (M-CC)

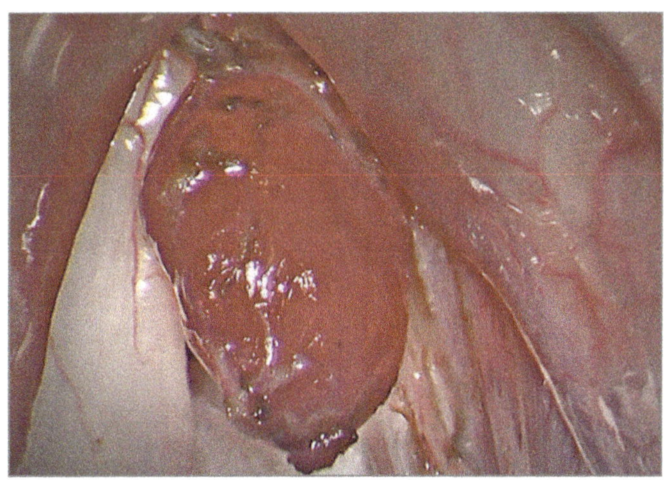

FIG. 5.66: Most of the overlying epithelium of the cyst is excised along with it, retaining only the infraglottic epithelium

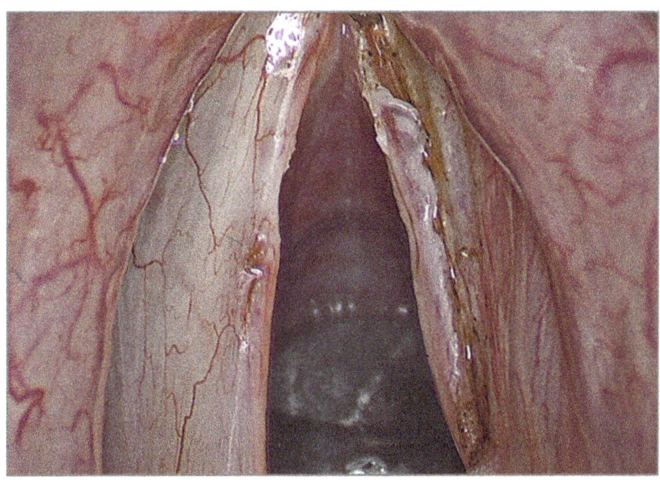

FIG. 5.67: Redraped infraglottic epithelium on the medial vibrating edge of the right vocal fold following complete excision of the cyst. (M-CC)

CASE 6

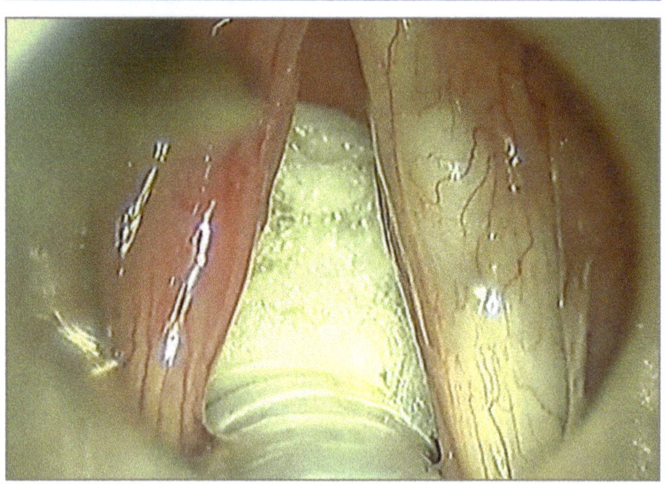

FIG. 5.68: Right subepithelial cyst with left vocal fold hemorrhage. (M-3 chip)

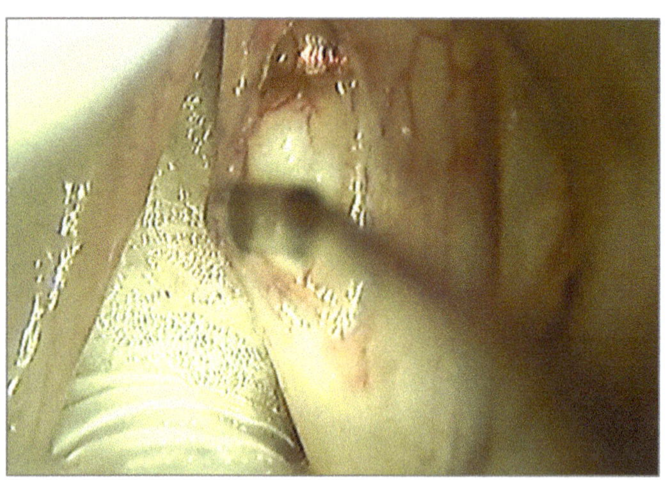

FIG. 5.69: CO_2 laser AcuBlade cutting the anterior fibrotic band. A blunt microflap elevator is being used to retract the medial edge of the epithelium to aid dissection of the cyst. (M-3 chip)

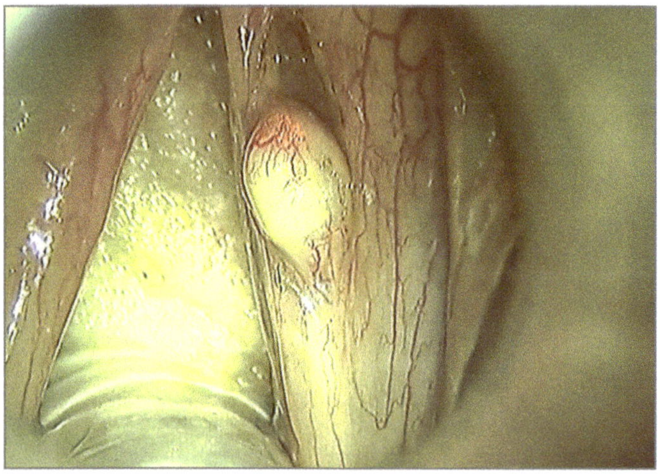

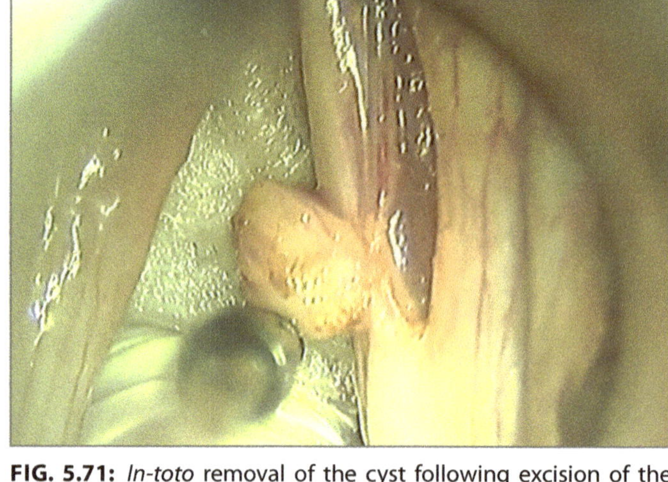

FIG. 5.71: *In-toto* removal of the cyst following excision of the posterior fibrotic band.

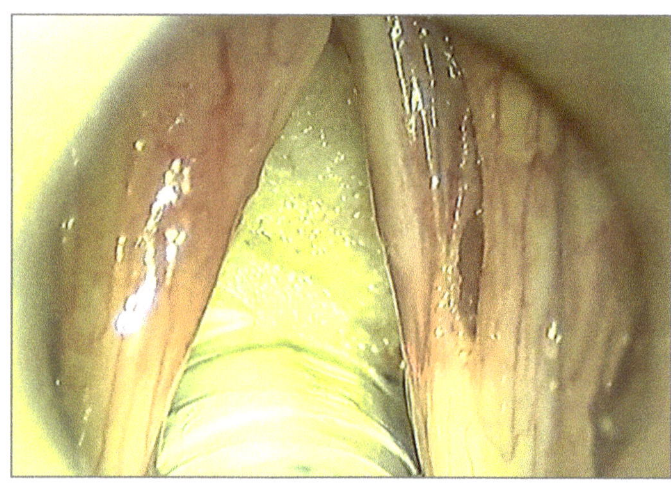

FIG. 5.72: Re-draping the epithelium on the medial vibrating edge. A small amount of epithelial loss is present posteriorly. (M-3 chip)

FIG. 5.70: The cyst has been released anteriorly. (M- 3 chip)

CASE 7

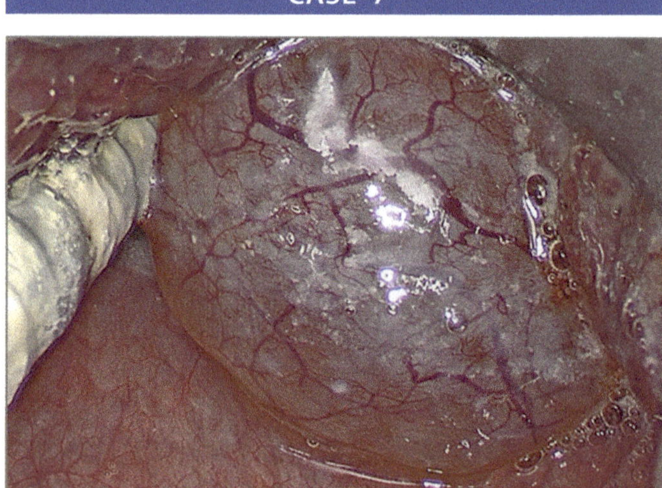

FIG. 5.73: A large right vallecular cyst. (E-CC)

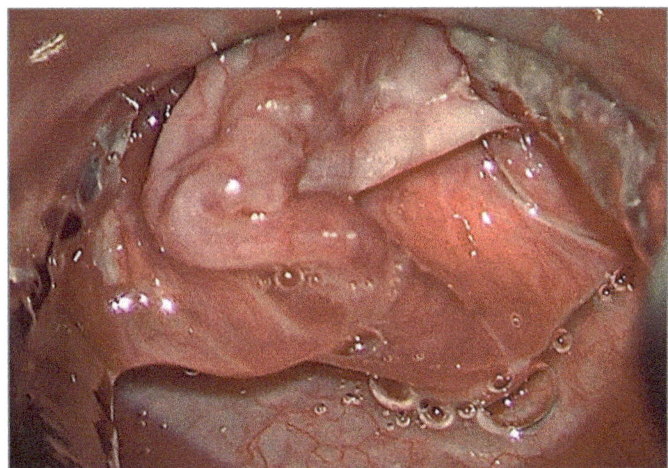

FIG. 5.74: Collapse of the cyst following aspiration of cyst contents. (M-CC)

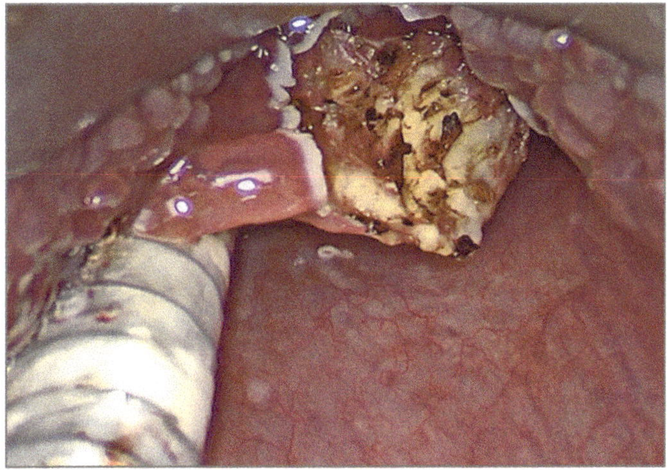

FIG. 5.75: Laser excision of the entire cyst wall, exposing the lingual surface of the epiglottic cartilage on the right side. (M-CC)

CASE 8

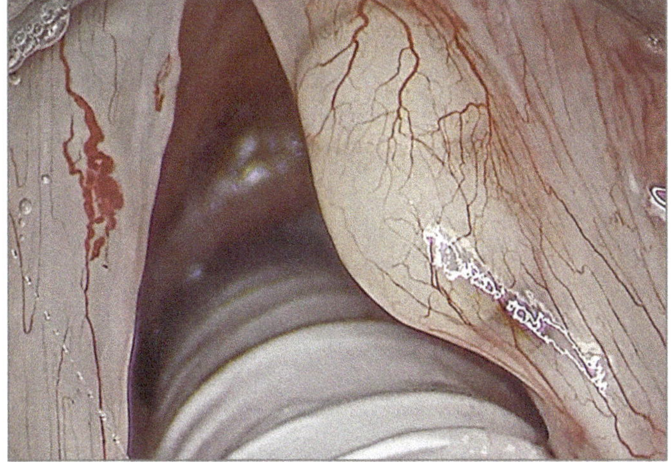

FIG. 5.76: A bilobed right subepithelial cyst with overlying blood vessels and left vocal fold ectasia. (E-CC)

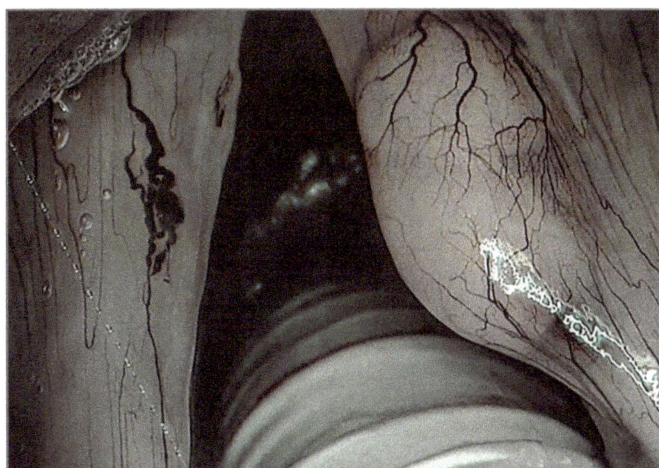

FIG. 5.77: Spectra A image of case 8 with blood vessels highlighted in cyan colour. (M-SA)

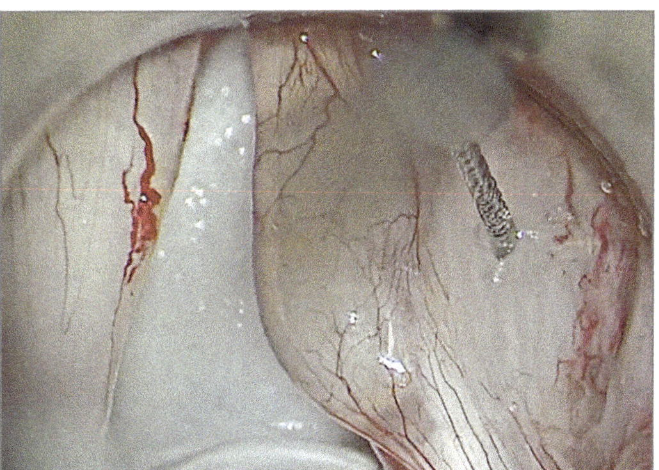

FIG. 5.78: Subepithelial infiltration technique being used on the right vocal fold using a 27 gauge needle. (M-CC)

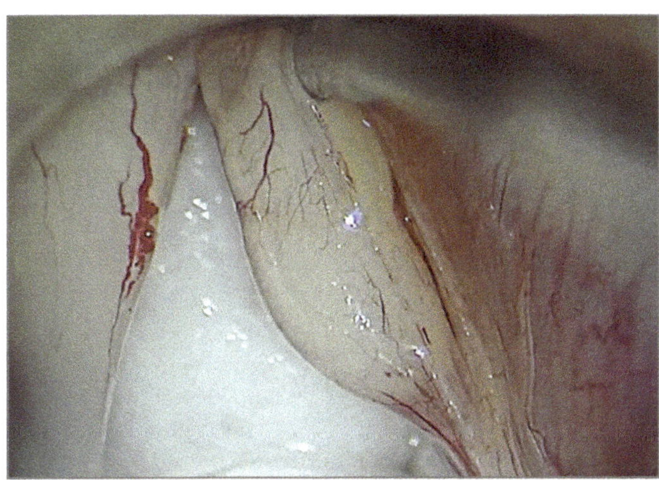

FIG. 5.79: Blunt dissection of the cyst from the overlying epithelium anteriorly. (M- CC)

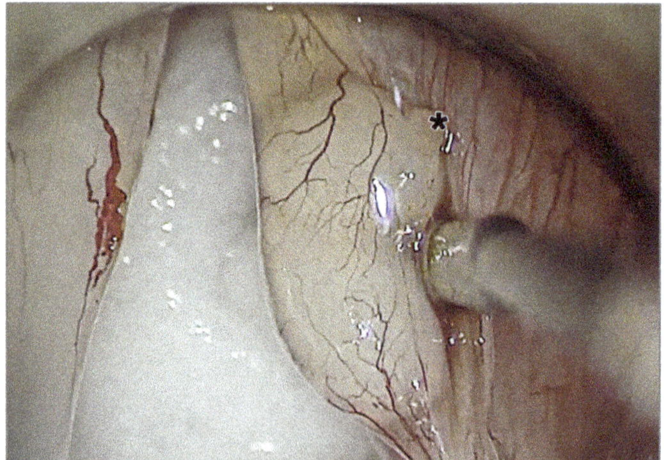

FIG. 5.80: An early leak of the cyst is seen (*), possibly caused at the time of incision. (M-CC)

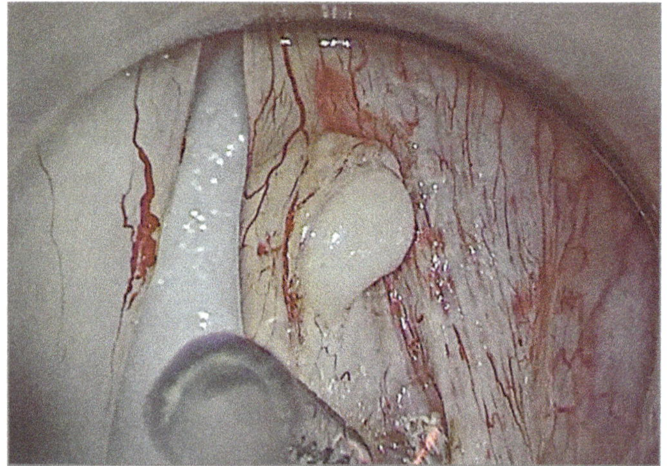

FIG. 5.81: Decision to excise the cyst with the overlying epithelium due to the leak in the cyst wall early on in the surgery when adequate dissection has not taken place. (M-CC)

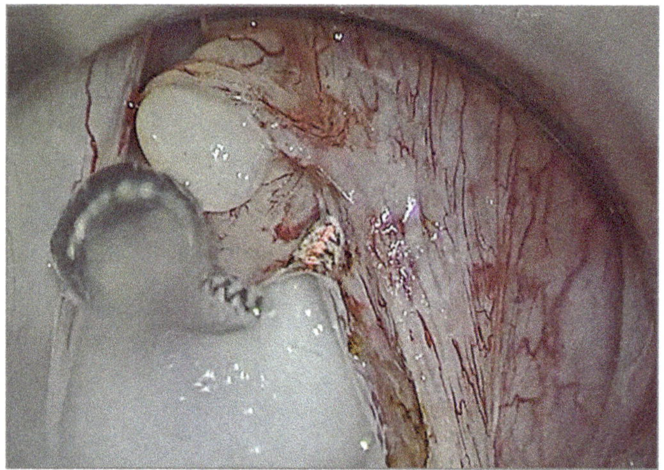

FIG. 5.82: Right crocodile holding the cyst with the overlying epithelium. CO_2 AcuBlade excision being performed from a posterior direction. (M-CC)

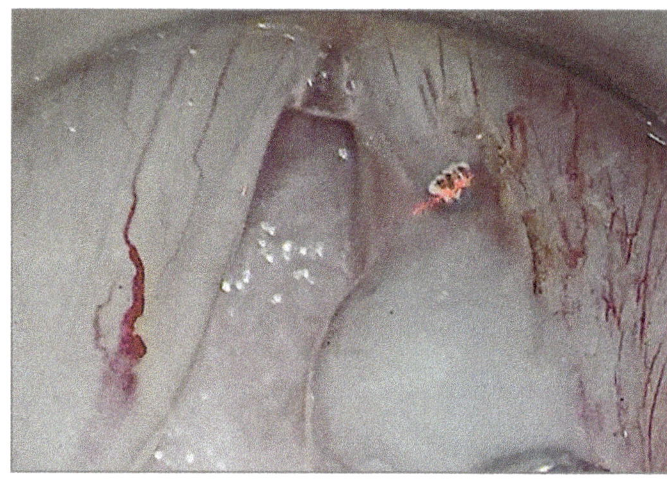

FIG. 5.83: The cyst is now lateralized to expose the epithelium anterior to the cyst where the final attachment is released with the AcuBlade. (M-CC)

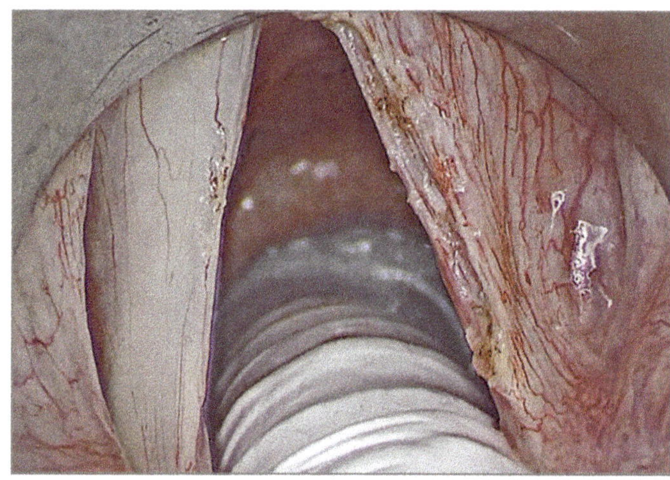

FIG. 5.84: Final postoperative picture, the healing will take longer due to epithelial loss. However, complete excision prevents recurrence and preservation of SLP promotes good healing. (E-CC)

CASE 9

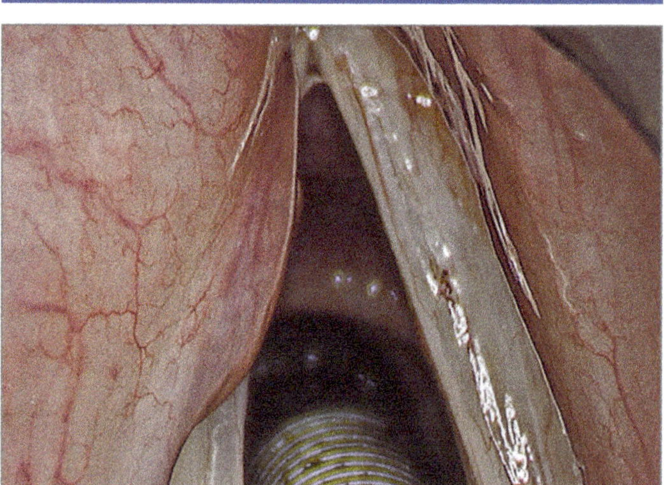

FIG. 5.85: A left ventricular cyst. (E-CC)

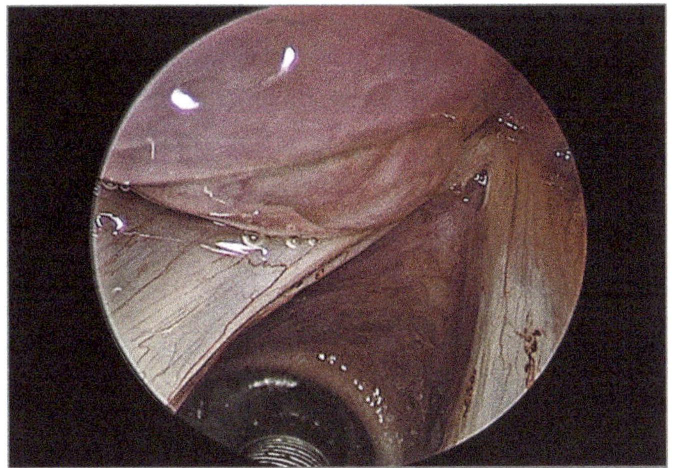

FIG. 5.86: Same cyst seen with a 30 degree telescope. (E-CC)

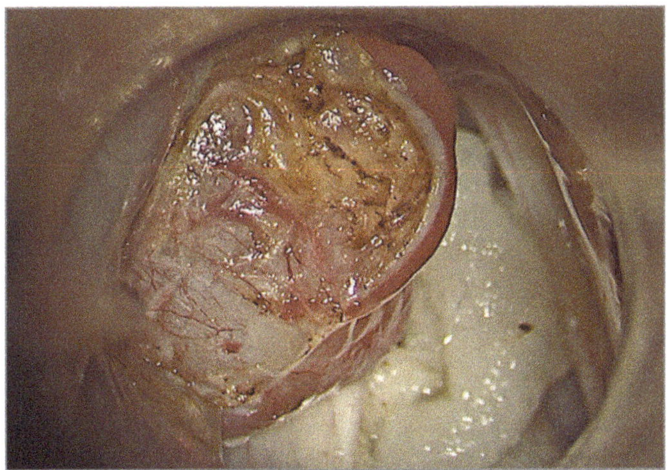

FIG. 5.87: Laser excision of the cyst. (M- CC)

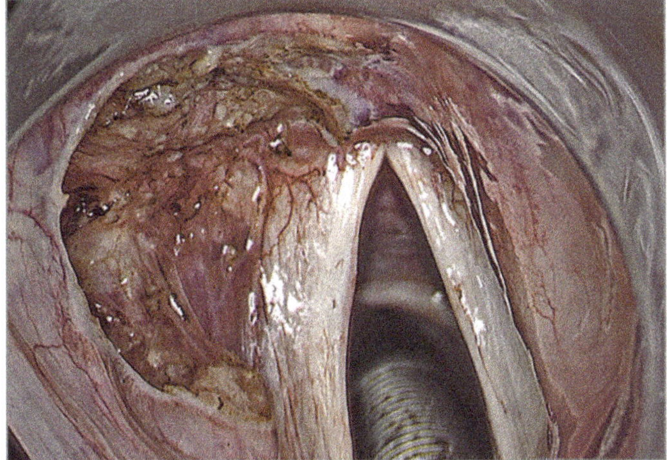

FIG. 5.88: Final postoperative picture following complete cyst excision. In the case of ventricular cysts, the overlying epithelium need not be retained. The true vocal fold is not operated upon. (E-CC)

CASE 10

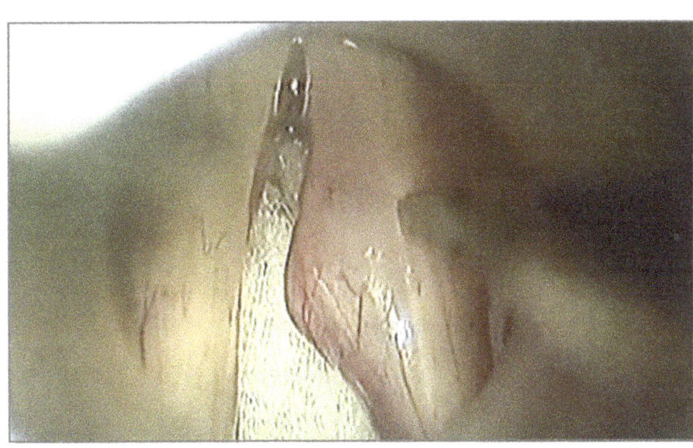

FIG. 5.89: Palpation of the lateral edge of the right subepithelial cyst. (M- 3 chip)

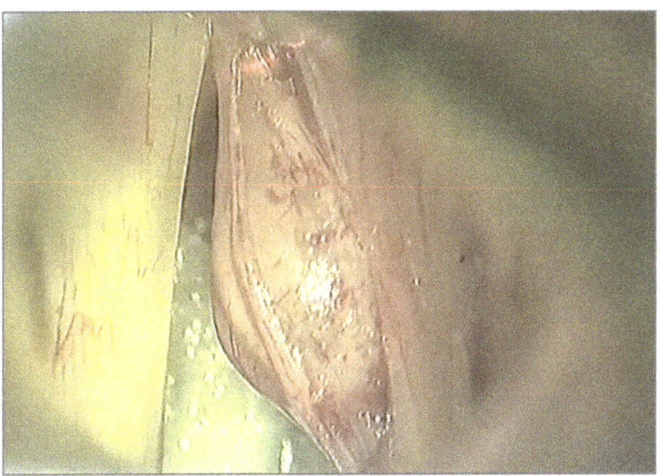

FIG. 5.90: Anterior fibrotic band being cut by the AcuBlade. (M- 3 chip)

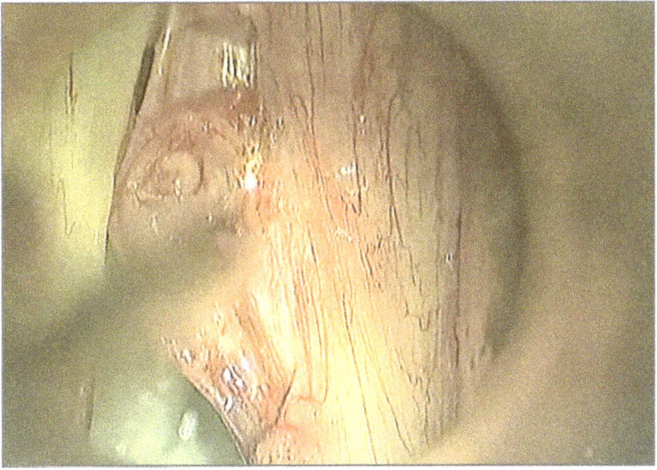

FIG. 5.91: During dissection of the cyst it is found attached to the ligament and the cyst opens up during this dissection. (M- 3 chip)

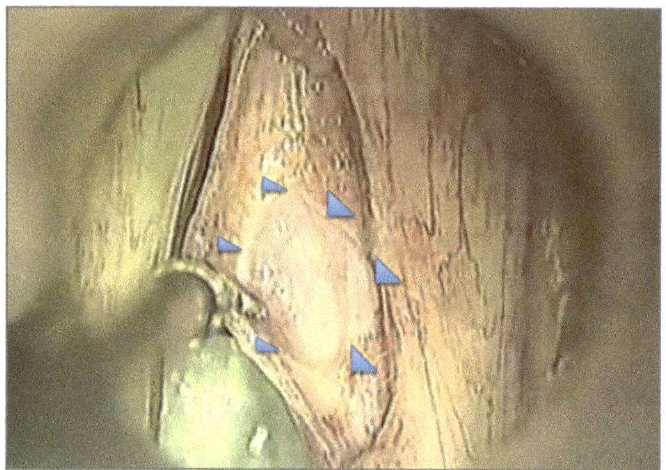

FIG. 5.92: Following excision of the cyst, inspection of the bed reveals residual cyst wall (in blue arrows) adherent to both the vocal ligament as well as part of overlying epithelium. (M-3 chip)

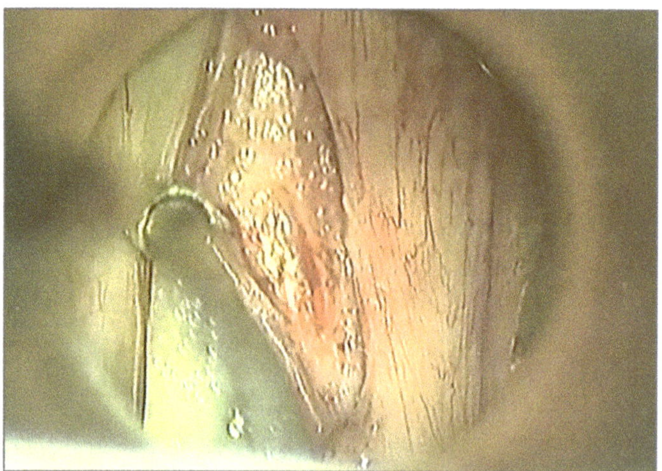

FIG. 5.93: The residual cyst wall is laserised with the CO_2 laser AcuBlade. (M-3 chip)

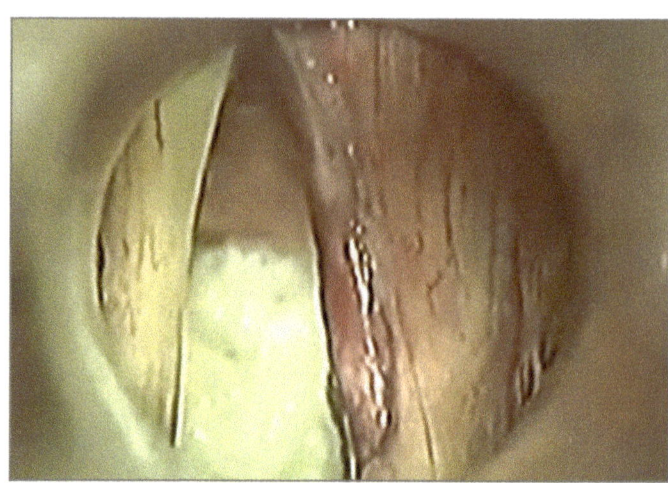

FIG. 5.94: The epithelial flap is reposited over the medial vibrating edge. (M-3 chip)

REFERENCES

1. Nupur KN. Cyst, sulci and mucosal bridge. In: Nupur KN, Amitabha R, editors. Textbook of laryngology: Official publication of the Association of Phonosurgeons of India. New Delhi: Jaypee Brothers Medical Publishers (P) Ltd.; 2017. pp. 155-70.
2. Rosen CA, Simpson CB. Pathological conditions of the vocal folds: Operative techniques in laryngology. Vol. 1. Berlin, Heidelgerg: Springer; 2008. pp. 21-8.
3. Nupur N, Sunita C. Sub epithelial vocal fold cyst-pearl on a string? Int J Phonosurg Laryngol. 2012;2(2):53-6.

CHAPTER 6

Sulcus

DEFINITION

Vocal fold sulcus is a linear invagination of epithelium along the medial edge of the vocal fold into or beyond the SLP. Depth of invagination generally correlates with symptom severity, as well as the prognosis for successful treatment.[1]

Sulci were originally thought to be always congenital with the patient giving a classical history of a hoarse voice from childhood. However, cases of sulci developing later on in life, probably due to vocal abuse and misuse or following upper respiratory tract infection are not uncommon.[2]

Garel, in 1923, first named the groove "vergeture," because it resembles the skin disorder of the same name ("vergeture" is the French term for stretch mark).[3]

Bouchayer and Cornut (1985) described 2 types of sulcus:

1. True sulcus, corresponding to an open epidermoid cyst with thickened epithelium where the bottom of the cystic pouch is adherent to or transgresses the vocal ligament
2. Sulcus vergeture, corresponding to atrophy of the mucosa covering the vocal ligament.[44]

Ford et al. (1996) have described a classification system for sulcus deformities.[5]

TYPE 1 (PHYSIOLOGICAL SULCUS)

A longitudinal depression of the epithelium into the SLP, but not up to the vocal ligament. This depression may extend from the anterior commissure to the vocal process. As the depth of invagination of the epithelium in a type 1 sulcus is shallow, the patient generally has no voice complaints and stroboscopy reveals a normal mucosal wave pattern. Such a sulcus warrants no intervention at all. A type 1 sulcus is also referred to as a physiological sulcus and it is typically picked up incidentally on stroboscopy.

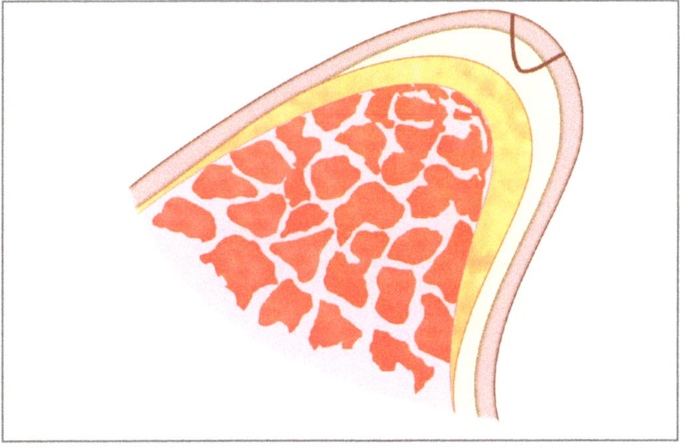

FIG. 6.1: Type 1: Physiological sulcus

TYPE 2: LINEAR VERGETURE/ SULCUS VERGETURE

A longitudinal depression of the epithelium into the SLP, reaching up to or going beyond the vocal ligament. This depression, like the type 1 sulcus, often extends from the anterior commissure to the vocal process. A type 2 sulcus is also referred to as a linear vergeture.

Both unilateral and bilateral linear vergeture usually result in an asymmetric spindle shaped phonatory gap.

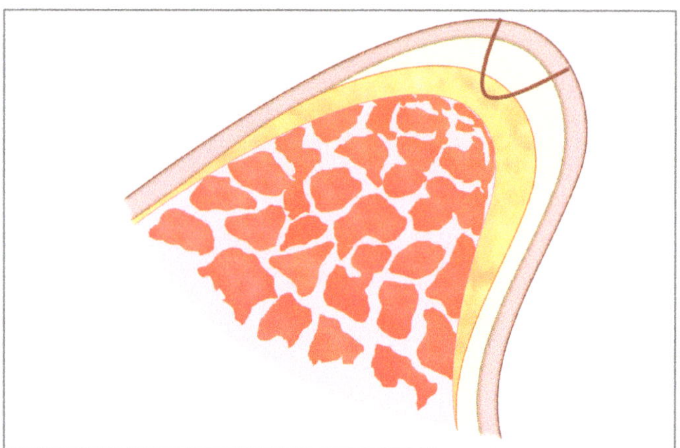

FIG. 6.2: Type 2: Linear vergeture/sulcus vergeture. Groove that runs along the free edge of the membranous vocal fold

TYPE 3 (FOCAL PIT/SULCUS VOCALIS)

A type 3 sulcus refers more to a localized area of depression also called a focal pit.

Hyperkeratosis is common near the deepest aspects of the sac or pocket. Some authors believe that this represents an open epidermal cyst.

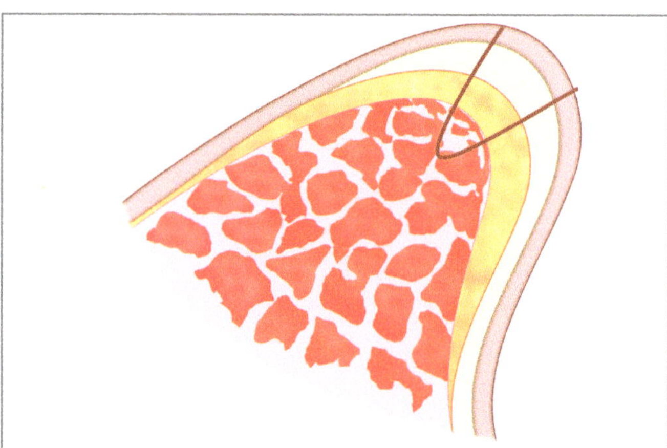

FIG. 6.3: Type 3: Focal pit/sulcus vocalis

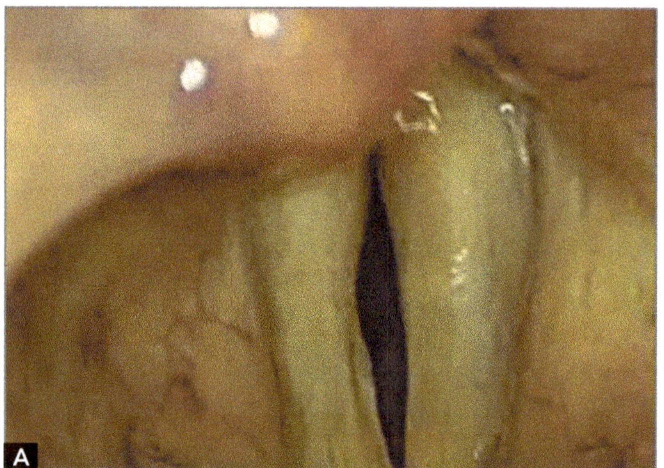

Continued

Continued

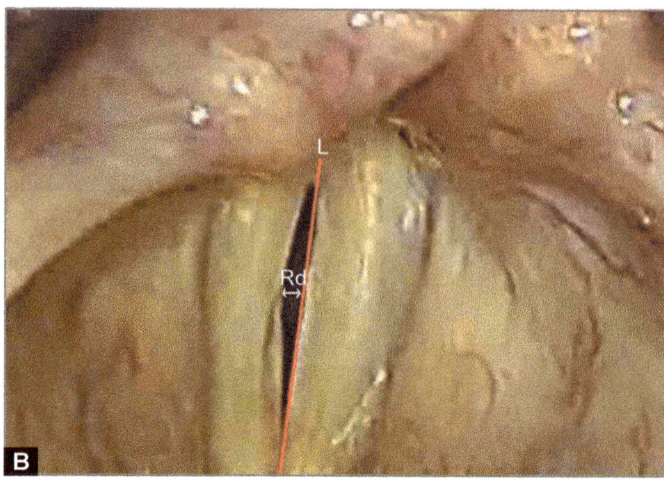

FIG. 6.4: An asymmetric phonatory gap is often seen in patients with a sulcus, even when the sulcus is bilateral. Any phonatory gap warrants a stroboscopic evaluation and sulci should be kept in mind, especially with asymmetric phonatory gaps[6]

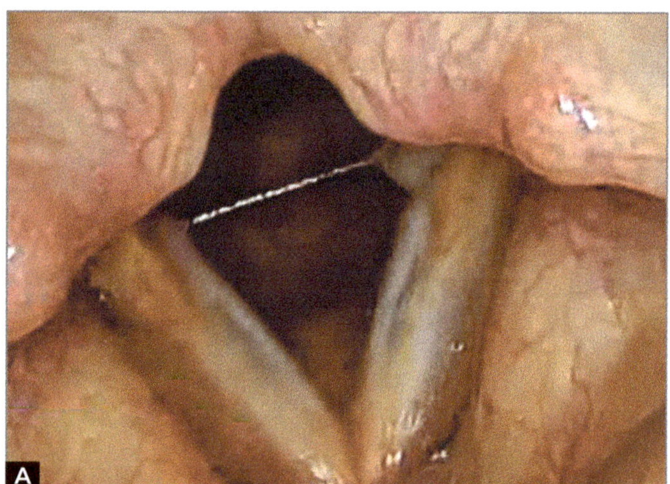

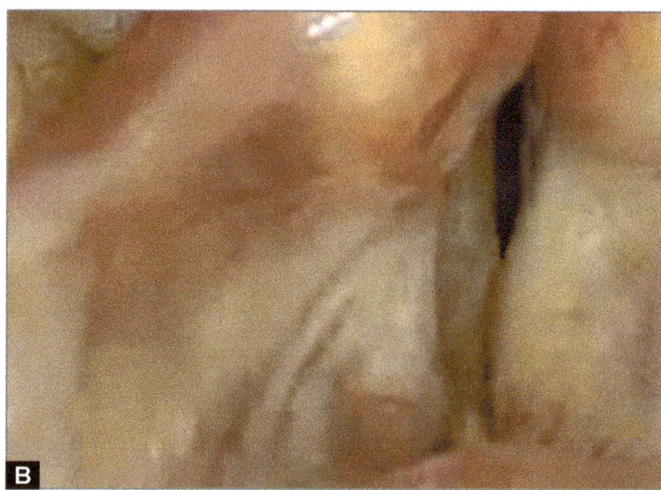

FIG. 6.5: A, Bilateral sulcus on white light laryngoscopy; **B,** Asymmetric phonatory gap with left ventricular compensatory phonation in the same patient

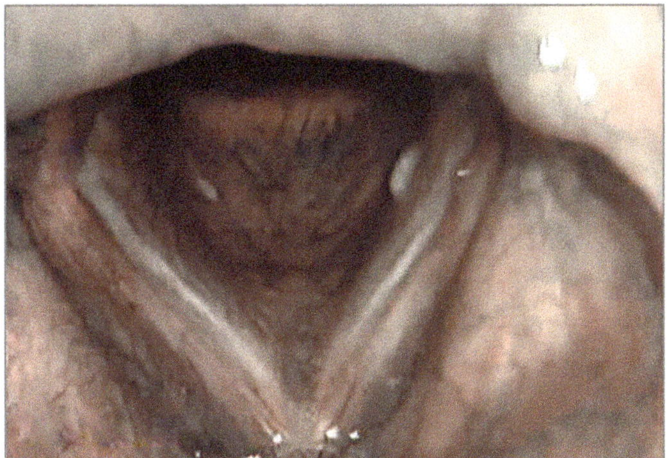

FIG. 6.6: Narrow band imaging (NBI) laryngoscopy of the same patient as above. Non-vascular lesions such as sulcus appear white in contrast to the surrounding normal mucosa which appears pinkish–gray on NBI

Many surgical procedures have been suggested for sulcus, primarily because no one procedure is clearly superior. As the results of surgery are not predictable, it is essential to exhaust voice therapy as a possible management option prior to performing surgery. Surgical candidates need to be counseled appropriately regarding the unpredictable postsurgical results and the need for possibly prolonged voice therapy once surgical healing takes place.

Depending on the length and depth of the sulcus, a variety of surgical options exist including fat injection, fat augmentation, excision of sulcus with suturing of fresh epithelial edges, Pontes procedure, medialisation thyroplasty, and Gray's mini thyrotomy.

CASE 1

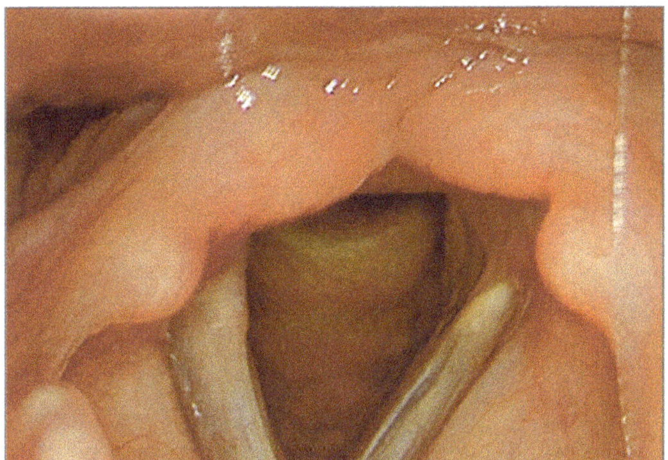

FIG. 6.7: A 70-degree laryngoscopic image revealing a sulcus on the left vocal fold in a 15-year-old girl who complained of longstanding hoarseness. Fat injection laryngoplasty under anesthesia was planned for her. (E-HD)

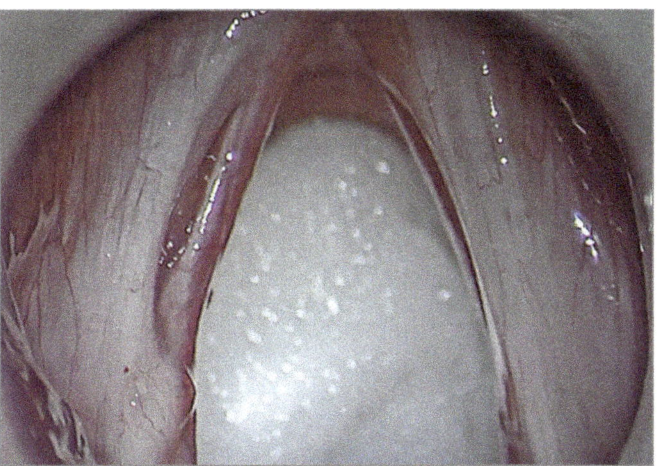

FIG. 6.8: On evaluating case 1 under anesthesia, a shallow sulcus was found even on the right vocal fold. This was left surgically untouched. (M-CC)

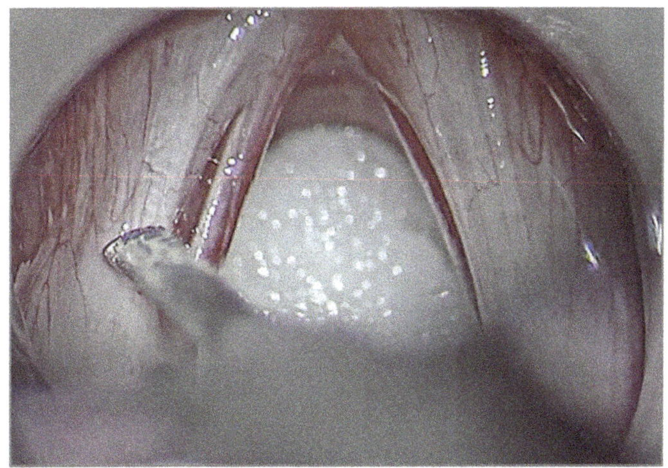

FIG. 6.9: 10 cc of fat was prepared from the lateral thigh. The fat was cut into small pieces, passed through the nozzle of a 5 cc syringe multiple times and washed in 2 L of saline to wash out the fatty acids. An 18-gauge scalp vein was used to inject the prepared fat in both the SLP as well as in the paraglottic space of the left vocal fold. The total fat injected was 1.5 cc. (M-CC)

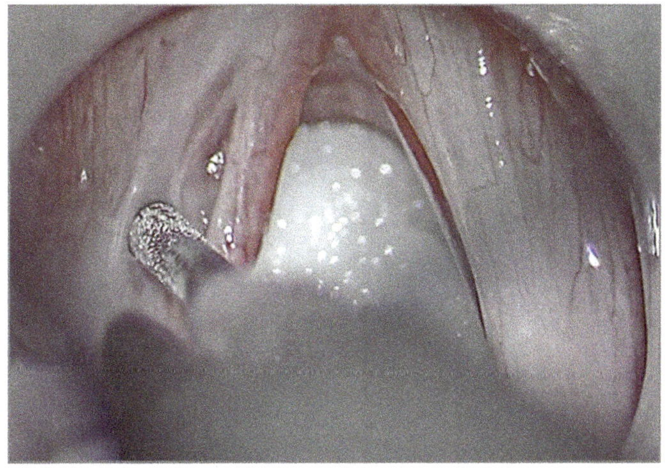

FIG. 6.10: Fat injection in the SLP of the left vocal fold. (M-CC)

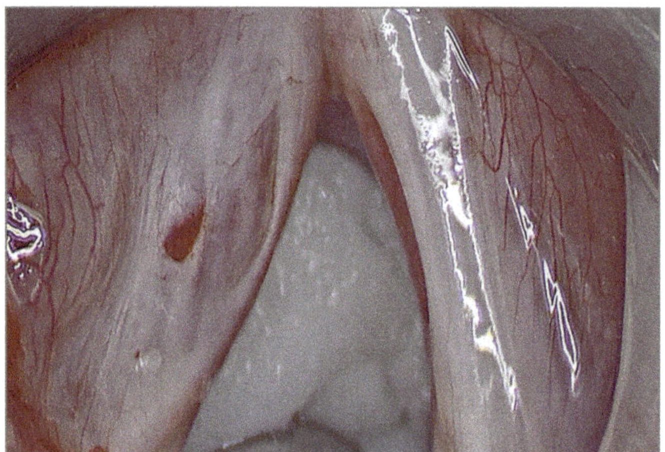

FIG. 6.11: Bulging of the left vocal fold following the fat injection in the SLP. The sulcus is seen opened up and flattened. (M-CC)

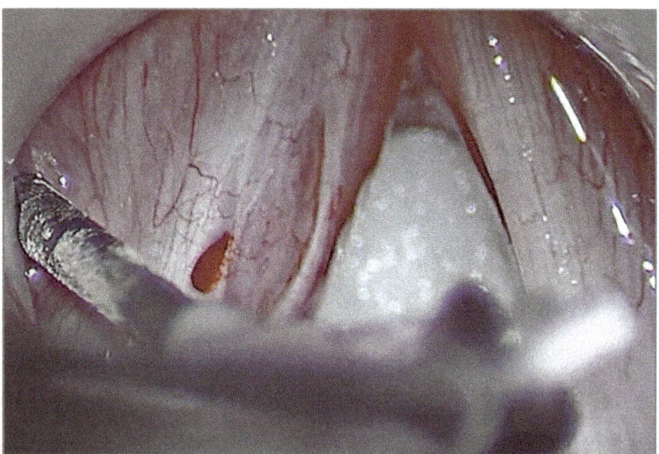

FIG. 6.12: Fat is now injected in the paraglottic space. Over-medialisation is the key as a variable amount of the fat is found to absorb over the next 6–12 weeks. (M-CC)

CASE 2

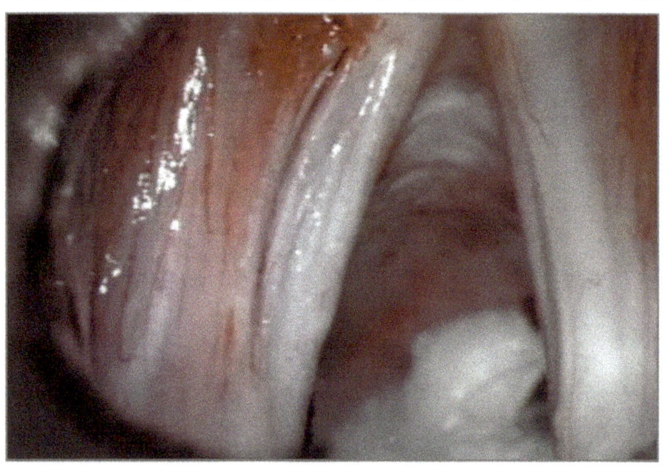

FIG. 6.13: Bilateral sulcus, left being deeper than the right, on palpation. The patient is planned for a left fat augmentation procedure. An epithelial cordotomy is performed immediately lateral to the lateral edge of the left sulcus following SEIT. (VLS-3 Chip)

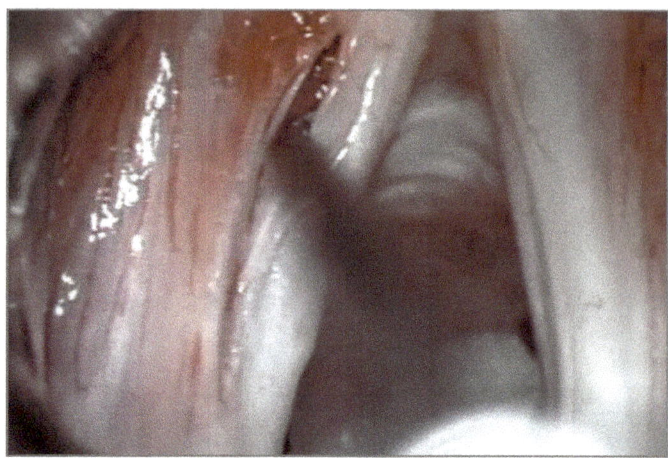

FIG. 6.14: A 90-degree, sharp, microflap elevator is used to separate the epithelium from the underlying vocalis muscle. Absence of vocal ligament suggests a sulcus vocalis on this side. (VLS-3 Chip)

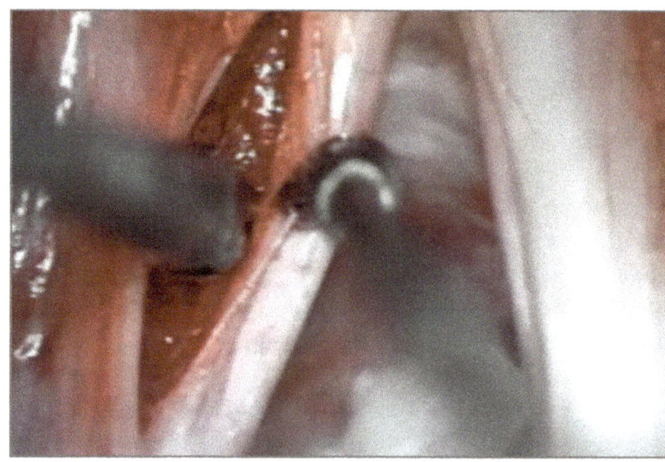

FIG. 6.15: A sharp scissors is now being used to separate the remaining epithelium of the sulcus vocalis from the underlying vocalis muscle. Care is taken not to puncture this epithelium, which is being held by a left crocodile. (VLS-3 chip)

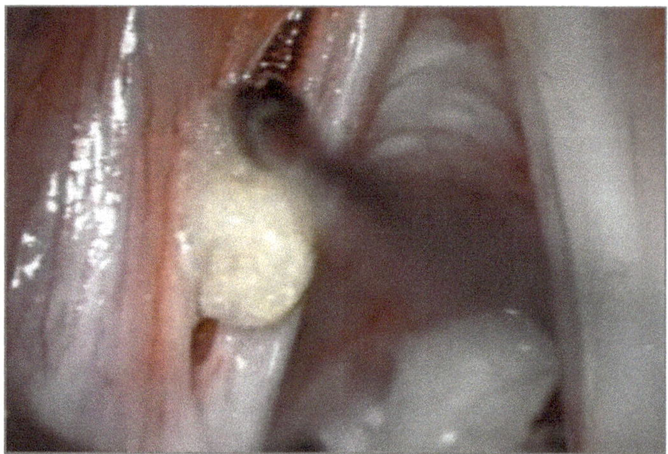

FIG. 6.16: Pieces of fat from the patient's thigh, which have been thoroughly washed in saline, are now packed into this subepithelial pocket. (E-VLS)

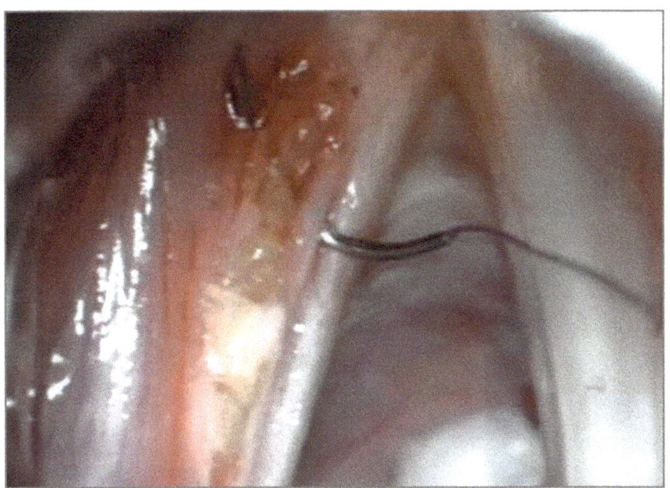

FIG. 6.17: A 5-0 vicryl is used to suture the edges of the epithelium so that the fat stays effectively within the pocket created. (E-VLS)

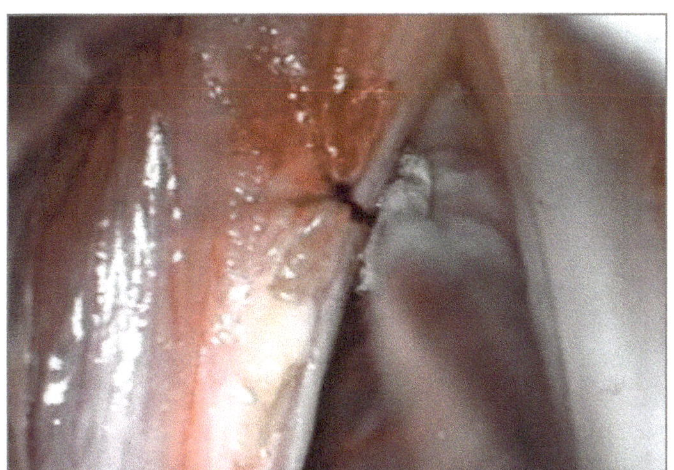

FIG. 6.18: Knot slider being used to slide the knot. (E-VLS)

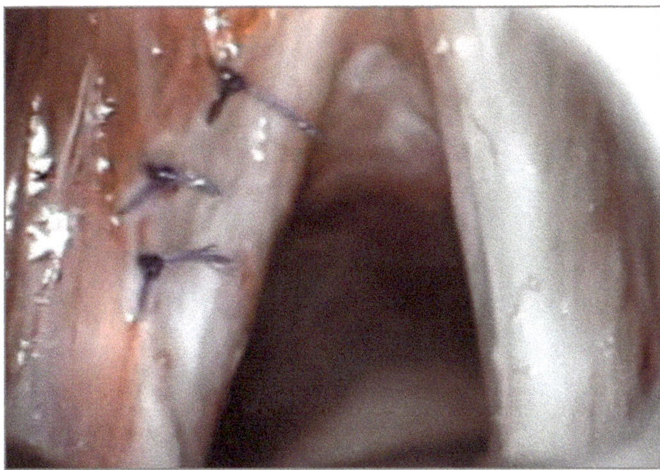

FIG. 6.19: The final postoperative picture. The right sulcus vergeture has not been operated upon at this time. (E-VLS)

CASE 3

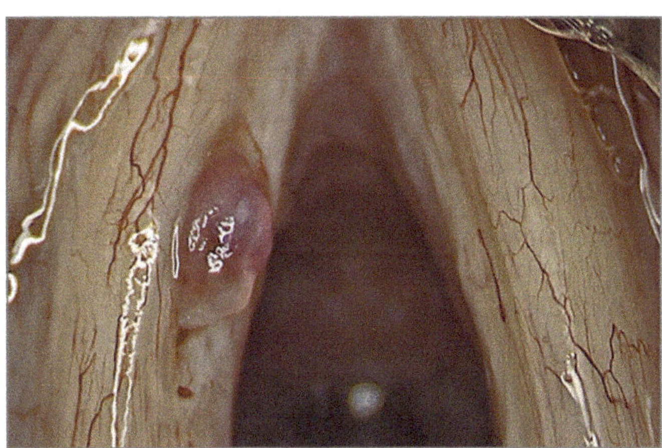

FIG. 6.20: A left vocal fold polyp is seen arising from within a focal pit. Such a polyp may be compensatory, developing as the body's response, to close the phonatory gap caused due to the focal pit. A shallow sulcus is seen on the right vocal fold. (E-CC)

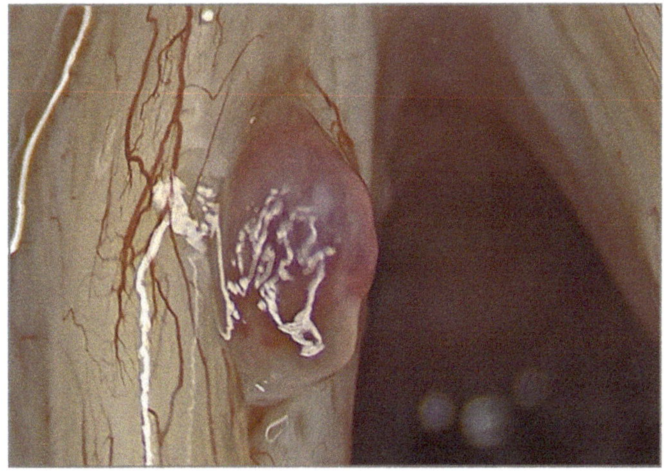

FIG. 6.21: Zoomed image of 6.20. (E-CC)

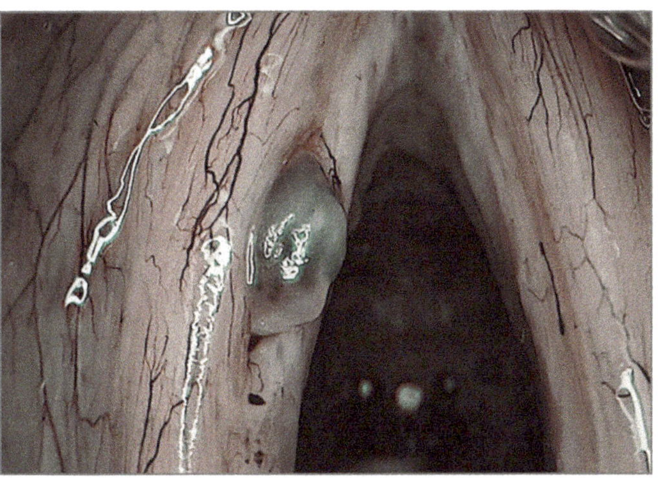

FIG. 6.22: Spectra A image of 6.20. The focal pit can be clearly appreciated . (E-SA)

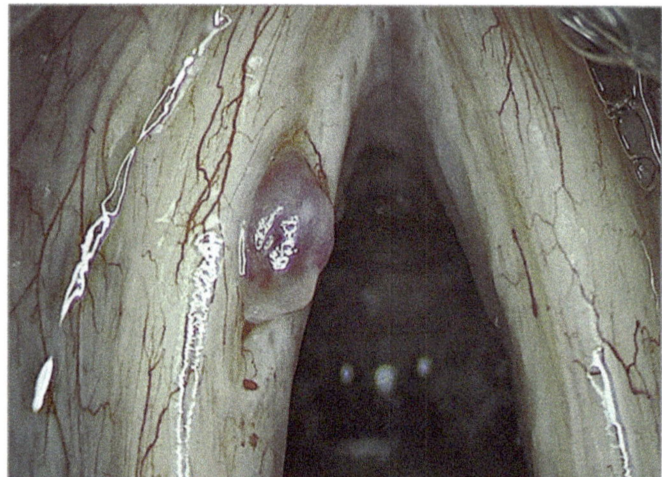

FIG. 6.23: Spectra B image of 6.20. (E-SB)

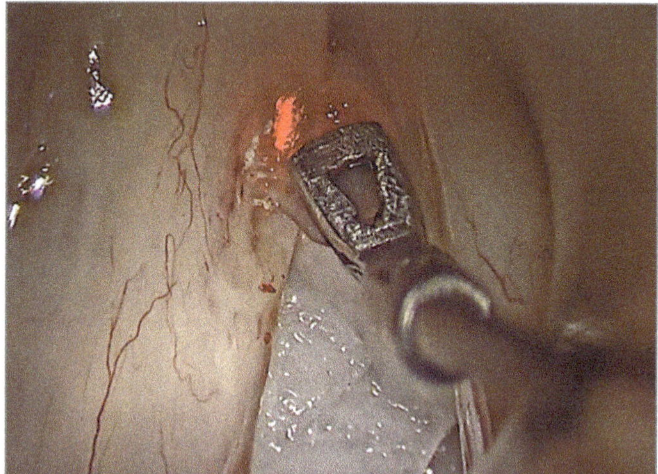

FIG. 6.24: CO_2 AcuBlade excision of the polyp

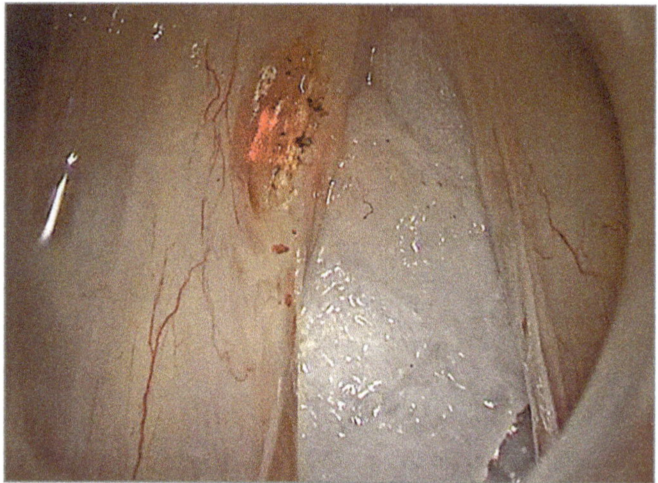

FIG. 6.25: The epithelium within the focal pit is excised with the CO_2 laser. (M-CC)

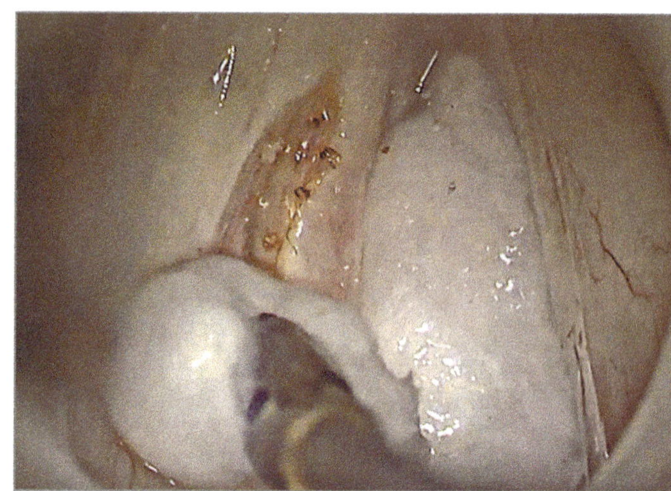

FIG. 6.26: The laser char is being wiped clean with a soaking cotton pledget. (M-CC)

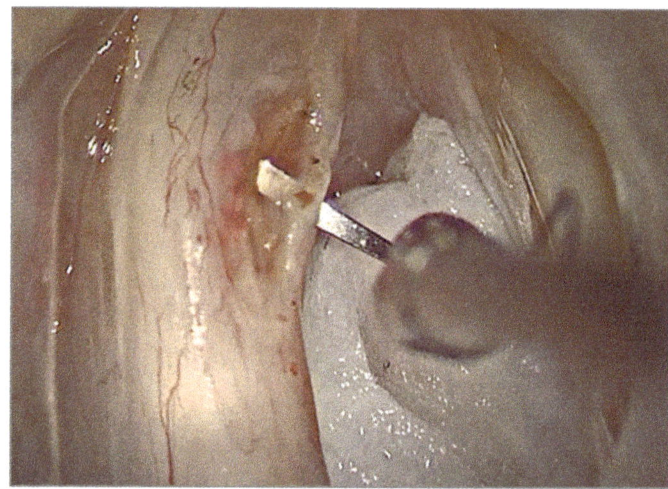

FIG. 6.27: The epithelial edges are sutured with 4-0 vicryl to get a good edge-to-edge approximation. (M-CC)

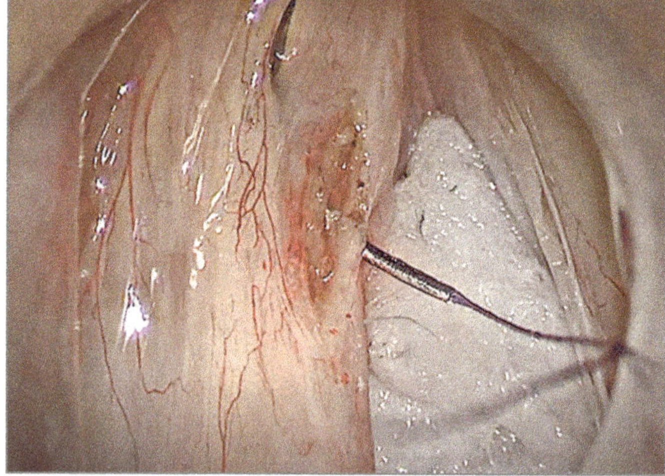

FIG. 6.28: The tip of the needle should be brought out in a clock wise direction as seen in 6.28, 6.29, and 6.30. (M-CC)

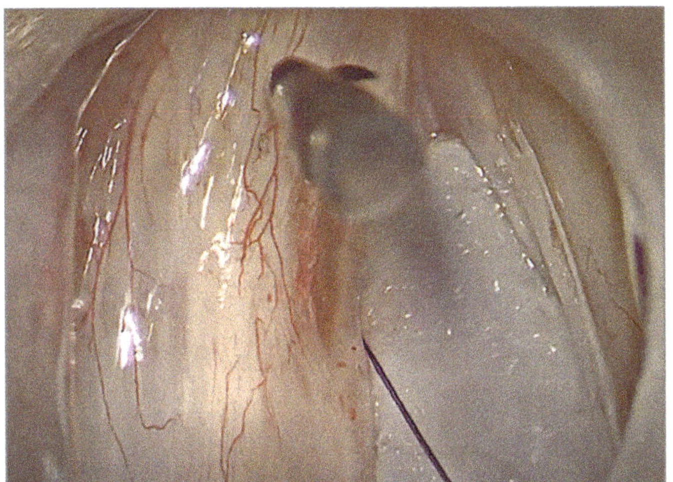

FIG. 6.29: Needle being removed in a clockwise direction.

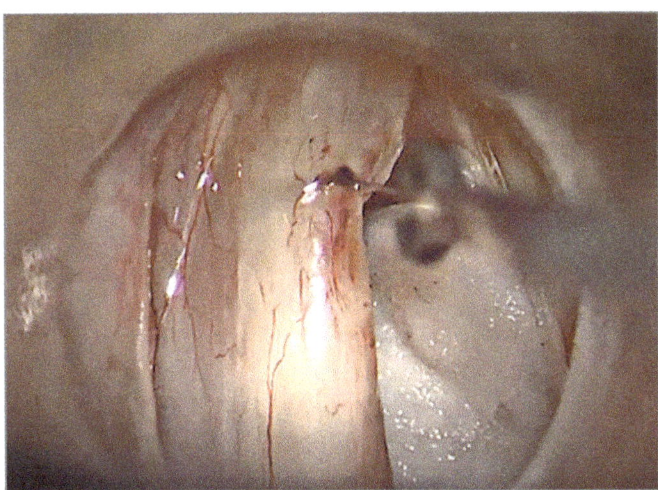

FIG. 6.32: 2 knots are safer than one to avoid opening-up of the knot. (M-CC)

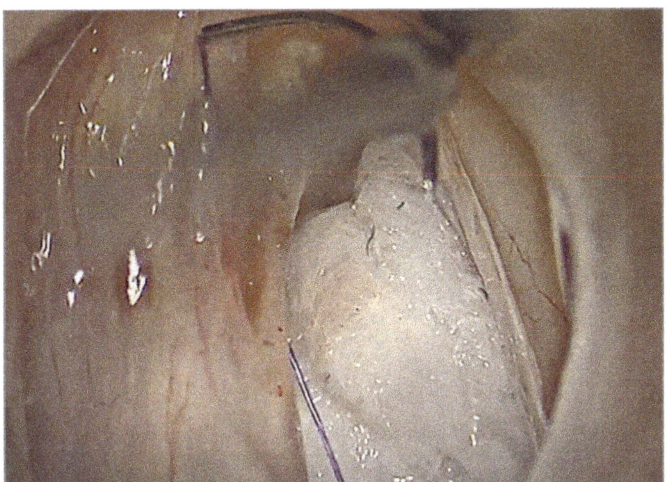

FIG. 6.30: Needle being removed in a clockwise direction.

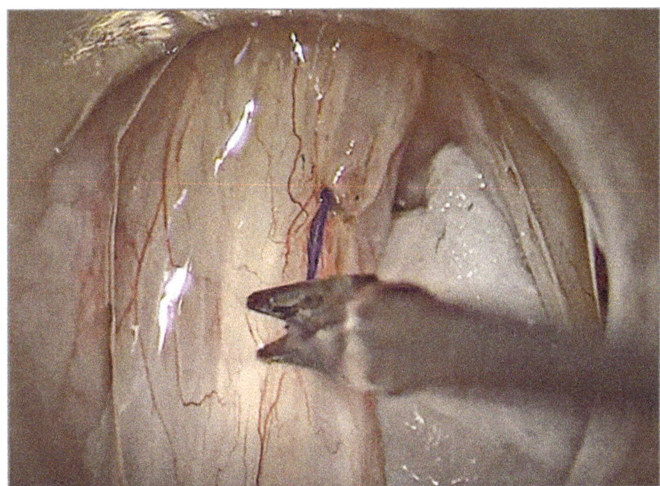

FIG. 6.33: A left scissors cutting the knot with adequately long threads left *in situ*. (M-CC)

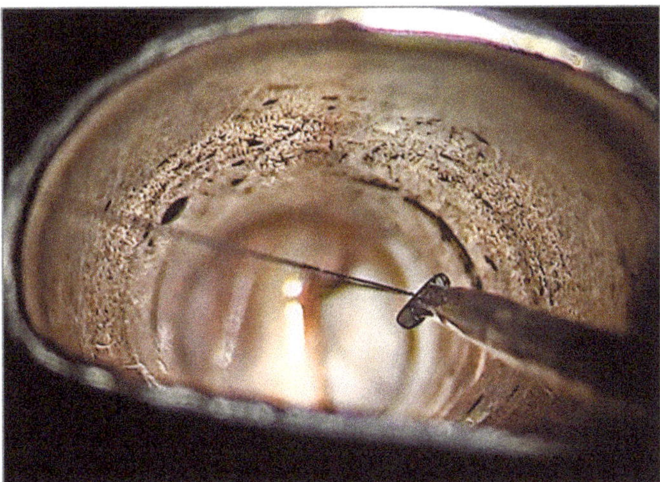

FIG. 6.31: The knot is tied outside the microlaryngoscope and then slid down with a knot slider. (M-CC)

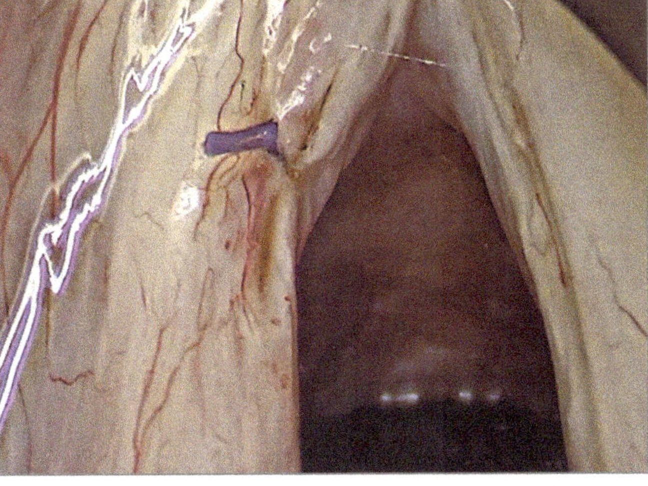

FIG. 6.34: Final postoperative image. The healing takes at least 6 weeks and the absorbable vicryl does not cause much discomfort to the patient. (M-CC)

CASE 4

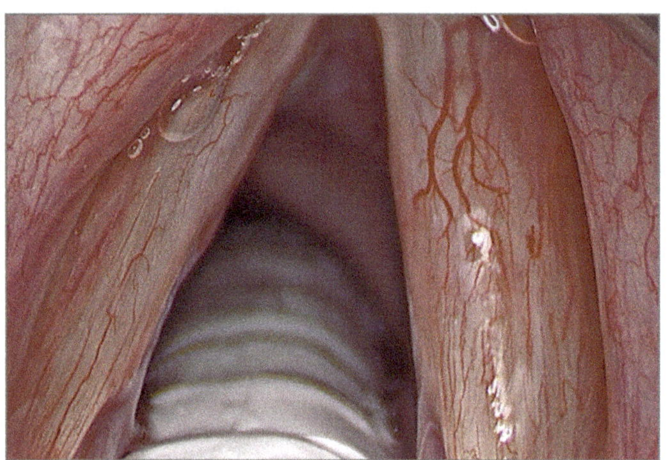

FIG. 6.35: An adult female patient suspected of having a right subepithelial cyst with overlying varices is taken up for surgical evaluation and excision. (E-CC)

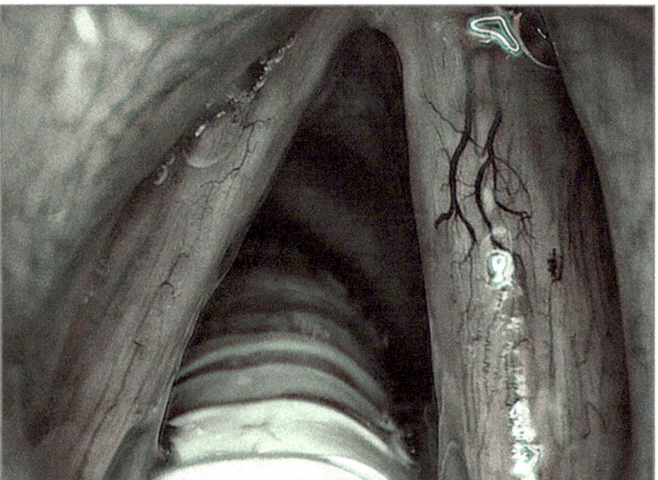

FIG. 6.36: Spectra A image of 6.35

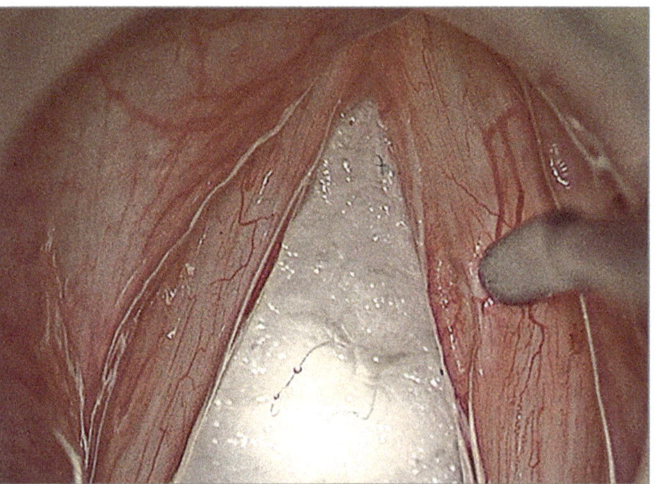

FIG. 6.37: Palpation under anesthesia with a blunt microflap elevator reveals a focal pit along the area of the lower lip of the vocal fold and absence of any cyst or fibrotic lesion. The varices seem directed towards this pit. (M-CC)

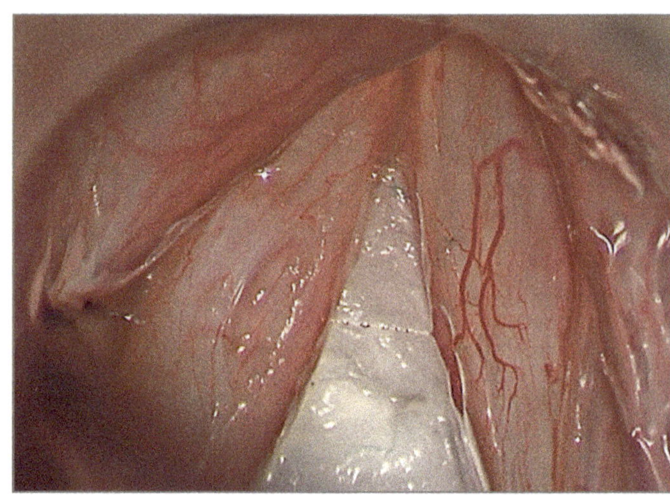

FIG. 6.38: The lower lip area of the left vocal fold also reveals a focal pit which is not as deep as the right side. (M-CC)

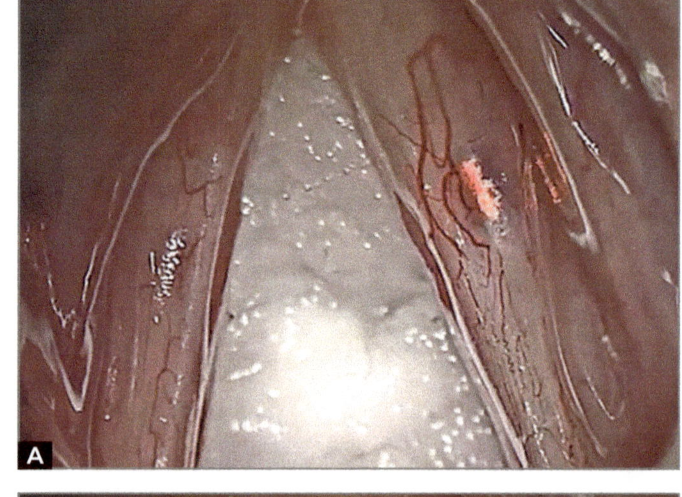

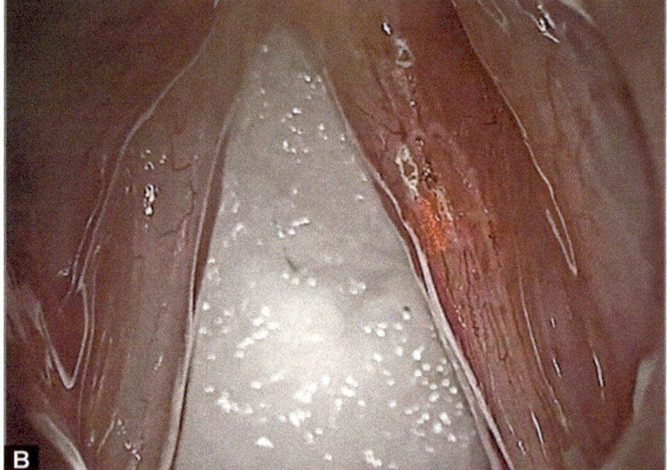

FIG. 6.39: The varices on the right vocal fold are laser ablated. (M-CC)

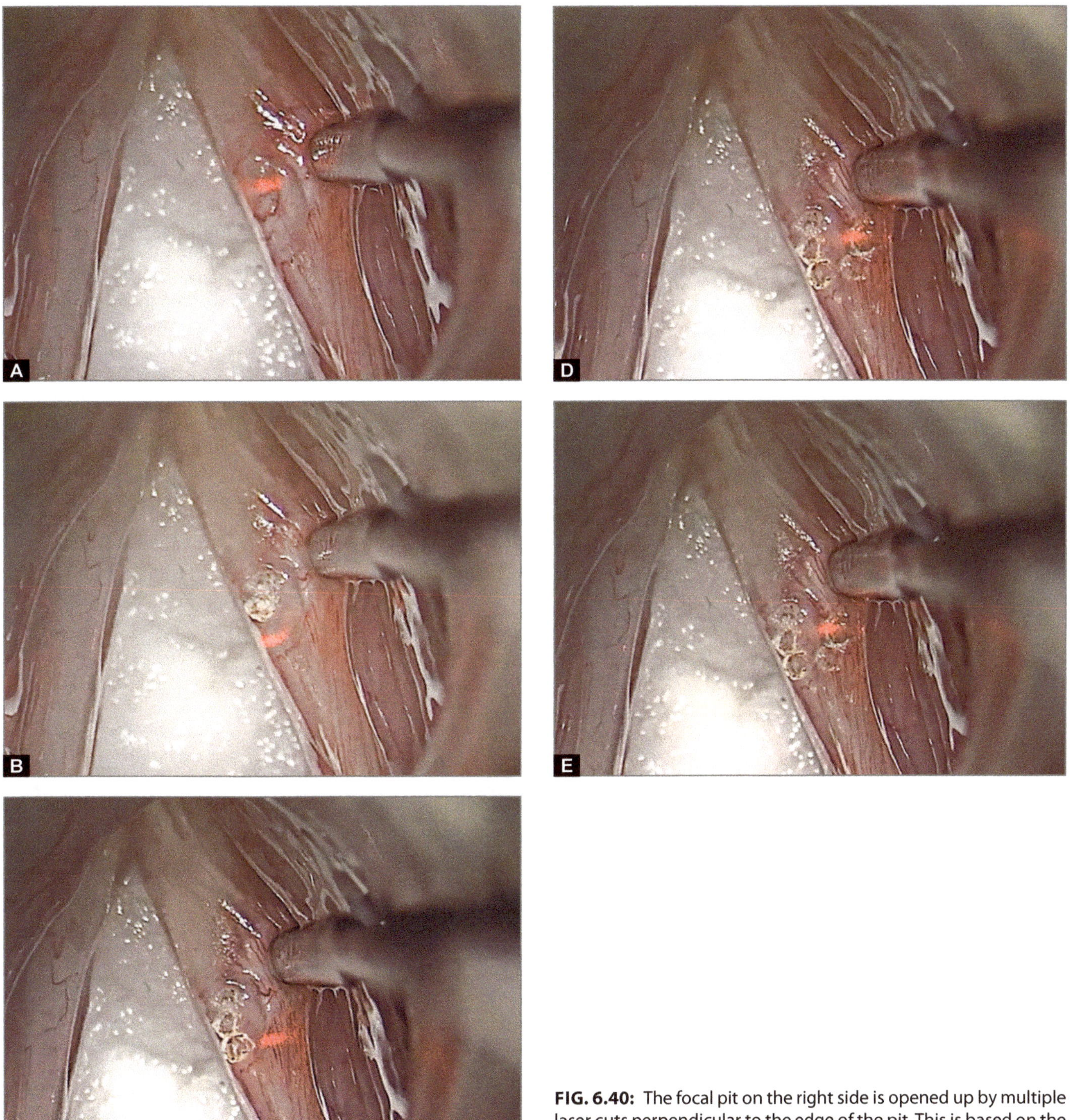

FIG. 6.40: The focal pit on the right side is opened up by multiple laser cuts perpendicular to the edge of the pit. This is based on the Pontes technique but differs in that the ligament is not elevated or incised. (M-CC)

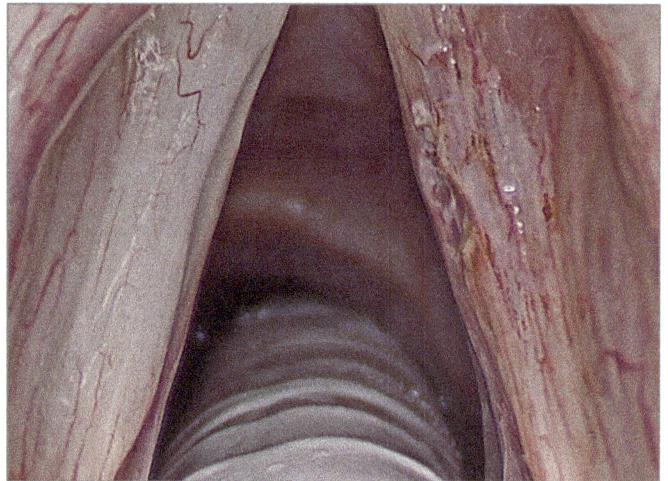

FIG. 6.41: Final postoperative appearance. (E-CC)

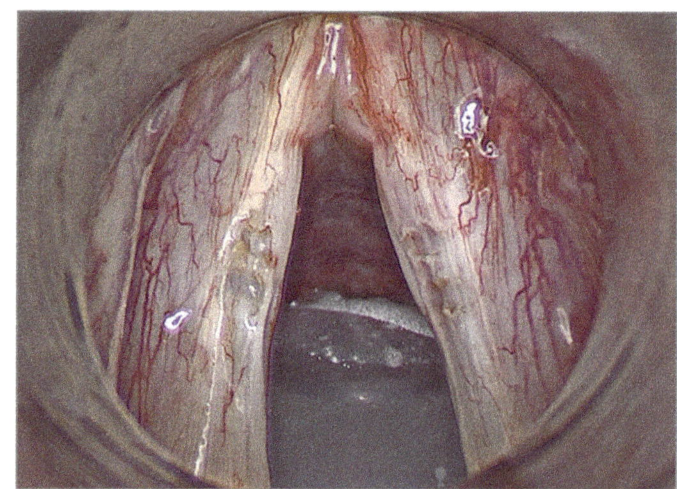

FIG. 6.44: A modified Pontes technique performed bilaterally as described for case 4

CASE 5

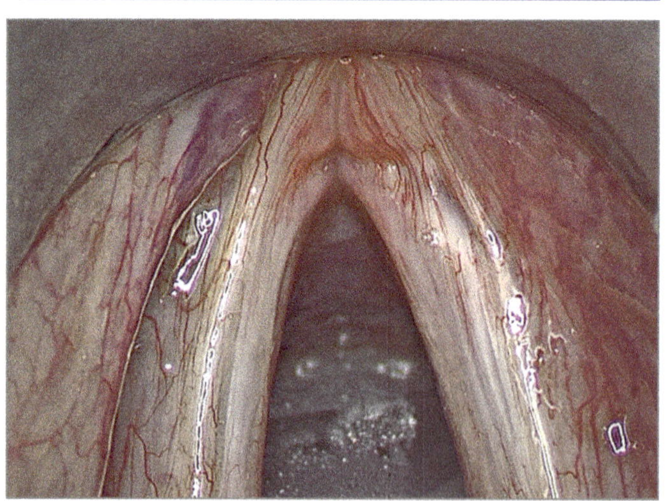

FIG. 6.42: Bilateral superficial sulci, two on the right and one on the left vocal fold. (E-CC)

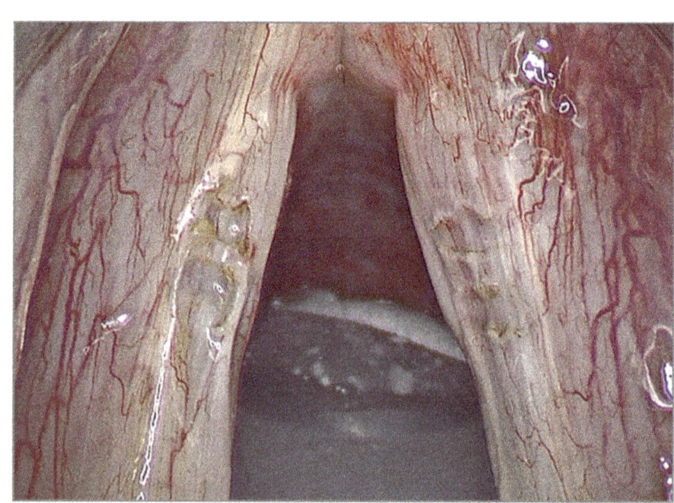

FIG. 6.45: Zoomed image of 6.44

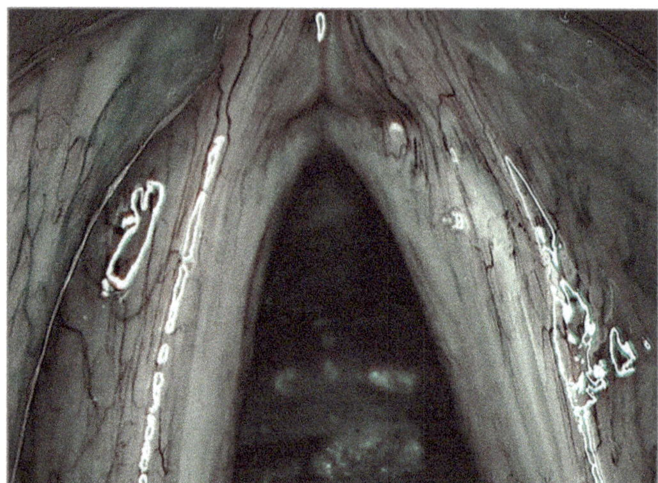

FIG. 6.43: Spectra A image of 6.42

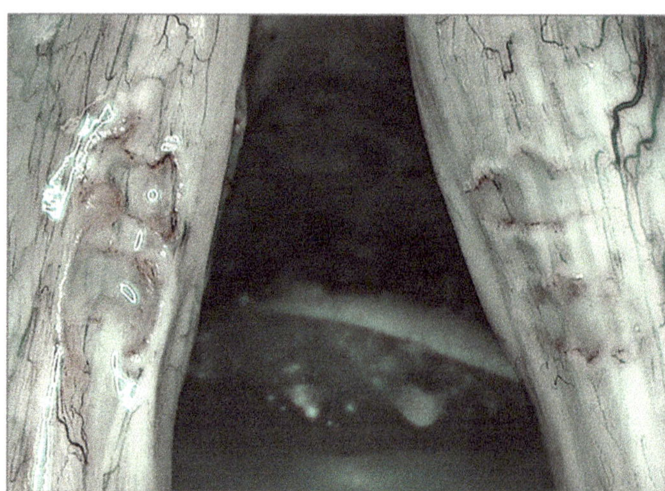

FIG. 6.46: Spectra A image of case 5 where the epithelial area can be appreciated.

REFERENCES

1. Franco RA, Andrus JG. Common diagnosis and treatments in professional voice users. Otolaryngol Clin North Am. 2007;40(5):1025-61.
2. Nupur KN. Cyst, sulci and mucosal bridge. In: Nupur KN, Amitabha R. Textbook of laryngology: Official publication of the Association of Phonosurgeons of India. New Delhi: Jaypee Brothers Medical Publishers (P) Ltd.; 2017. pp. 155-70.
3. Remacle M, Hantzakos A, Matar N, et al. Laser surgery for common laryngeal pathology. In: Oswal V, Remacle M, editors. Principles and practice of lasers in otorhinolaryngology and head and neck surgery, 2nd ed. Amsterdam: Kugler Publications; 2014. pp. 117-31.
4. Bouchayer M, Cornut G, Witzig E, et al. Epidermoid cysts, sulci and mucosal bridges of the true vocal cord: A report of 157 cases. Laryngoscope. 1985;95(9 Pt 1):1087-94.
5. Ford CN, Inagi K, Khidr A, et al. Sulcus vocalis: a rational analytical approach to diagnosis and management. Ann Otol Rhinol Laryngol. 1996; 105:189-200.
6. Nupur N, Harsh G, Ajay S. Diagnostic challenge of sulcus vocalis made easier. Int J Phonosurg Laryngol. 2015;5(2):39-41.

CHAPTER 7

Mucosal Bridge

DEFINITION

A mucosal bridge is an epithelial strip lying free over the vocal fold epithelium, attached only anteriorly and posteriorly.

According to the theory of Bouchayer and Cornut (1985),[1] a mucosal bridge arises from two apertures in a single epidermoid cyst—superior and inferior—since the mucosal bridge between the two apertures is always thick and hyperkeratotic. Some of them could develop from vocal fold microtrauma.[2]

Whenever two linear sulci are observed on stroboscopy or during microlaryngeal surgery, a mucosal bridge should also be looked for. When the patient is under anesthesia, a blunt flat elevator may be used to confirm the presence of the mucosal bridge.[3]

There exists a dichotomy of opinion among laryngologists as to the necessity to excise this mucosal bridge or let it remain. The author believes in its excision when it is thin and epithelial so as to avoid having two epithelial surfaces vibrating as separate entities during phonation. However, in the authors' opinion, thick mucosal bridges are best not removed for fear of decreasing the bulk of the vocal fold significantly.

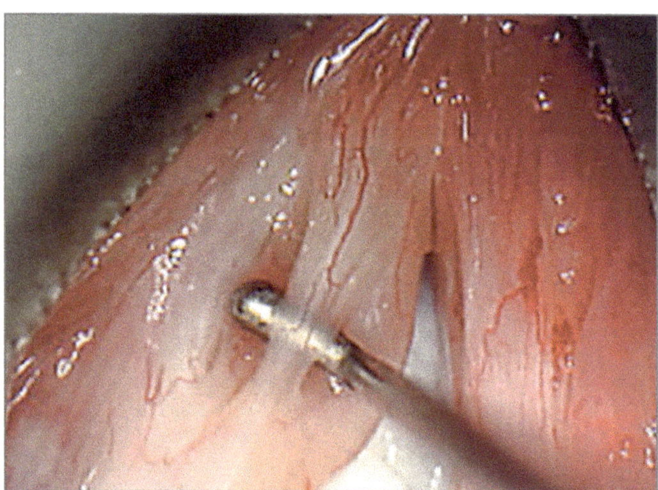

FIG. 7.1: Left mucosal bridge. (E-CC)

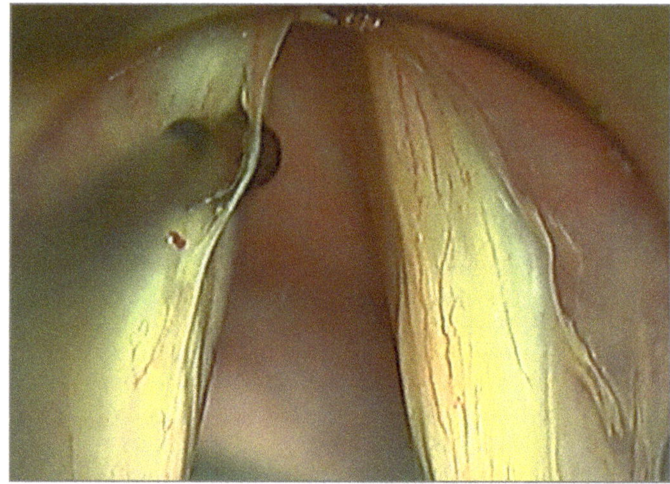

FIG. 7.2: Left thin epithelial mucosal bridge

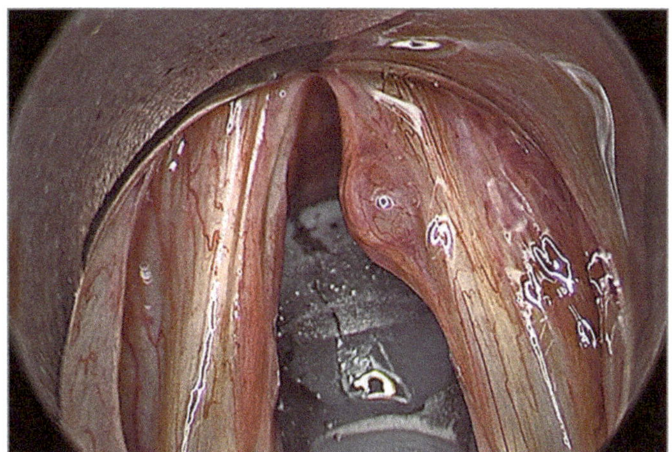

FIG. 7.3: A patient is taken up for surgical excision of a right polyp. Also seen are two parallel sulci on the left vocal fold. This appearance of two parallel sulci can often suggest the presence of a mucosal bridge overlying a single sulcus, the lateral edges of this single sulcus may be visible, giving the appearance of two sulci

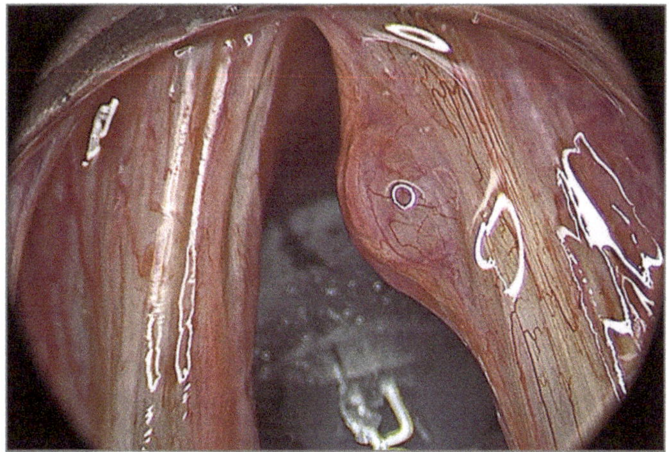

FIG. 7.4: Magnified image of 7.3

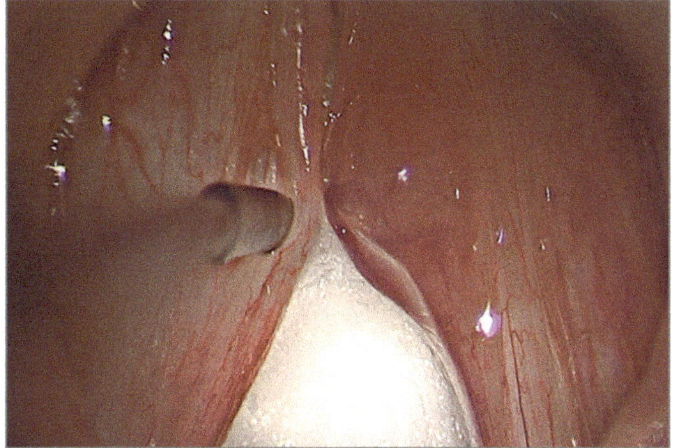

FIG. 7.5: Mucosal bridge of the left vocal fold overlying a single sulcus

CASE 1

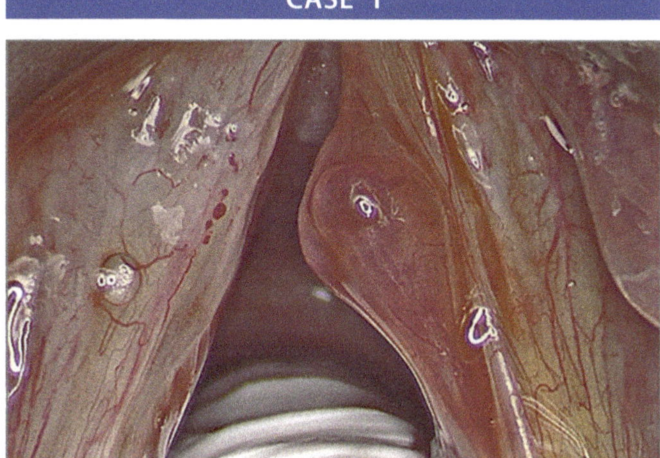

FIG. 7.6: A young female patient on treatment for pulmonary tuberculosis develops hoarseness over 1 month. Stroboscopy reveals a right hemorrhagic polyp for which surgical excision is planned. Contact varices are observed on the left vocal fold, striking zone, along with resolving SEH of the right vocal fold. (E-CC)

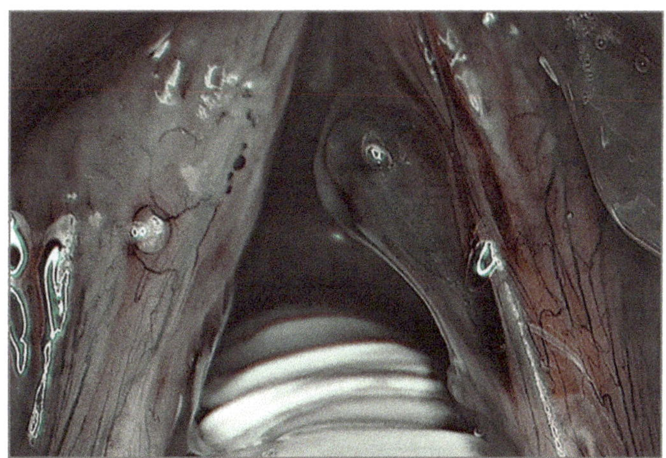

FIG. 7.7: Spectra A image of 7.6

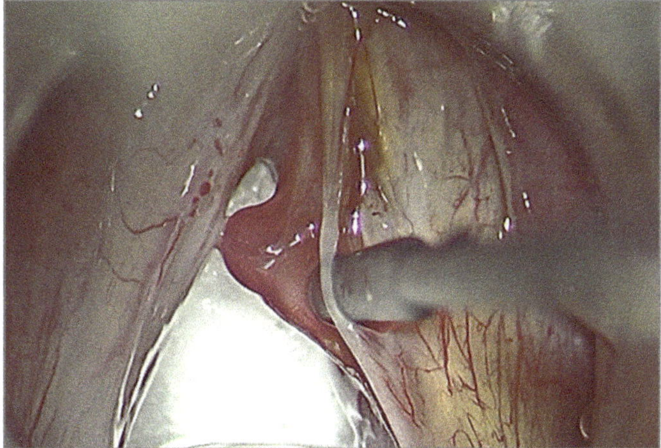

FIG. 7.8: Palpation of the right vocal fold reveals a thin epithelial mucosal bridge just lateral to the hemorrhagic polyp overlying a shallow sulcus. Retrospective evaluation of the laryngostroboscopy does reveal a tethering band just lateral to the right polyp. (M-CC)

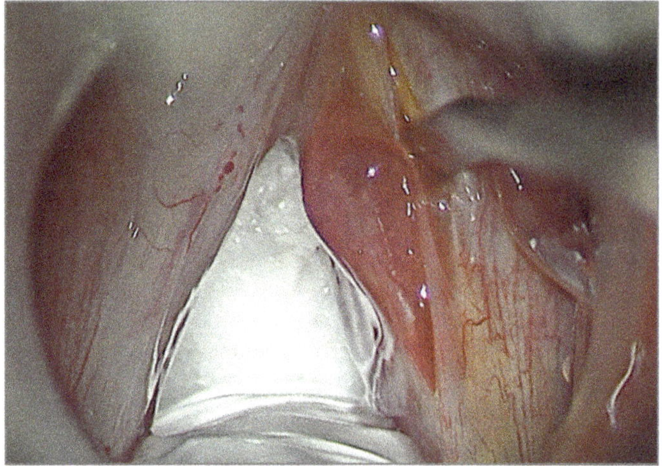

FIG. 7.9: A blunt microflap elevator is seen palpating the sulcus, underlying the mucosal bridge. (M-CC)

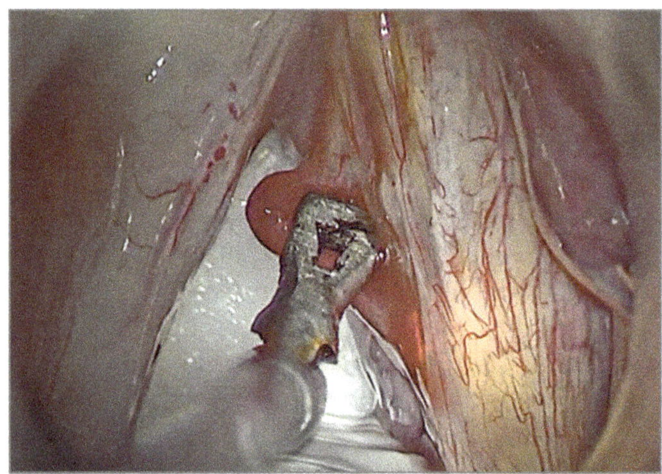

FIG. 7.10: An upward Bouchayer forceps is holding the polyp. (M-CC)

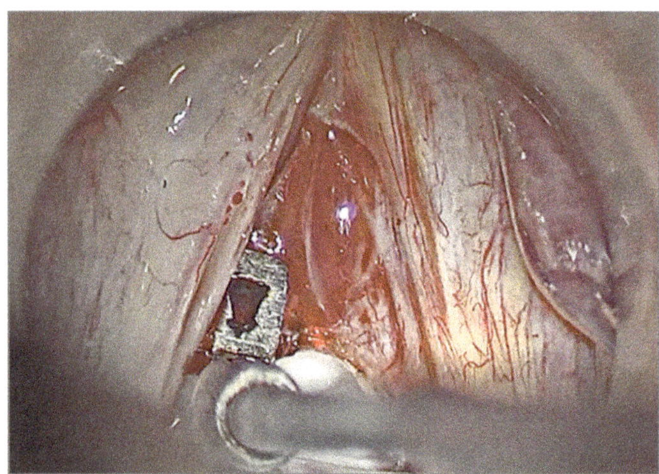

FIG. 7.11: CO_2 AcuBlade laser being used to excise the polyp such that the infraglottic epithelium is preserved. (M-CC)

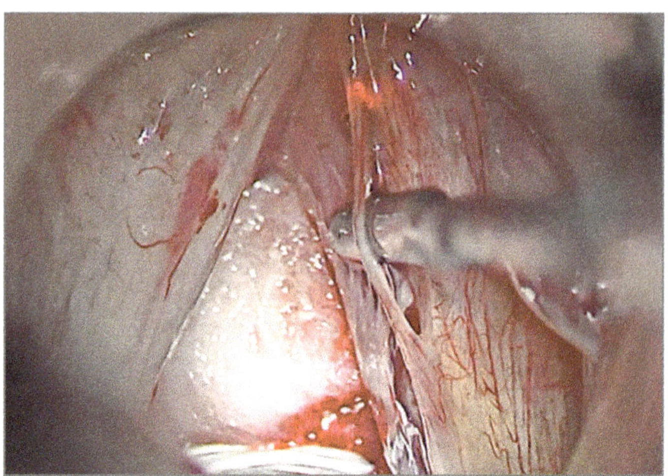

FIG. 7.12: Following polyp excision the infraglottic epithelium is seen redraping the medial vibrating edge. The thin epithelial mucosal bridge is being excised so as to prevent tethering and interruption of the mucosal wave propagation. (M-CC)

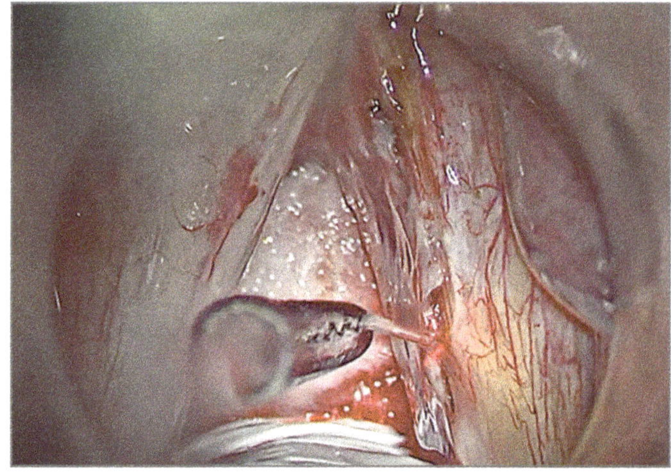

FIG. 7.13: Excision of the posterior attachment of the mucosal bridge. (M-CC)

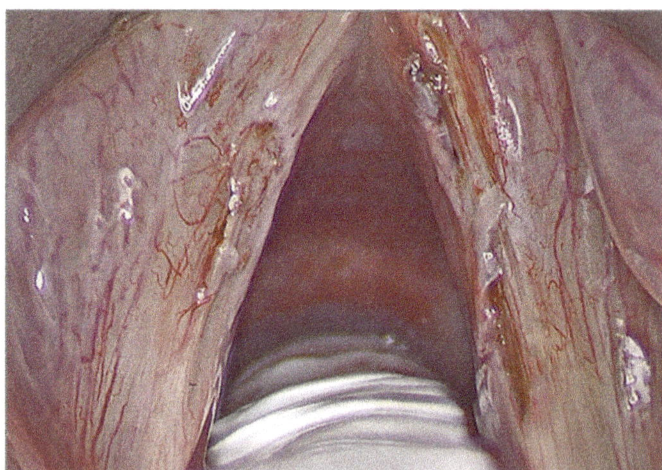

FIG. 7.14: Final postoperative image. (E-CC)

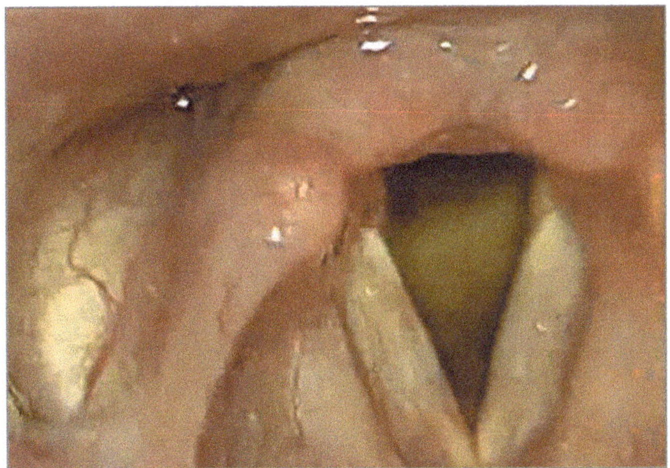

FIG. 7.15: Four weeks postoperative stroboscopy image. (E-HD)

CASE 2

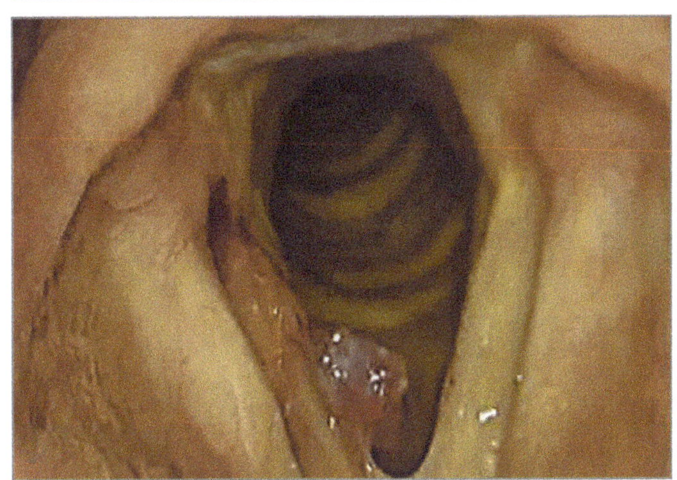

FIG. 7.16: Laryngostroboscopy revealing a right hemorrhagic polyp with what appears to be a varix lateral to it. (E-HD)

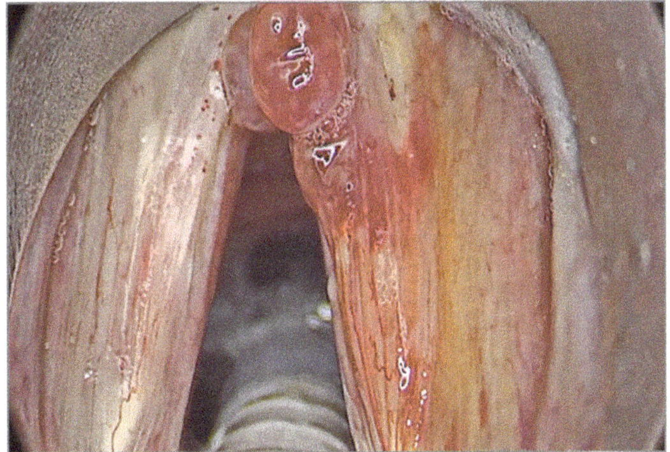

FIG. 7.17: Under anesthesia the polyp has a bilobed appearance with some SEH posteriorly. No varix is seen lateral to the polyp. (E-CC)

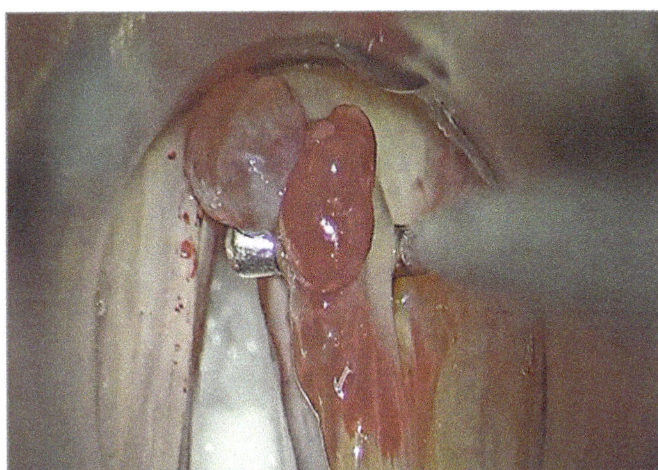

FIG. 7.18: Palpation of the right vocal fold identifies a thick mucosal bridge onto which the pedicle of the bilobed polyp is attached. (E-CC)

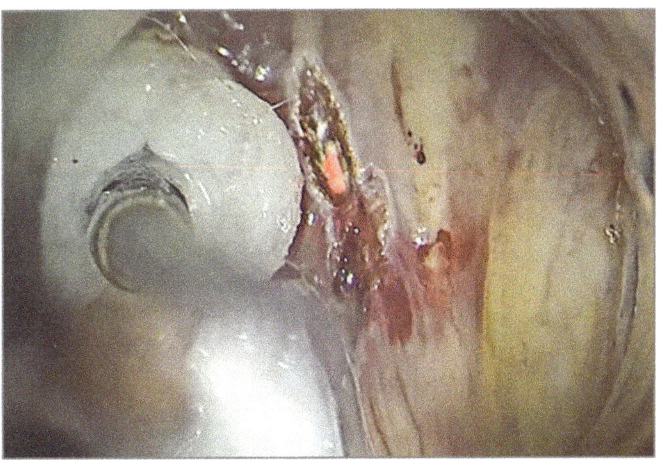

FIG. 7.19: CO_2 laser AcuBlade excision of the bilobed polyp from the thick mucosal bridge is performed. A moist cotton ball is medialising the polyp. (M-CC)

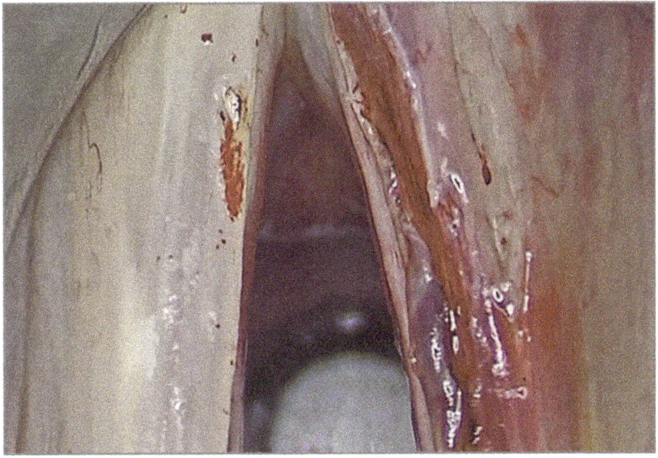

FIG. 7.20: The final postoperative image following excision of the right polyp and laser ablation of the varices of the left vocal fold. A decision is taken not to excise the thick right mucosal bridge, as that would cause a resultant large phonatory gap consequent to thinning of the right vocal fold. (E-CC)

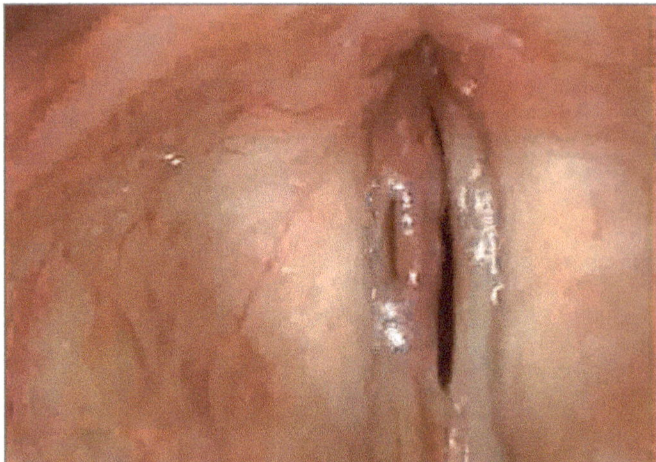

FIG. 7.21: One week postoperative video laryngoscopy clearly reveals the slit in the right vocal fold delineating the right mucosal bridge from the right vocal fold. The thickness of this bridge can be appreciated. (E-SD)

CASE 3

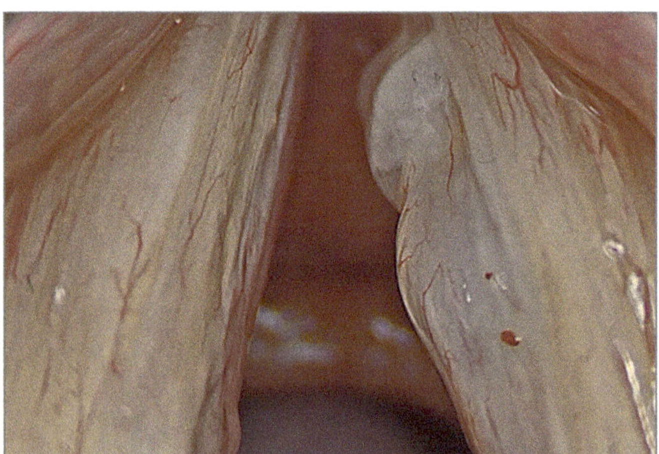

FIG. 7.22: Right bilobed subepithelial cyst and the appearance of two parallel sulci on the left vocal fold. (E-CC)

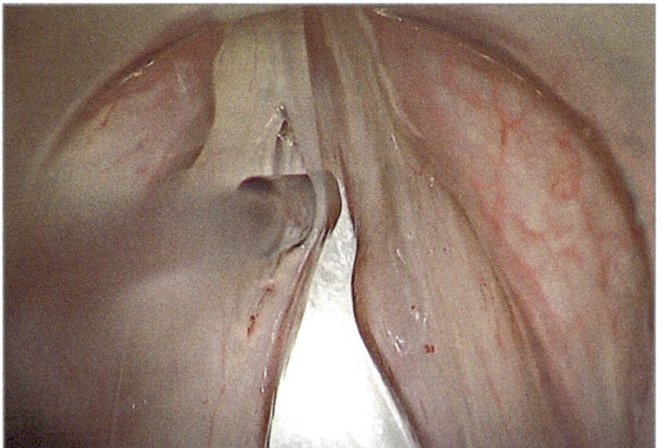

FIG. 7.23: Two parallel sulci may often represent a mucosal bridge covering a single sulcus. The lateral edges of that single

Continued

Continued

sulcus are often not hidden by the mucosal bridge and thus seen as two parallel sulci.

However, in this patient (case 3) the mucosal bridge appears on palpation to be incomplete, stopping just short of opening up at its medial edge. Thus, the blunt microflap elevator just stops short of entry at the medial side. Such an incomplete mucosal bridge may be considered to be a variant of a focal pit in the author's opinion, best described as an epithelial pocket parallel to the epithelial surface.

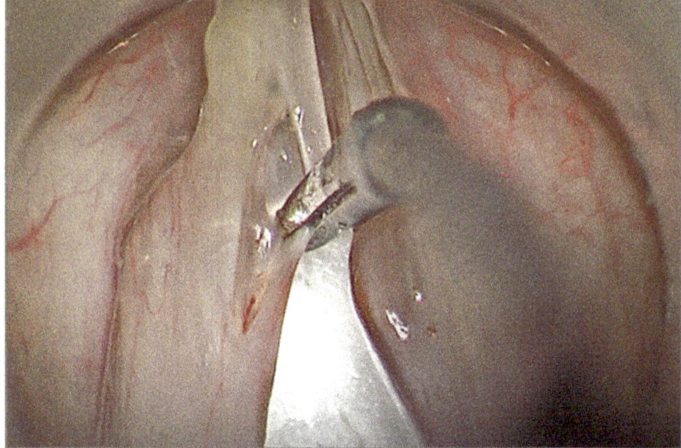

FIG. 7.24: A left crocodile is gently medially retracting the incomplete mucosal bridge (M-CC)

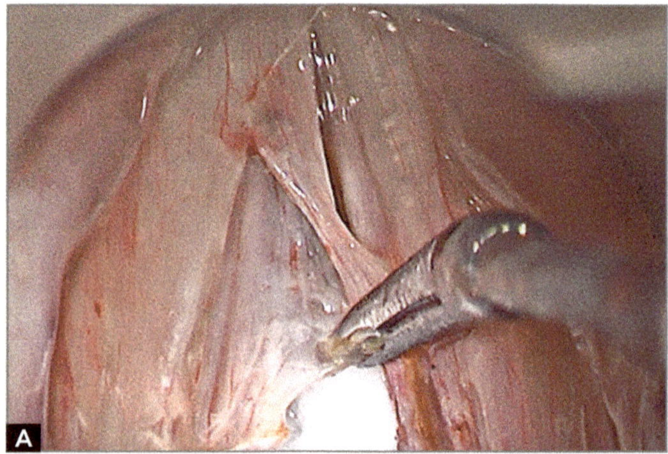

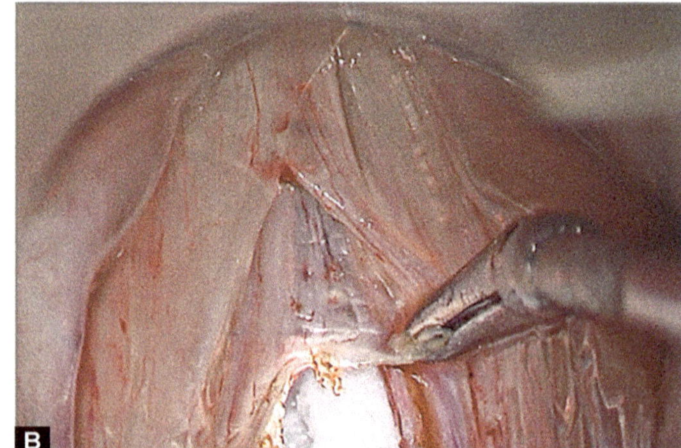

Continued

Continued

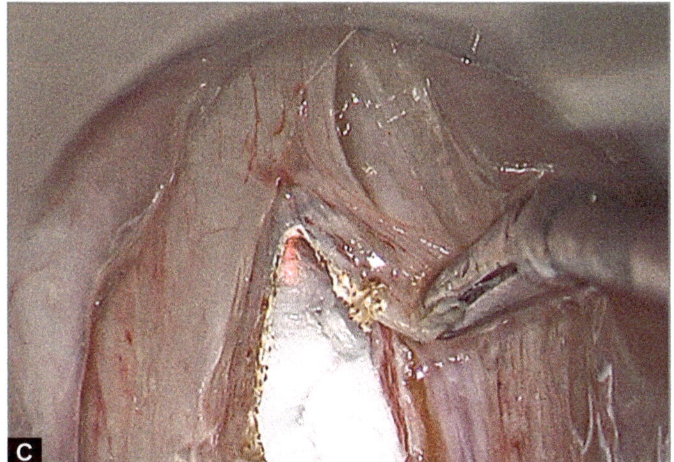

FIG. 7.25: The right subepithelial cyst has been excised. The left incomplete mucosal bridge is being excised by the CO_2 laser AcuBlade. (M-CC)

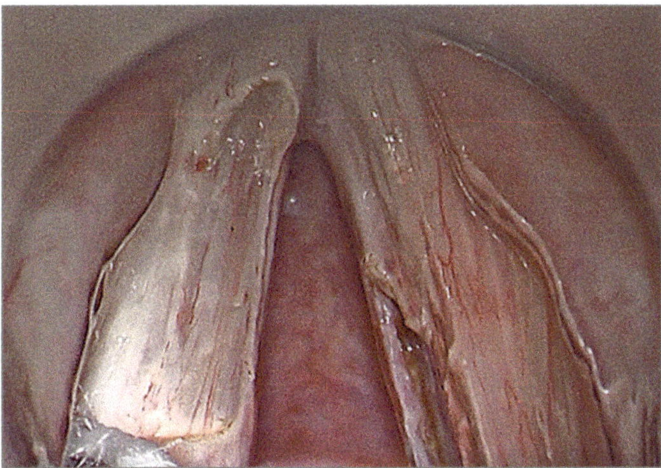

FIG. 7.26: The final postoperative image. The left vocal fold has a thin epithelial cover and the right vocal fold has a slit epithelial loss following cyst excision. (E-CC)

REFERENCES

1. Bouchayer M, Cornut G, Witzig E, et al. Epidermoid cysts, sulci and mucosal bridges of the true vocal cord: A report of 157 cases. Laryngoscope. 1985;95(9 Pt 1):1087-94.
2. Man LX, Statham MM, Rosen CA. Mucosal bridge and pitting of the true vocal fold: An unusual complication of cidofovir injection. Ann Otol Rhinol Laryngol. 2010;119(4):236-8.
3. Nerurkar NK. Cysts, sulci and mucosal bridge. In: Nerurkar NK, Roychoudhury A. Textbook of laryngology: Official textbook of Association of Phonosurgeons of India. New Delhi: Jaypee Brothers Medical Publishers (P) Ltd.; 2017. pp. 155-70.

CHAPTER 8

Reinke's Edema

DEFINITION

Reinke's edema is also termed polypoid corditis and is characterized by excessive myxomatous tissue in the superficial lamina propria (SLP). The myxomatous tissue extends bilaterally along the entire length of the membranous vocal folds.[1]

Grades of Reinke's Edema

Depending on the volume of the excessive myxomatous tissue in the SLP, Reinke's edema may be graded based on the results of laryngoscopy, as suggested by Yonekawa which are given below:[2]

- Grade I: Lesions contact the anterior third of the vocal fold
- Grade II: Lesions contact the anterior two-thirds of the vocal fold
- Grade III: Lesions contact the entirety of the vocal fold.

ETIOLOGY

It is commonly caused by smoking, gastroesophageal reflux disease, and vocal abuse.[1] Although polypoid degeneration of the vocal folds can be seen with severe hypothyroidism, most patients have normal thyroid function.[3]

Smoking cessation is an essential first step in the treatment and many patients will have normalization of voice within 6 months to 1 year after stopping cigarettes.[4]

However, grade II and II, and occasionally even grade I, Reinke's edema does need surgical excision of the excess myxomatous SLP.

Care has to be taken during surgery not to cause a raw area at the anterior commissure with consequent webbing. If the epithelium of one vocal fold has been damaged, it is safer to stage the opposite side rather than risk glottic stenosis.

While operating on male patients, one should be cautious about excessive removal of the SLP, with consequent thinning of the vocal folds, which may result in an unacceptable high pitched voice.

CASE 1

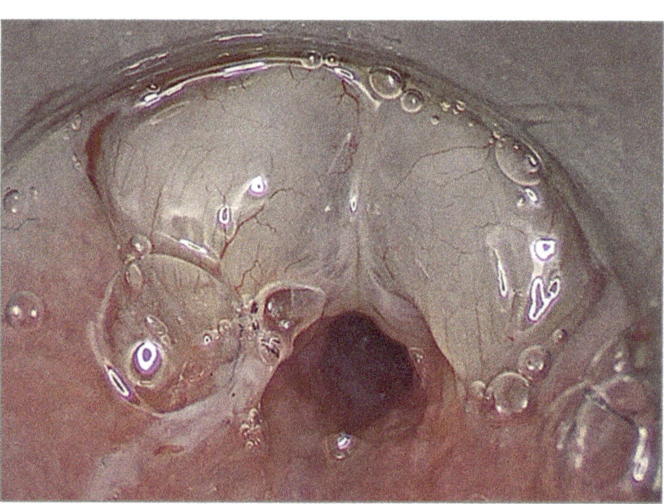

FIG. 8.1: Bilateral Grade II Reinke's edema. (E-CC)

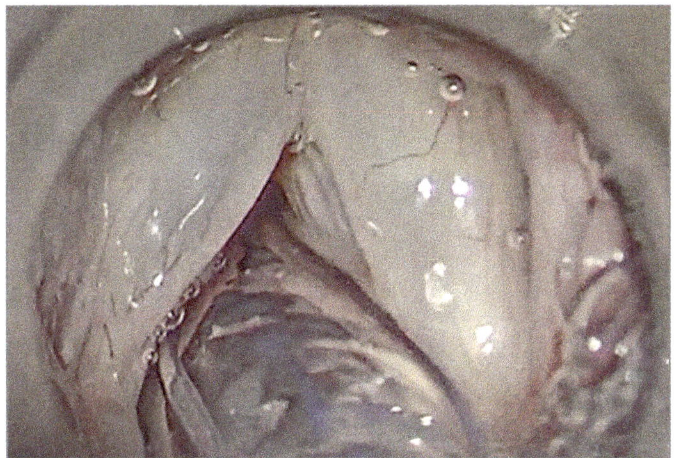

FIG. 8.2: Patient intubated with a 5 endotracheal tube. (M-CC)

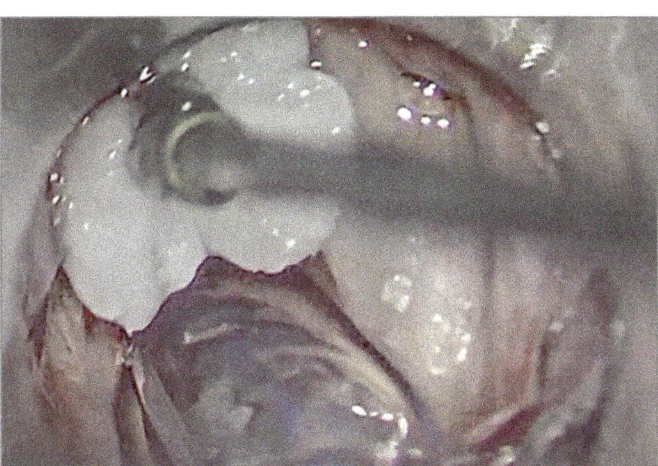

FIG. 8.5: The myxomatous material of the Reinke's edema is very stubborn and needs to be sucked out with a strong suction or squeezed out with cotton pledgets or occasionally even removed with a cup forceps or the CO_2 laser. (M-CC)

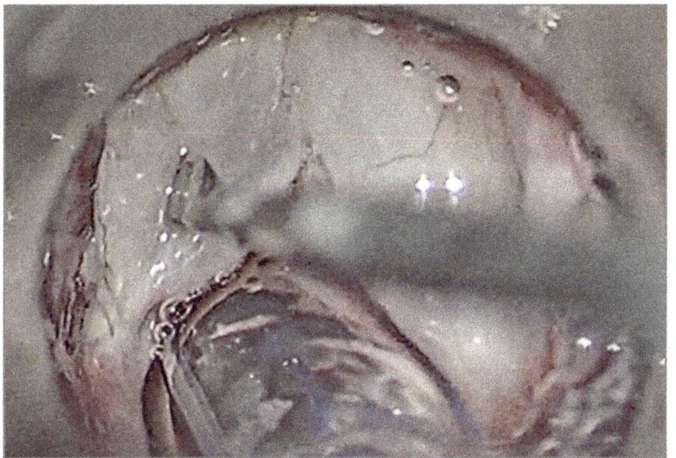

FIG. 8.3: An epithelial cordotomy being performed with an upward directed sickle knife on the superior surface of the left vocal fold. (M-CC)

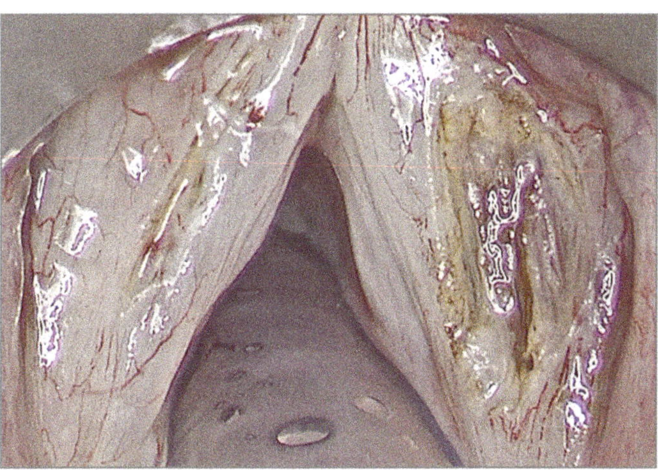

FIG. 8.6: Final postoperative image following bilateral surgery. The anterior commissure has not been made raw and the incisions have been made on the superior surface of the vocal folds bilaterally. (E-CC)

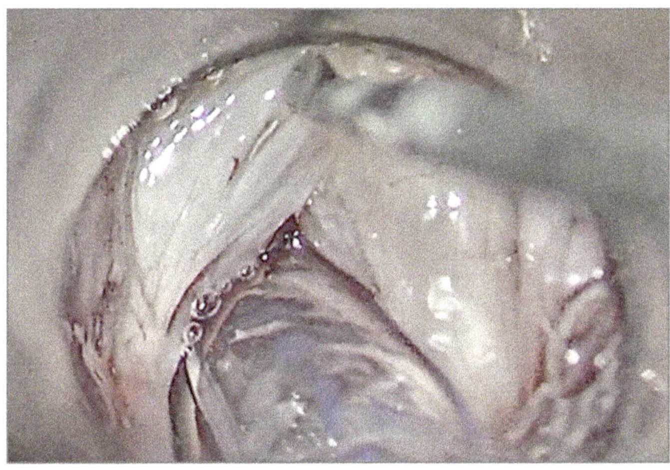

FIG. 8.4: Extension of the epithelial cordotomy anteriorly. (M-CC)

CASE 2

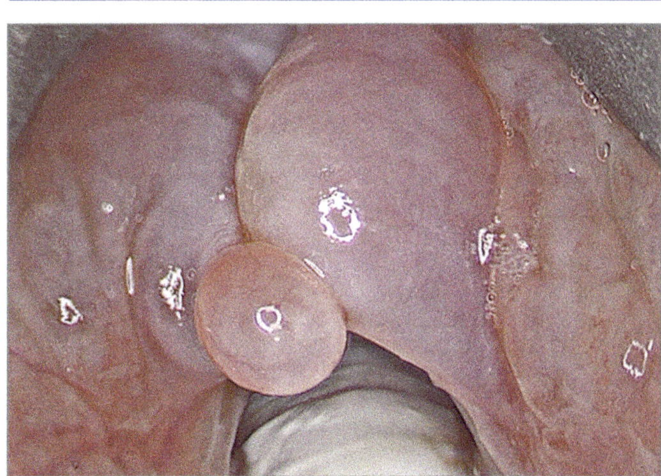

FIG. 8.7: Grade 3 Reinke's edema with a 5.5 laser tube *in situ*. (E-CC)

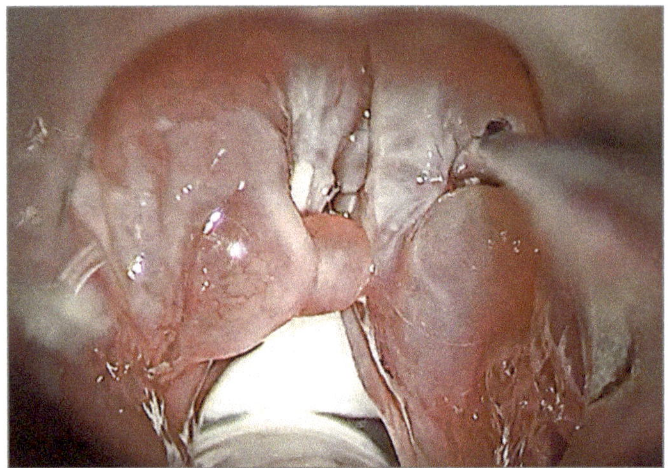

FIG. 8.8: Palpation of both the vocal folds and lateral retraction of the vocal fold so as to inspect the infraglottis. A cotton pledget has been placed in the subglottis. (M-CC)

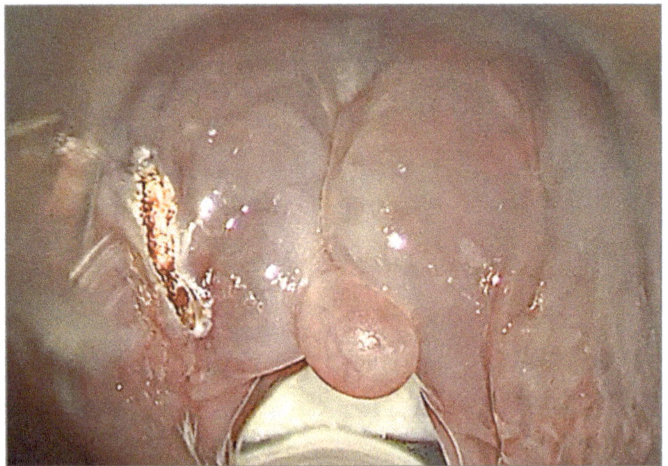

FIG. 8.9: An epithelial cordotomy being performed on the left vocal fold superior surface with the CO_2 laser AcuBlade. (M-CC)

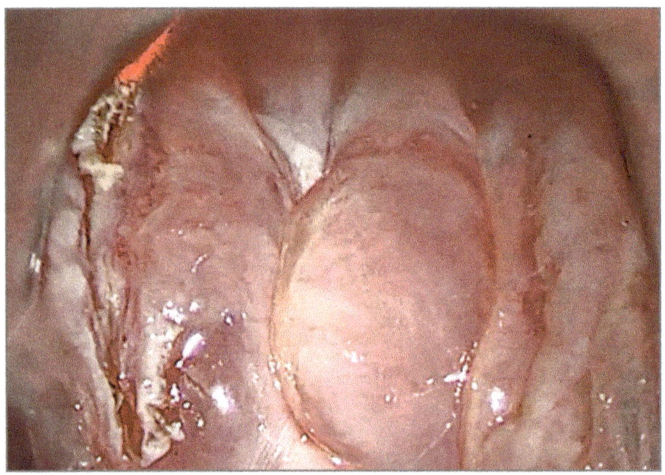

FIG. 8.10: Extension of the left epithelial cordotomy anteriorly. (M-CC)

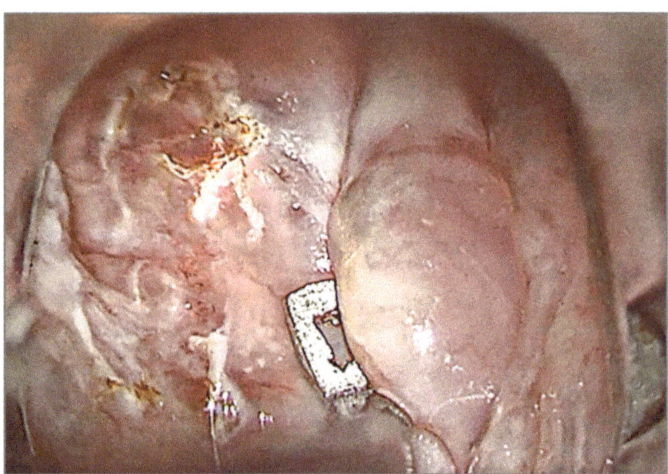

FIG. 8.11: An upward Bouchayer holding the left polypoid corditis to provide some traction during laser excision. (M-CC)

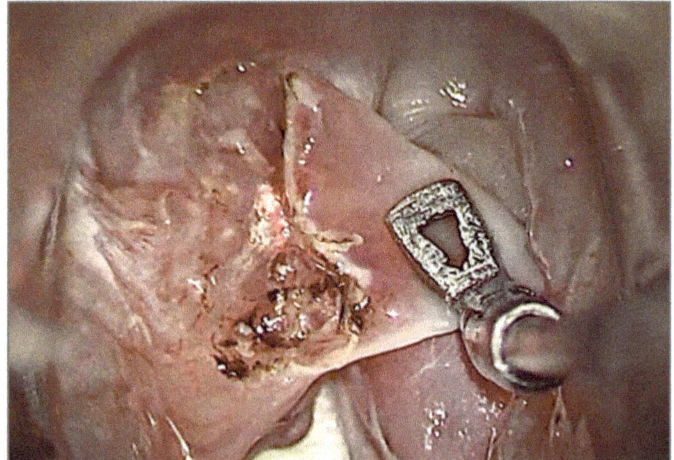

FIG. 8.12: The excess SLP as well as excess epithelium is excised taking care to leave behind adequate SLP as well as an untouched anterior commissure (M-CC)

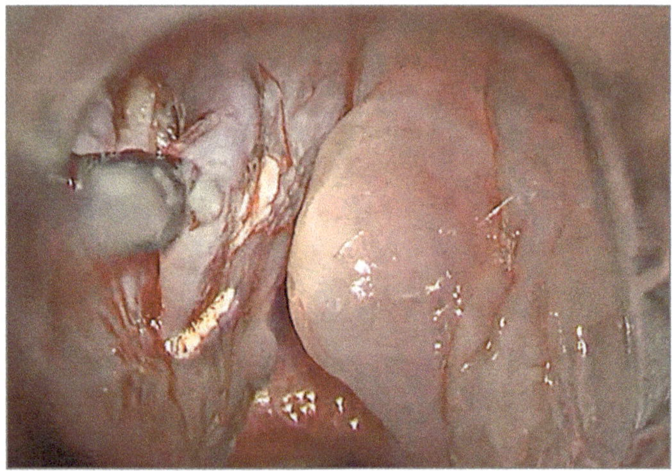

FIG. 8.13: Making the laser cut on the infraglottic surface of the left vocal fold(M-CC)

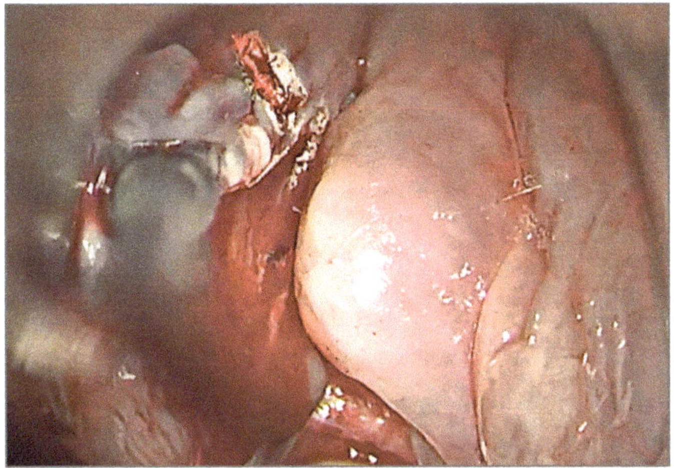

FIG. 8.14: Final anterior epithelial cut to remove the left polypoid corditis. (M-CC)

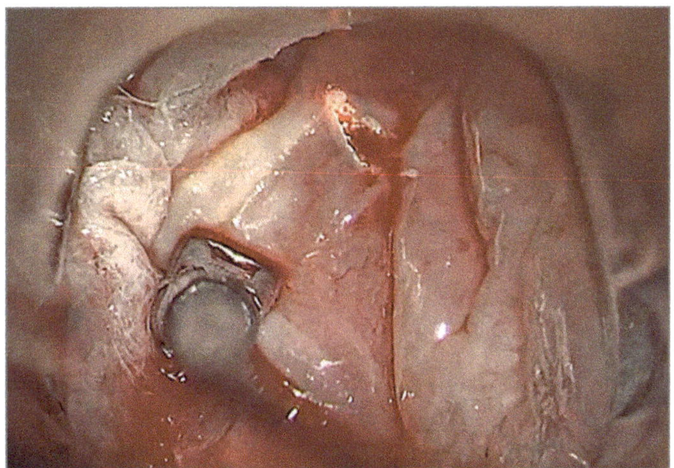

FIG. 8.15: Grasping the right polypoid corditis with a straight Bouchayer and initiation of the left epithelial cordotomy. (M-CC)

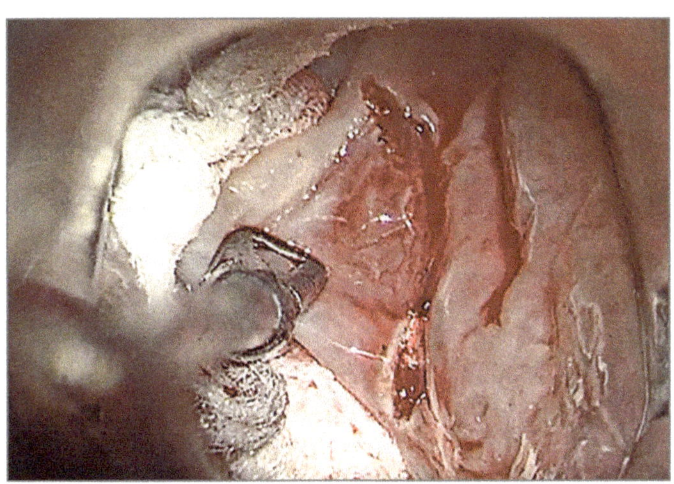

FIG. 8.16: Completing the laser epithelial cordotomy. (M-CC)

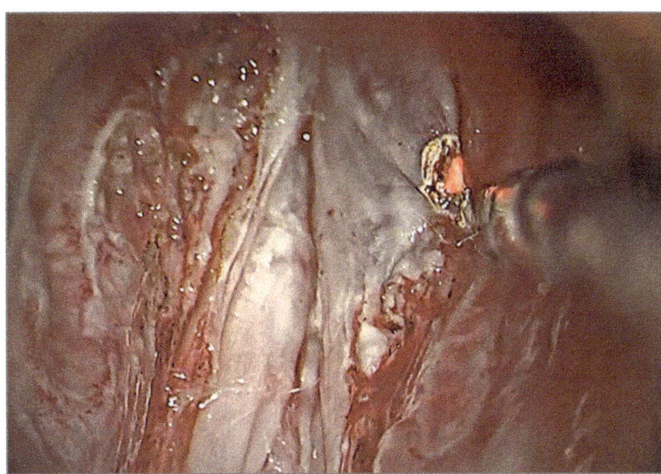

FIG. 8.17: The infraglottic incision being made for the polypoid corditis of the right vocal fold. (M-CC)

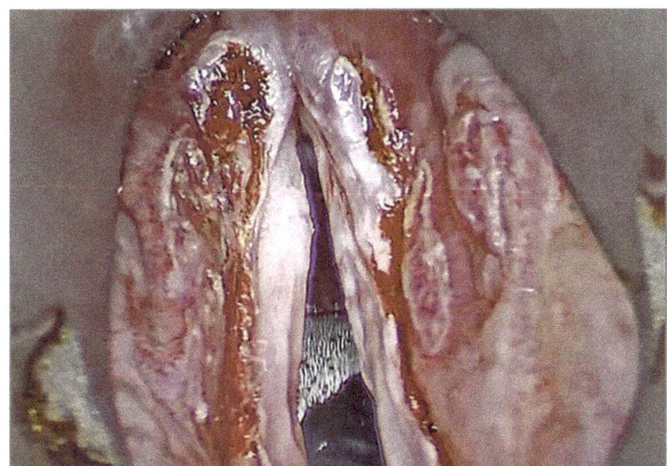

FIG. 8.18: Final postoperative image revealing an untouched anterior commissure (anteriormost 3 mms of the vocal folds bilaterally). (E-CC)

REFERENCES

1. Simpson CB, Ossoff RH. Surgical principles of microlaryngoscopy: Principles and techniques of operative laryngoscopy: In: Ossoff RH, Shapshay SM, Woodson G, et al., editors. The larynx. Lippincott Williams & Wilkins; 2003. pp. 111-23.
2. Yonekawa H. A clinical study of Reinke's edema. Auris Nasus Larynx. 1988;15 (1): p. 57-78.
3. White A, Sim DW, Maran AG. Reinke's edema and thyroid function. J Laryngol Otol. 1991;105(4):291-2.
4. Anderson T. Benign lesions of the larynx. In: Merati A, Bielamowicz S, editors. Textbook of laryngology. San Diego, CA: Plural Publishing Inc; 2006. pp 303-22.

CHAPTER 9

Nodules

DEFINITION

Vocal fold nodules are benign, small, and nodular swellings on the medial edge of vocal folds. Classically, they are located at the junction of anterior and middle thirds (striking zone) of the vocal fold due to maximum phonotrauma at this site.[1]

ETIOLOGY

Vocal abuse and misuse are the major contributory factors to the development of nodules. It has also been noted that an abnormal vibratory pattern may be more damaging than a high-intensity vibration.[2]

Nodules develop over a period of time due to repeated collision at the striking zone and an initial localized congestion with edema gradually leads to basement membrane zone (BMZ) injury. This leads to epithelial hyperplasia and thickening of the BMZ with increased deposition of type IV collagen and fibronectin. Continued phonotrauma over the early nodule thus formed leads to fibrosis and callus formation in the long run, resulting in hard, permanent nodules.[3,4]

MANAGEMENT PHILOSOPHY

Treatment of vocal fold nodules is voice rest followed by voice therapy. Perseverance with voice therapy should be the hallmark of management of vocal fold nodules. Surgery is only indicated when the nodules are extremely hard and nonresponsive to prolonged voice therapy or have converted into large polyps. Presurgical therapy is a must and will always aid in the postsurgical therapy compliance, thus decreasing the chances of recurrence of nodules.

Surgical excision of nodules in singers has to be a decision well thought out and discussed as it may result in changing the very character of voice the singer is famous for and may also result in suboptimal vocal outcomes in terms of the singing voice.

Both the case studies illustrated in this chapter were patients who had received over 3 months of therapy and had been extremely compliant with it.

CASE 1

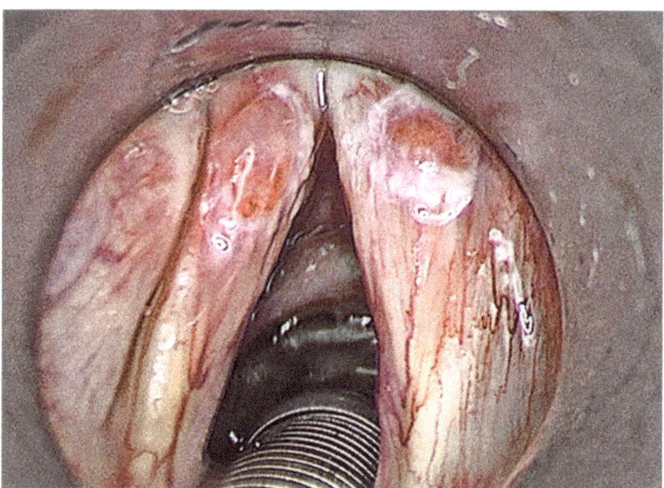

FIG. 9.1: Bilateral, firm, and nodular lesions on the striking zone of the vocal folds. There is some keratosis seen surrounding the nodules and increased vascularity of both the vocal folds. (E-CC)

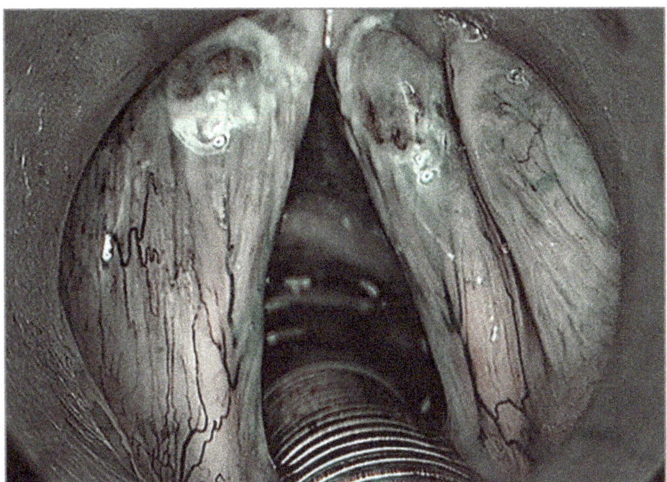

FIG. 9.2: Spectra A image of 9.1. The keratosis surrounding the nodules is clearly seen as whitish-gray. The subepithelial veins are seen as cyan (blue) in color. (E-SA)

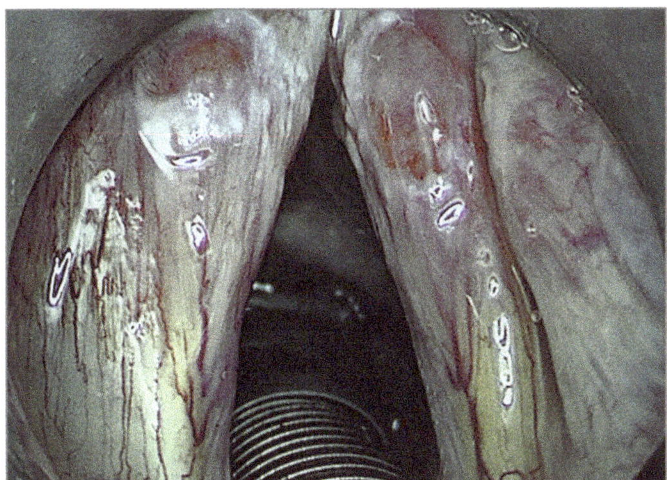

FIG. 9.3: Spectra B image of 9.1

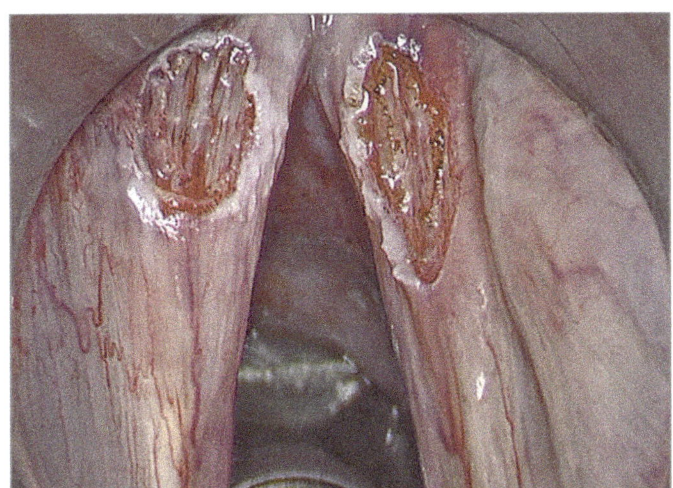

FIG. 9.4: The nodules are excised bilaterally as the anterior commissure is uninvolved. No epithelium is preserved, as nodules are epithelial lesions. The histopathology of this patient revealed mild dysplasia

CASE 2

A teacher who had a long-standing hoarseness with a more recent complaint of odynophonia and severe vocal fatigue was planned for surgical excision of her polypoidal nodules after a 3 month course of voice therapy.

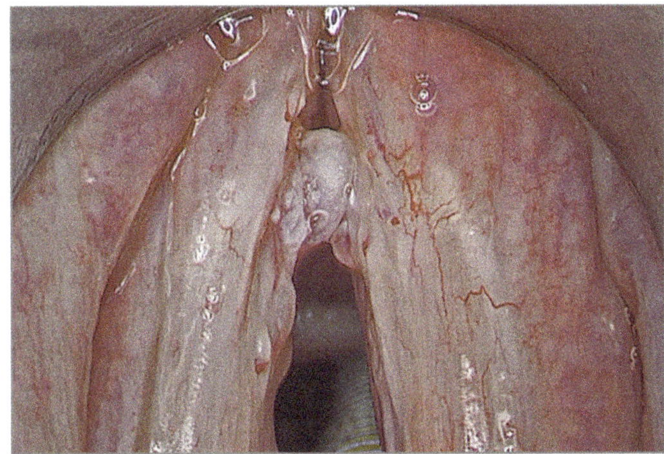

FIG. 9.5: Bilateral kissing polypoidal nodules are seen with a surrounding area of edema and increased vascularity. (E-CC)

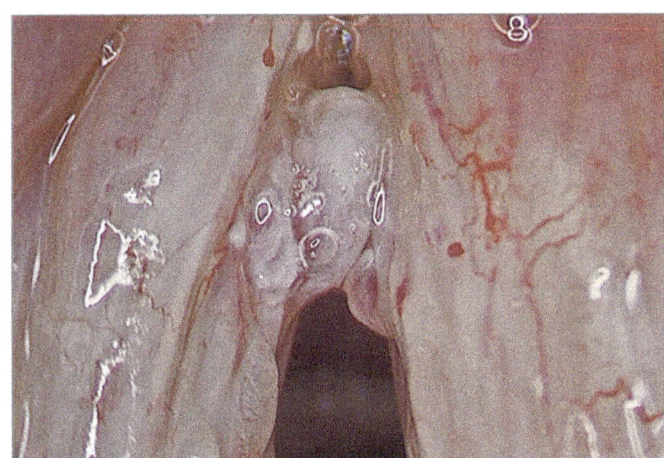

FIG. 9.6: Zoomed image of 9.5. (E-CC)

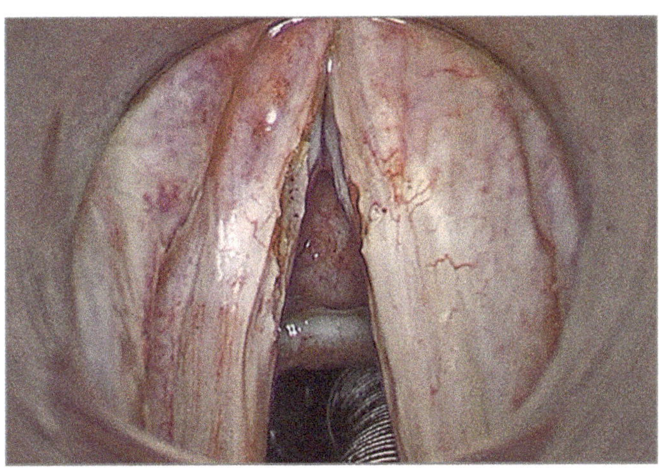

FIG. 9.7: Final postoperative image following bilateral laser excision with a CO_2 laser AcuBlade after SEIT. (E-CC)

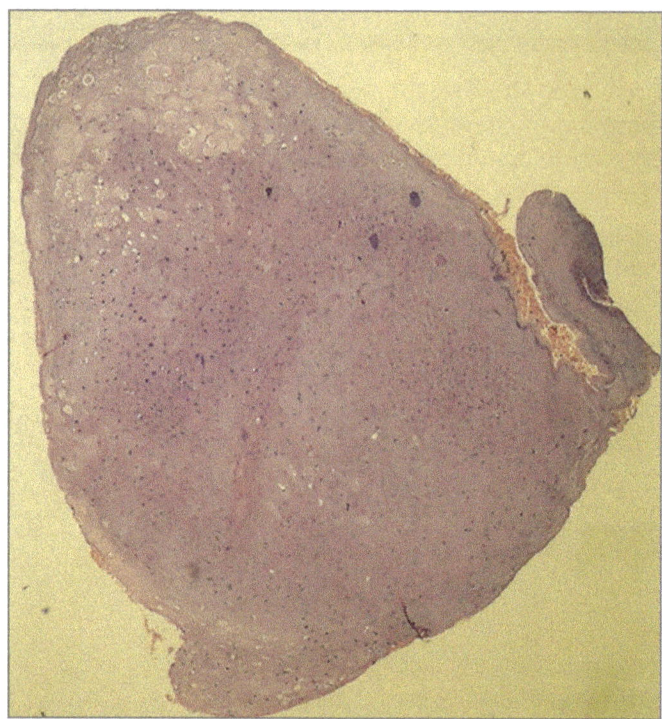

FIG. 9.8: Histopathology of an excised vocal fold nodule in H&E staining revealing a thick basement membrane of epithelium

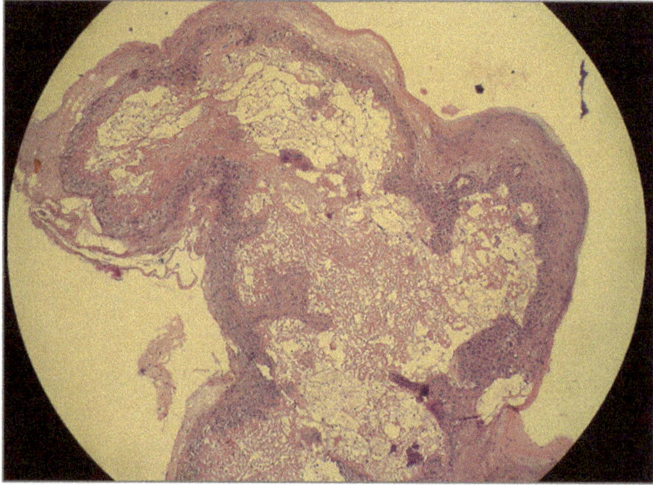

FIG. 9.9: Histopathology of an excised vocal fold polyp in H&E staining revealing a normal epithelium and excessive gelatinous material in the SLP

REFERENCES

1. Amitabha R. Nodules and polyps. In: Nerurkar NK, Roychoudhury A. Textbook of laryngology: Official textbook of Association of Phonosurgeons of India. New Delhi: Jaypee Brothers Medical Publishers (P) Ltd.; 2017. pp. 147-54.
2. Jiang JJ, Diaz CE, Hanson DJ. Finite element modeling of vocal fold vibration in normal phonation and hyperfunctional dysphonia: Implications for the pathogenesis of vocal nodules. Annals Otol Rhinol Laryngol. 1988; 107:603-10.
3. Altman KW. Vocal fold masses. Otolaryngol Clin North Am. 2007; 40: 1091-108.
4. Aronson AE, Bless DM. Clinical voice disorders. 4th ed. New York: Thieme Medical Publishers; 2009. pp. 174-5.

CHAPTER 10

Glottic Web

DEFINITION

An epithelial covered layer spanning the vocal folds, glottic webs can occur at any point of the larynx and are divided into anterior, posterior, and complete webs.[1,2]

ETIOLOGY

In the mid to late 1800s, infectious diseases such as diphtheria, syphillis, and tuberculosis were all typical causes of glottic web formation due to extensive epithelial sloughing on opposing vocal folds, giving rise to thick, fibrous scar formation and epithelialization.[3,4] Since the mid-20th century, endotracheal intubation is the most significant etiologic factor for all glottic webs.[4]

Anterior glottic webs are the most common type, often the result of trauma and less commonly congenital in origin.

COHEN'S CLASSIFICATION FOR LARYNGEAL WEBS[5]

Cohens Classification

- Type I: Involves less than 35% of the glottis, usually thin and uniform in thickness with no subglottic extension
- Type II: The web involves 35–50% of the glottis and can be thin or thick, but the vocal folds can usually be seen within the web. These may be associated with some subglottic extension of stenosis
- This type involves 50–75% of the glottis, is usually thick anteriorly, and may thin out posteriorly. The true vocal folds may or may not be visible within the web; these almost always have a subglottic component to them
- Type IV: Involves 75–90% of the glottis and the vocal folds are not identifiable within the web and may be one continuous, thick band. Almost always requires an emergency tracheotomy.

MANAGEMENT PHILOSOPHY FOR ANTERIOR GLOTTIC WEBS

Small glottic webs (Cohen's type 1) may often be picked up incidentally. The patient may have mild hoarseness with a slightly high-pitched voice and these webs are best left alone.

Cohen's type 2 and 3 webs cause a moderate to severe hoarseness with a variable amount of dyspnea on exertion. Prior to any surgical intervention, radiologic documentation of the subglottic extent and cricoid development is essential in treatment planning.

Cohen's type 4 webs would need a tracheostomy almost always due to stridor and surgical management if planned would be open airway surgery.

Endoscopic management of anterior glottic webs faces the constant challenge of restenosis due to the close approximation of the raw epithelial edges of the operated vocal folds at the anterior commissure.

In order to prevent this, many surgeries have been described such as cutting the web followed by regular clean ups, temporary stent placement postoperatively, and flap surgeries.

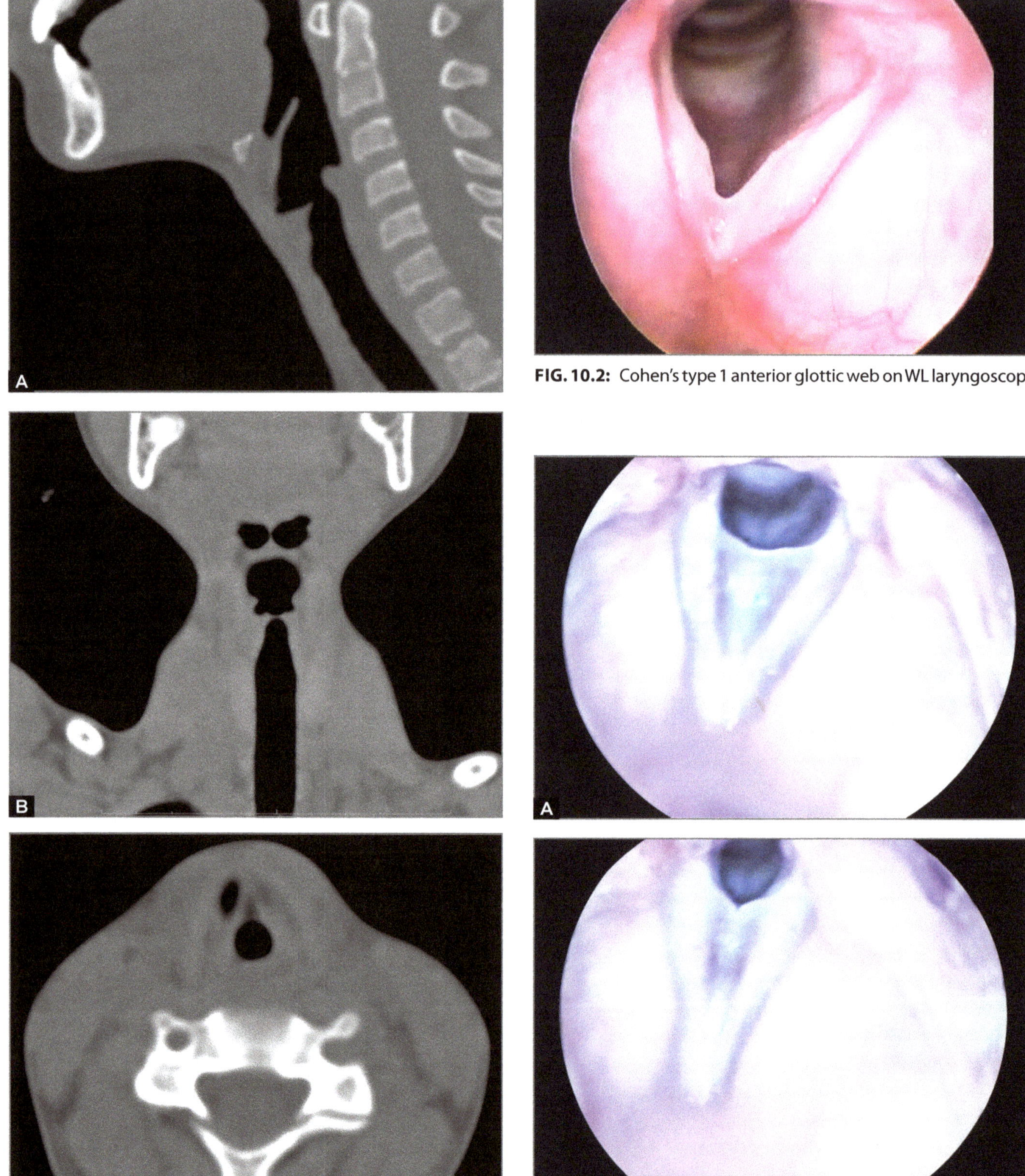

FIG. 10.1: Cohen's type 2 glottic web seen on sagittal, coronal, and axial CT images

FIG. 10.2: Cohen's type 1 anterior glottic web on WL laryngoscopy

FIG. 10.3: Cohen's type 2 anterior glottic web on WL laryngoscopy in **A,** abduction and **B,** adduction, revealing good vocal fold motion. The vocal folds can be appreciated through the web

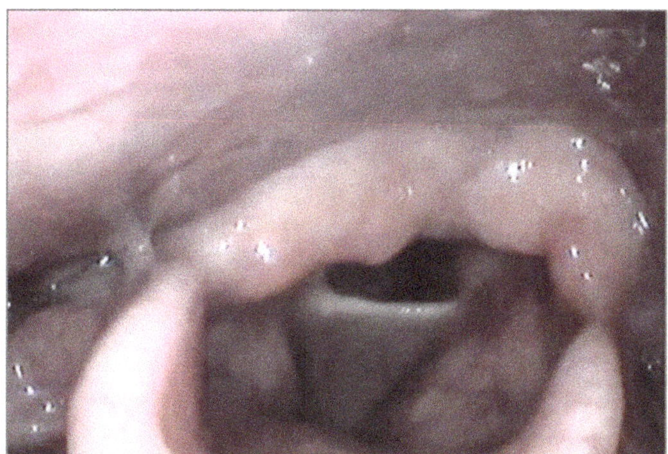

FIG. 10.4: Cohens type 3 anterior glottic web on WL laryngoscopy, the vocal folds are not identifiable and a thick sheet of the web is seen

CASE 1: COHEN'S TYPE 2—CONGENITAL

Cohen's type 2 congenital anterior glottic web operated by midline laser excision and subsequent slough cleaning under anesthesia after 10 days.

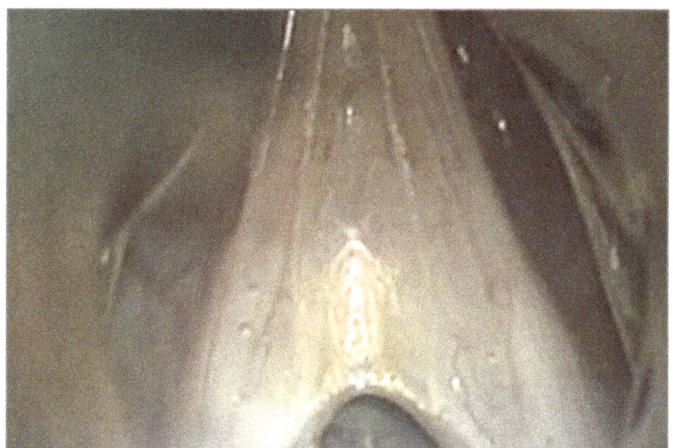

FIG. 10.5: AcuBlade CO_2 laser being used to cut a congenital Cohen's type 2 web in the midline

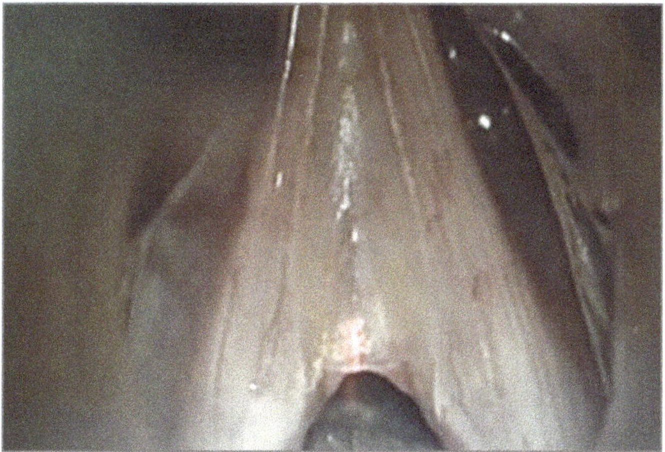

FIG. 10.6: The bilateral prominent ventricles seen are a result of the glottic web

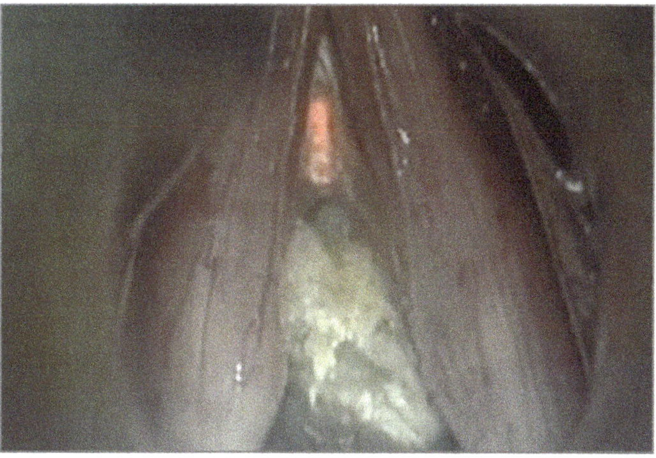

FIG. 10.7: The web is being cut from a posterior to anterior direction. A subglottic moist cotton pledget is seen protecting the endotracheal tube cuff. The anterior most part of the web has some amount of subglottic component which is being excised by the AcuBlade

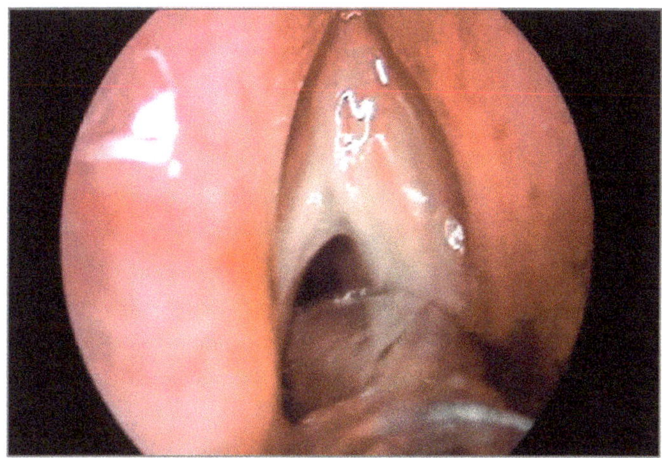

FIG. 10.8: This is the image 10 days postsurgery where slough has substituted the web. If this slough is not gently removed, it promotes the formation of the rewebbing

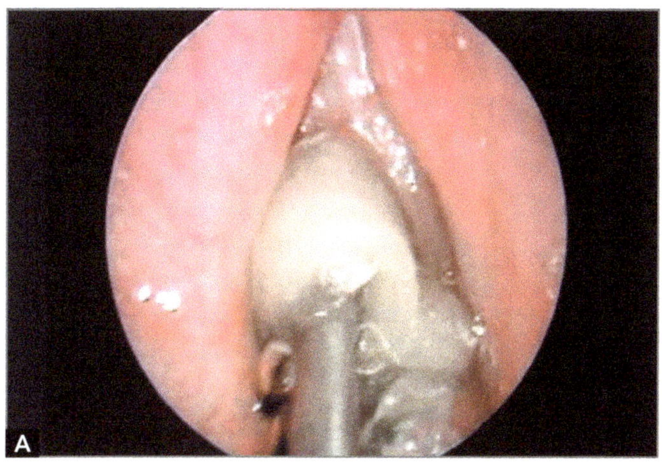

Continued

Continued

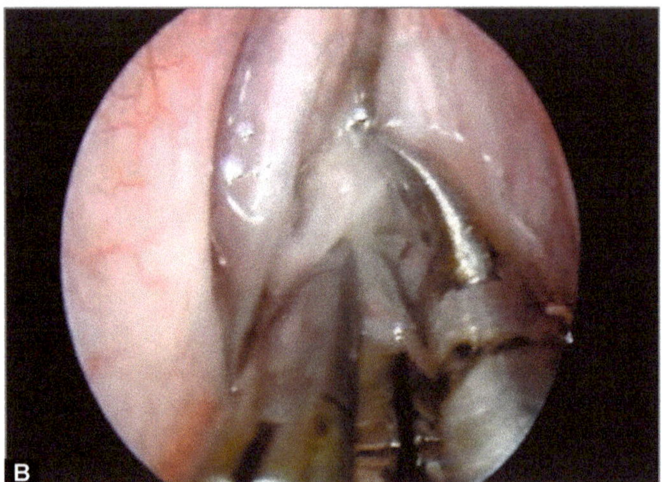

FIG. 10.9: The slough is removed with **A,** a soaking cotton pledget, and if necessary, with **B,** scissors, without any bleeding. If required, this clean-up can be repeated once or twice in another 10 days to 2 weeks till neo-epithelisation takes place

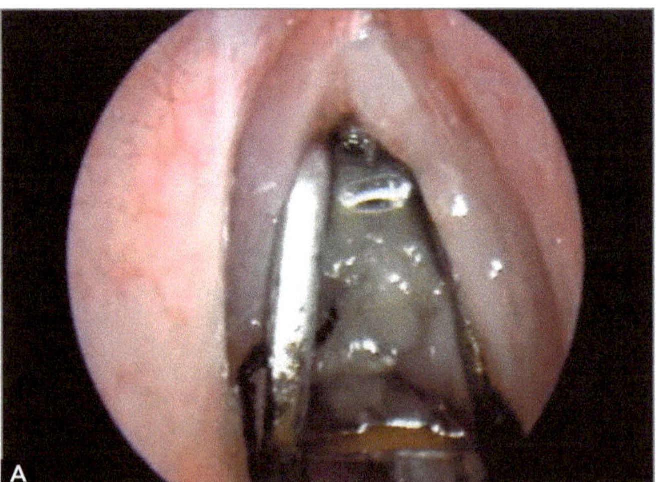

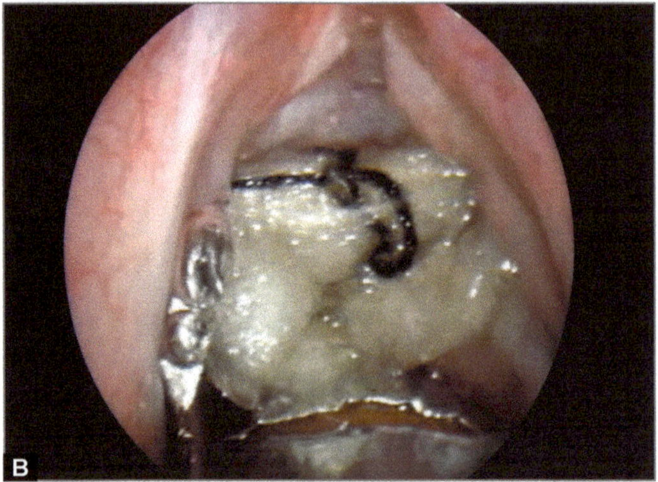

FIG. 10.10: A vocal fold separator may be used to effectively to break any anterior attachments at this stage

CASE 2: COHEN'S TYPE 2—IATROGENIC

Cohen's type 2, iatrogenic web following type 6 cordectomy for invasive squamous cell carcinoma, operated by flap technique.

Since the primary problem in anterior glottic web surgery is the close proximity of 2 raw surfaces, the microflap surgery is a technique meant to circumvent this problem by creating one epithelized vocal fold.

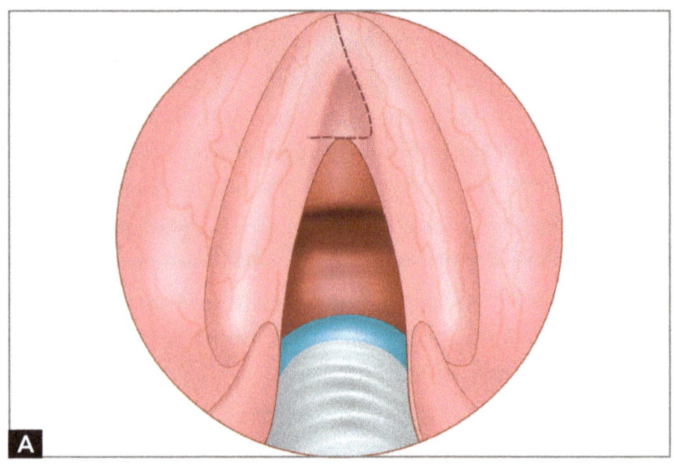

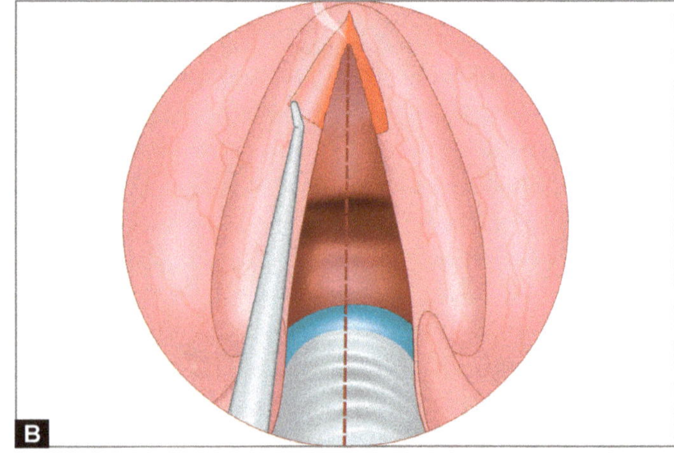

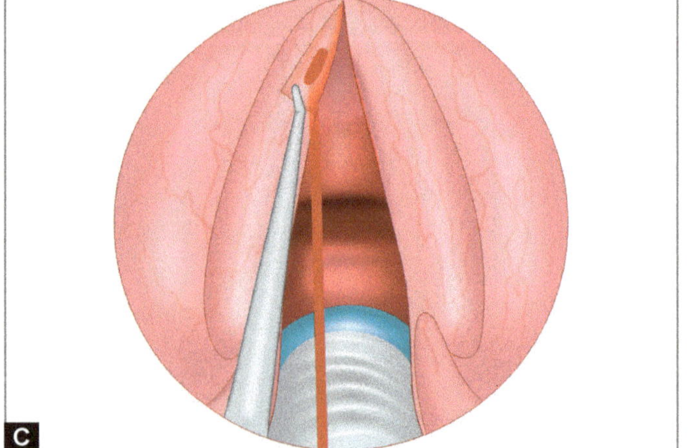

Continued

Continued

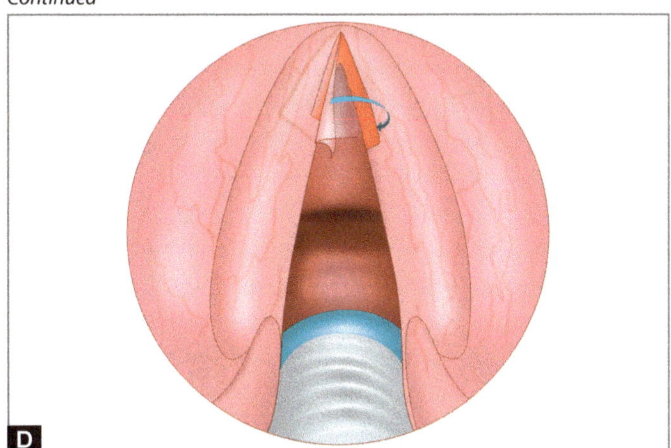

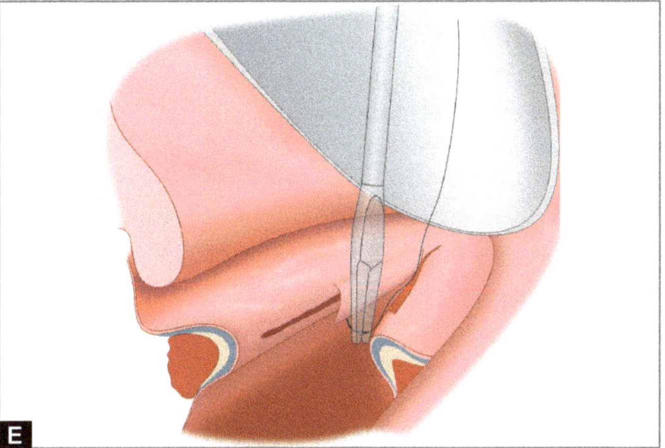

FIG. 10.11: A and B, An incision is made along the proposed margin of one vocal fold cutting the web such that a triangular tissue is obtained attached to the contralateral vocal fold; **C,** The undersurface of this triangular epithelium which is the web tissue is made raw; **D and E,** This is now sutured to or glued to the infraglottic surface of this contralateral vocal fold. Thus, one vocal fold now has epithelial cover

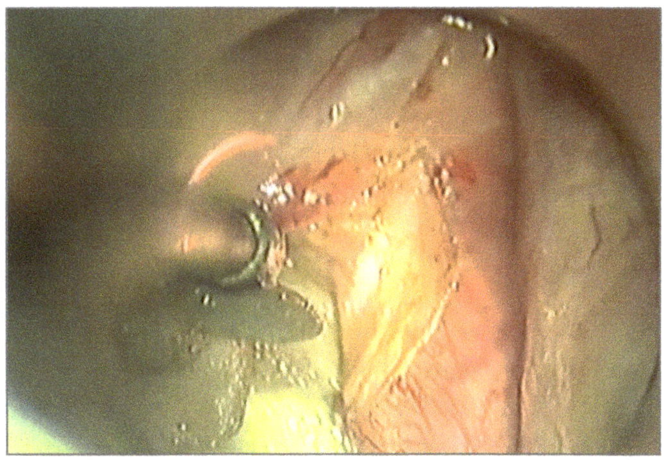

FIG. 10.13: Web tissue attached to the left vocal fold is being preserved

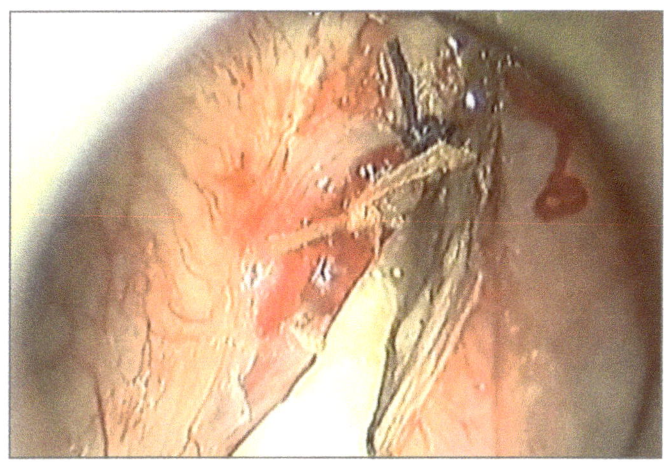

FIG. 10.14: After making the undersurface of this tissue raw it is sutured to the infraglottic surface of the left vocal fold with 4-0 vicryl. Two sutures have been taken

FIG. 10.12: CO_2 acuBlade laser incision along the proposed right vocal fold edge, from posterior to anterior

CASE 3: COHENS'S TYPE 2—MALIGNANT

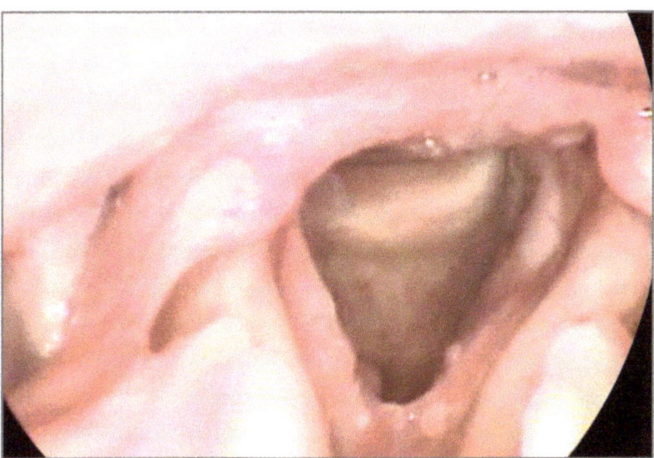

FIG. 10.15: Cohen's type 2 web with granulomatous lesions over it, in an adult male nonsmoker

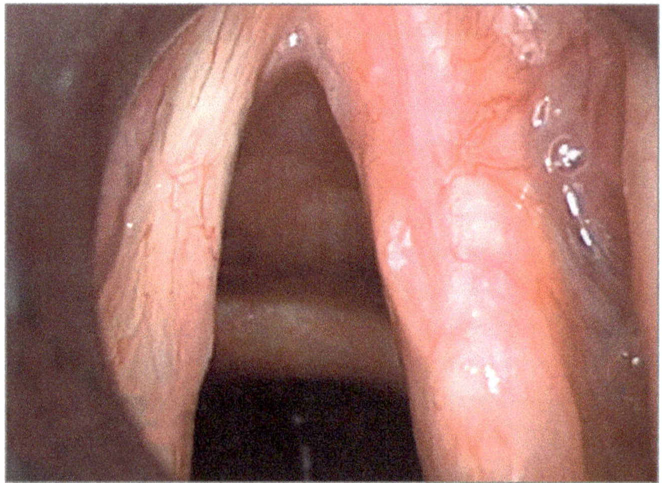

FIG. 10.16: A staged surgery was planned for this patient who had an anterior glottic web with granulomatous lesions over both the vocal folds and the web. The left vocal fold epithelium and SLP was removed in the first stage upto the anterior commissure. The frozen was carcinoma *in situ*. Fig 10.16 is the image 4 weeks after the first stage showing good left vocal fold healing

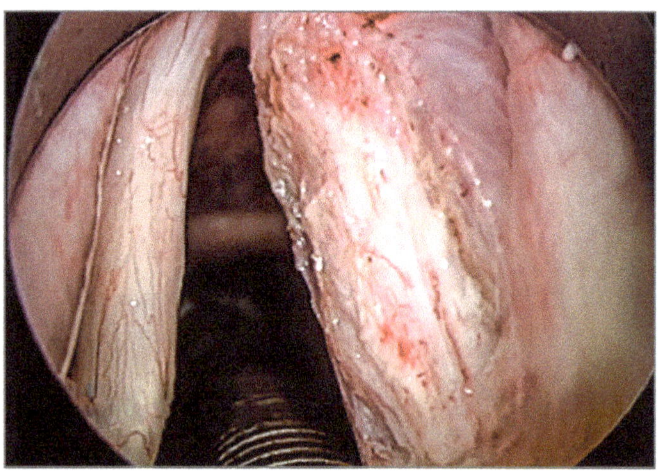

FIG. 10.17: The right vocal fold epithelium and SLP is now excised

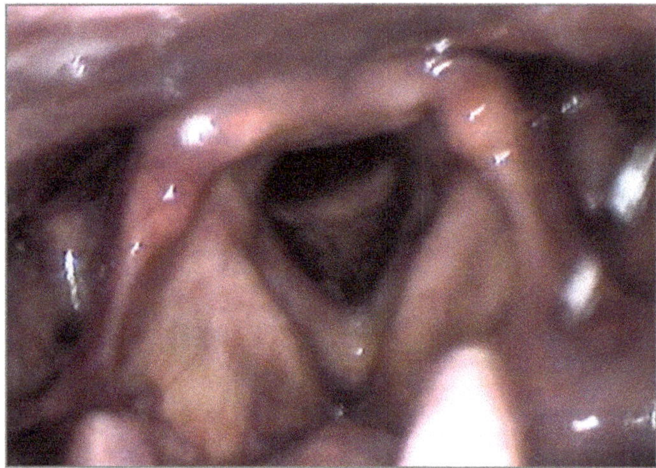

FIG. 10.18: Final flexible laryngoscopic image of the patient after complete healing

CASE 4: COHENS TYPE 2—TRAUMATIC

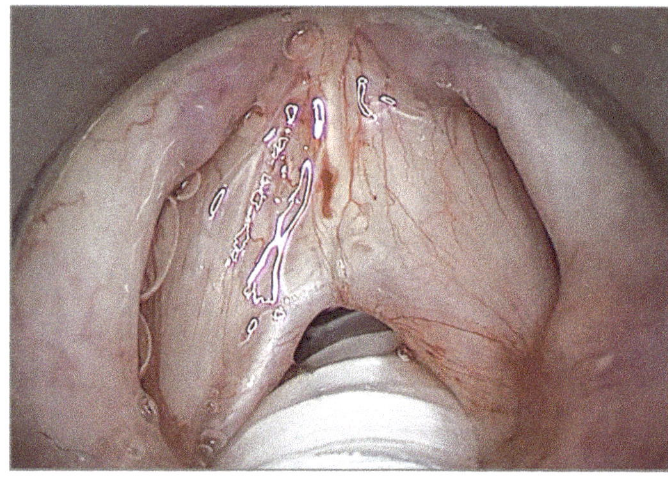

FIG. 10.19: Post vehicular accident traumatic anterior glottic Cohens type 2 web in a young female patient

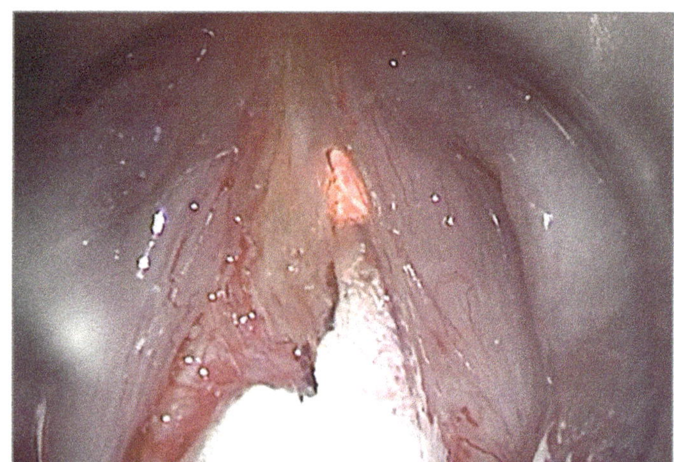

FIG. 10.20: Microflap surgery with suturing is planned for this web. A laser cut is made along the proposed edge of the right vocal fold from a posterior to anterior direction

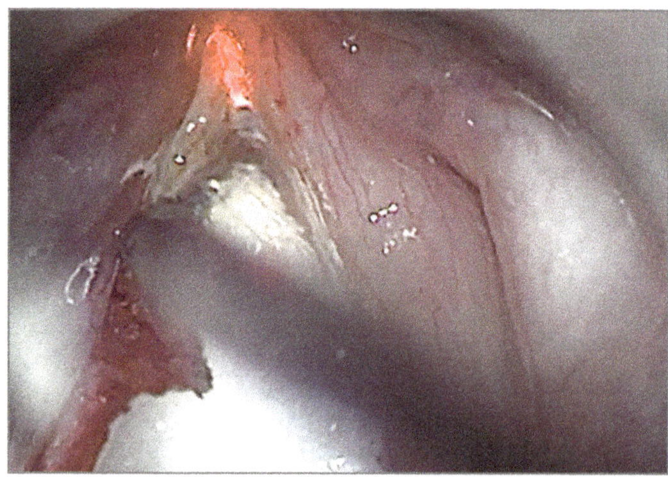

FIG. 10.21: Anterior completion of the web incision

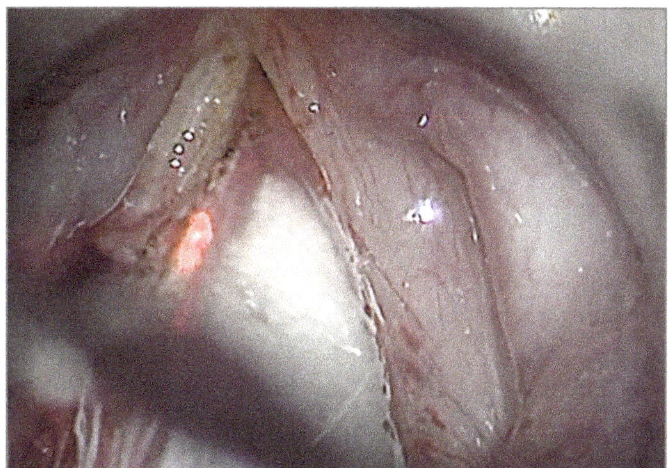

FIG. 10.22: Making the undersurface of the web epithelium raw with the CO_2 laser

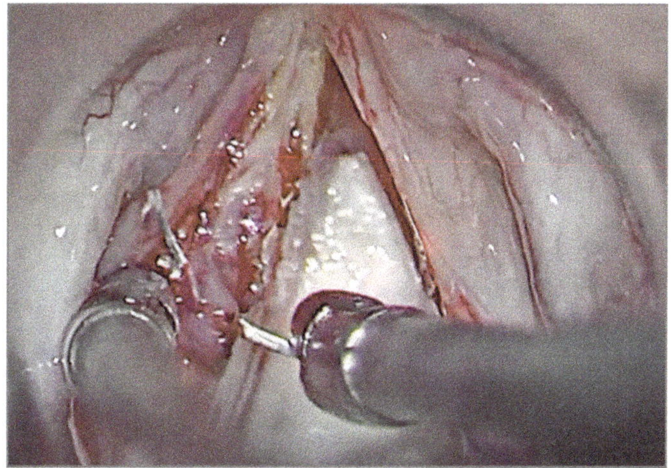

FIG. 10.23: Suturing the infraglottic surface of the vocal fold to the triangular flap of web tissue with 4-0 vicryl

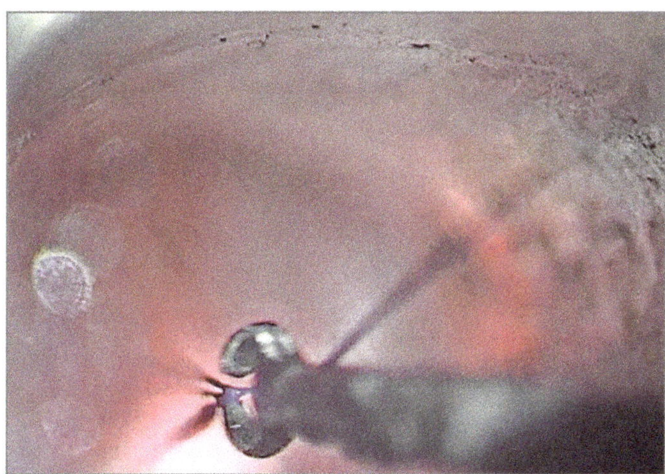

FIG. 10.24: Sliding the knot with a knot slider

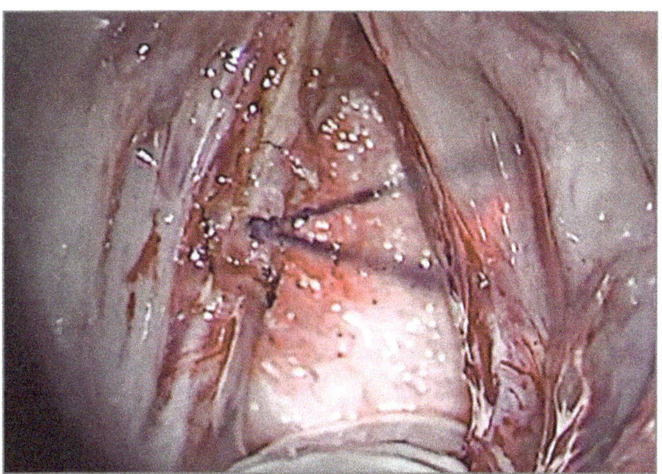

FIG. 10.25: Knot in place, allowing the epithelium to cover the left vocal fold medial edge

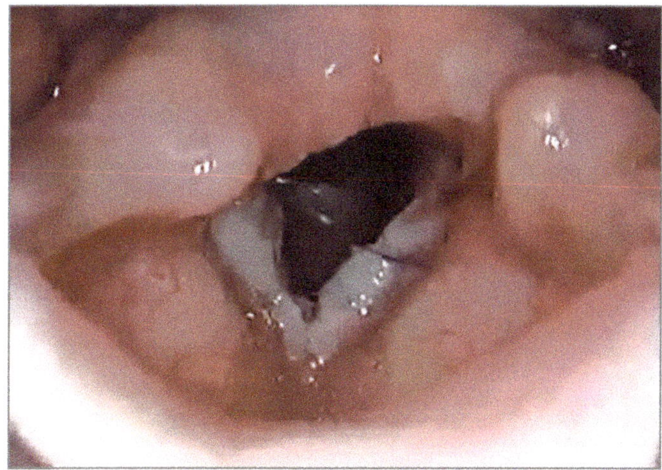

FIG. 10.26: Postoperative WL laryngoscopy at 2 weeks. The vicryl can still be seen in situ with a sharp anterior commissure.

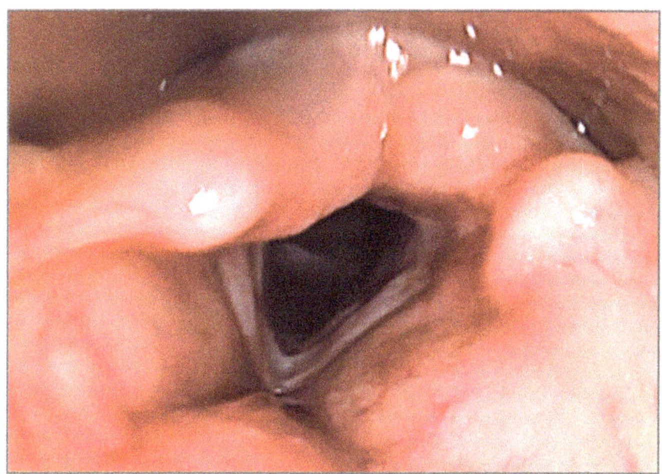

FIG. 10.27: Postoperative image of the patients vocal folds after 1 year

CASE 5: COHEN'S TYPE 3—CONGENITAL WEB

Keeping in mind the subglottic extension of the stenosis anteriorly in a Cohen's type 3 web, it is preferable to place a keel between the cut edges of the vocal folds and in the subglottis for 3–6 weeks till new epithelium has a chance to grow. This keel may be introduced via a laryngofissure or endoscopically.

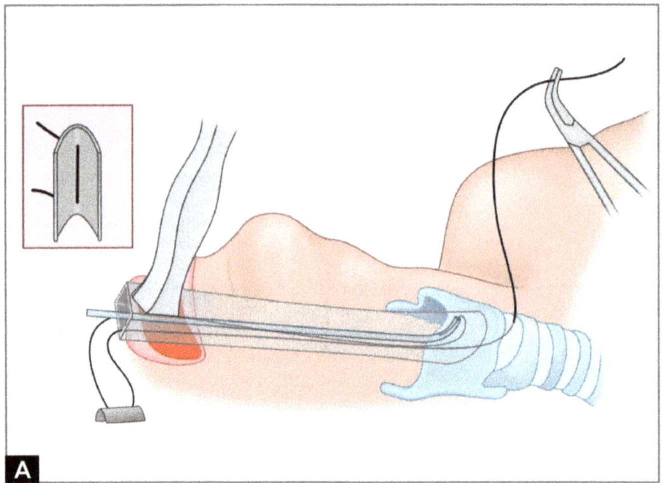

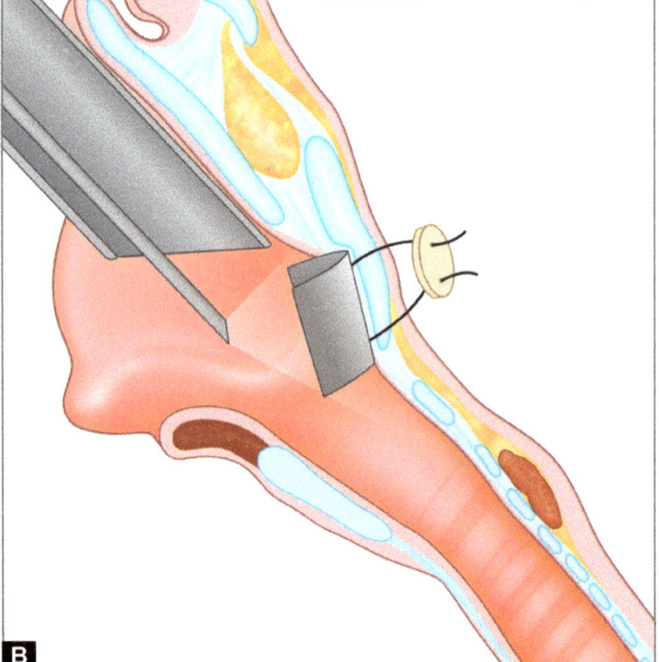

FIG. 10.28: This is a diagrammatic representation of an endoscopic keel placement. The keel is typically made from an oval cutout of a thin Silastic sheet, which is bent in the center to form two wings. An infant feeding tube may be sutured or glued into this bend in the Silastic in which case the anchoring thread runs through the infant feeding tube with less chance of a cut through of the stitch. The keel is placed at the anterior commissure and anchored to the neck with the help of a Lichtenberger needle or by looping threads through a number 18 intravenous catheter

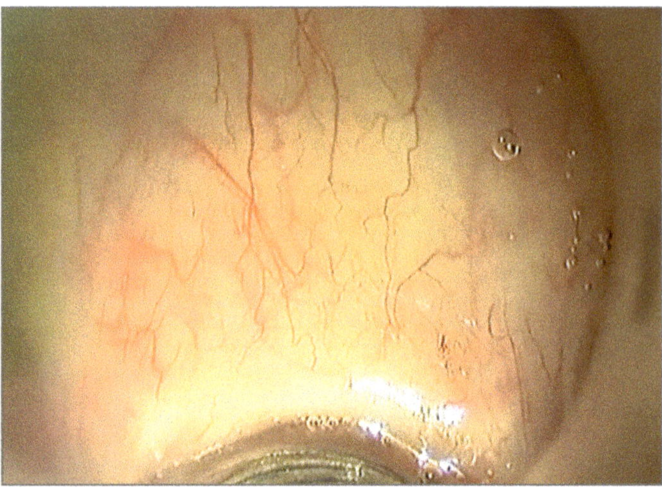

FIG. 10.29: A congenital grade 3 Cohen's anterior glottic web

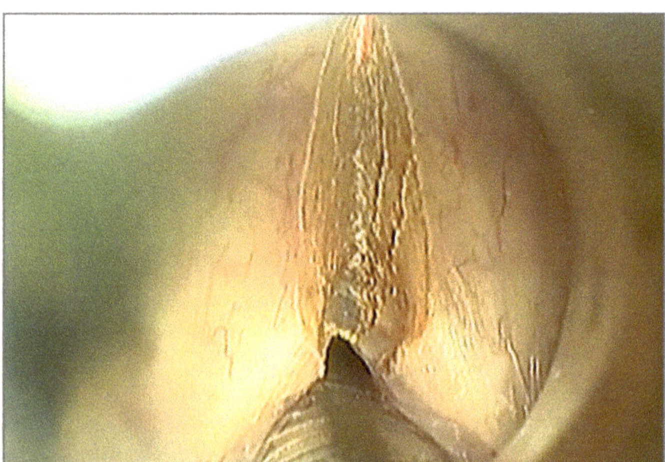

FIG. 10.30: CO_2 laser AcuBlade cutting the web in the midline from posterior to anterior

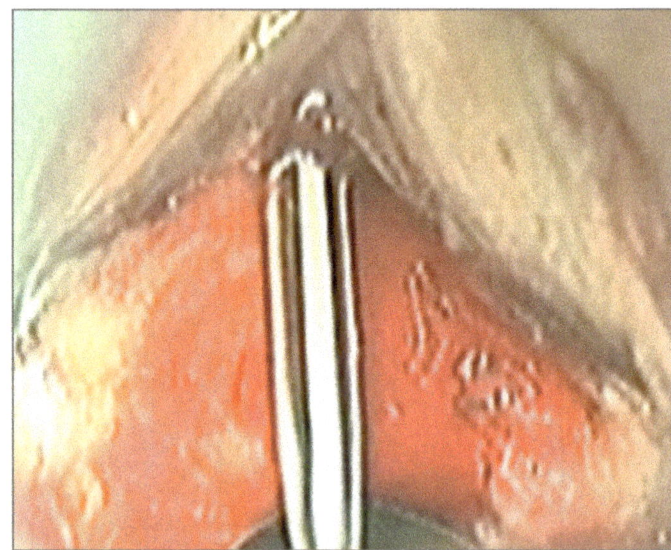

FIG. 10.31: An 18 gauge intravenous catheter passed from the midline of the neck into the subglottic area. A 1-0 prolene is passed through it and then threaded into the infant feeding tube of the keel

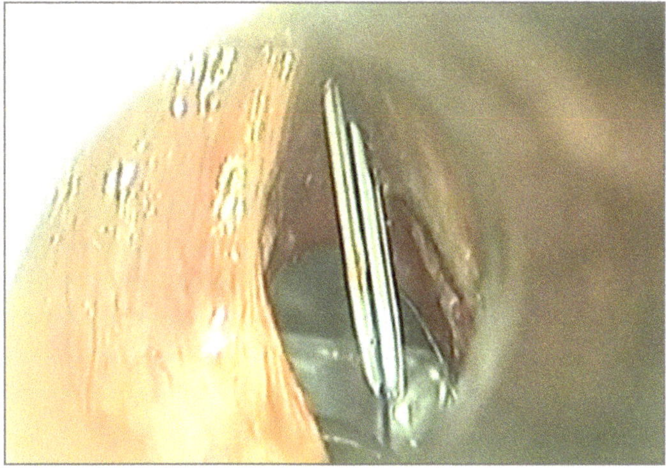

FIG. 10.32: A 1-0 prolene suture passed through another 18 gauge IV catheter that has been passed from the neck midline into the supraglottis

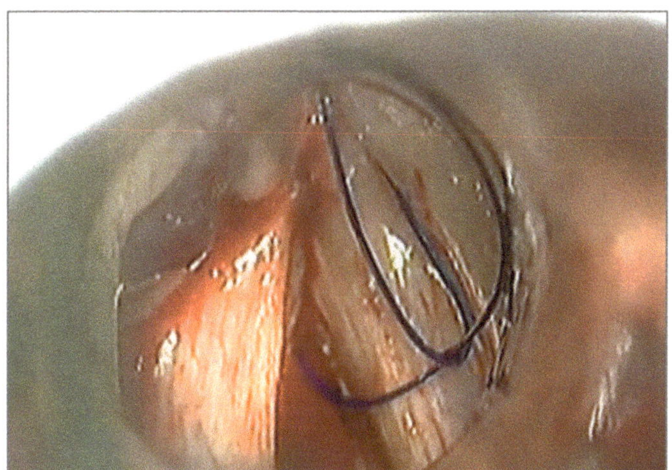

FIG. 10.33: The prolene threads are looped into one another and one is pulled out of the neck such that the Silastic keel is now on only one thread which is anchored to the neck

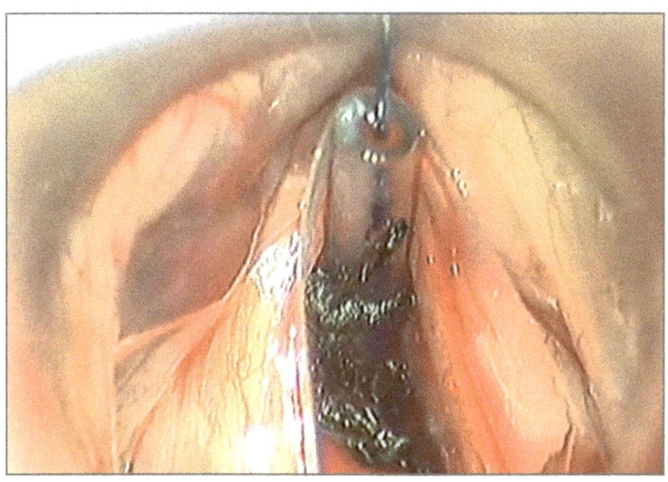

FIG. 10.34: The Silastic keel with the infant feeding tube seen at the anterior commissure with the 1-0 prolene thread anchoring it in the neck

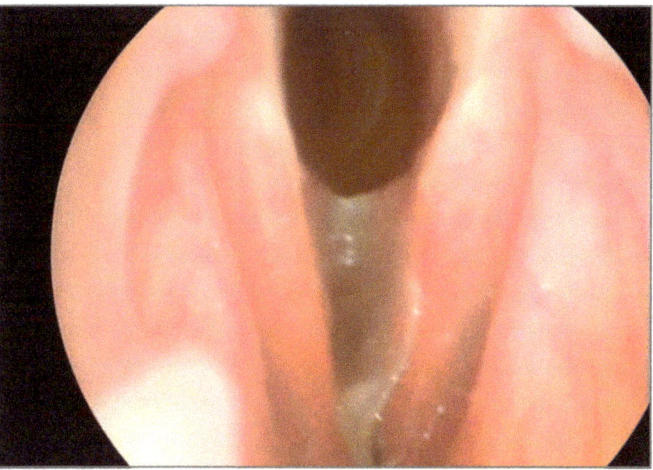

FIG. 10.35: Postoperative laryngoscopy image showing the Silastic keel *in situ*

CASE 6: COHENS TYPE 3—CONGENITAL ANTERIOR GLOTTIC WEB

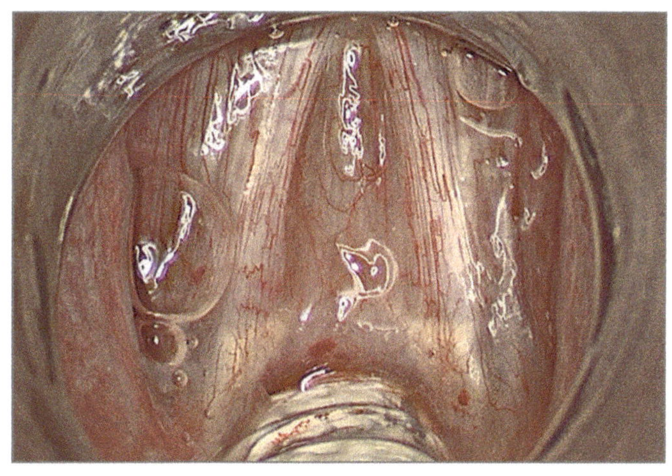

FIG. 10.36: Cohen's type 3—congenital anterior glottic web with anterior subglottic extension and 50–60 % of the glottic length involved

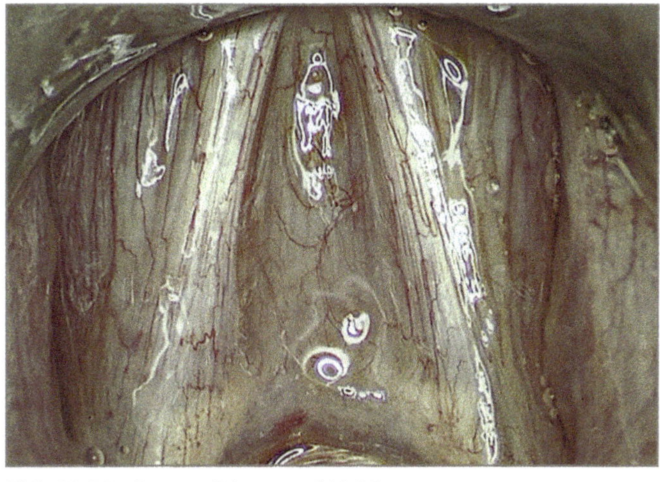

FIG. 10.37: Spectra B image of 10.36

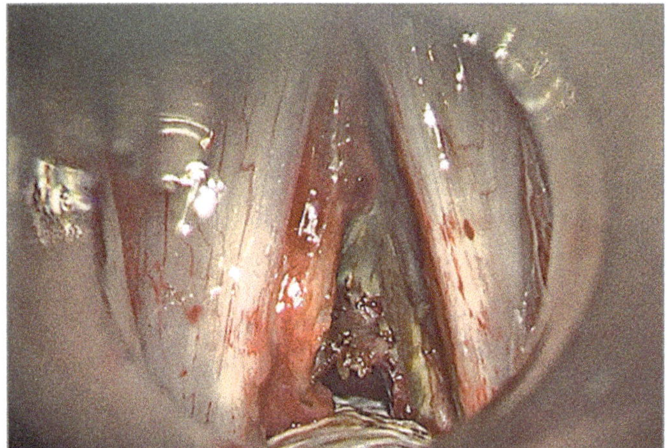

FIG. 10.38: CO_2 acuBlade cut made along the right vocal fold perceived edge, however, dense thyroid and cricoid cartilage encountered in the infraglottic area. In the CT scan, the cricoid was not seen as it was not ossified and the length of the stenosis anteriorly was reported as less than 1 cm

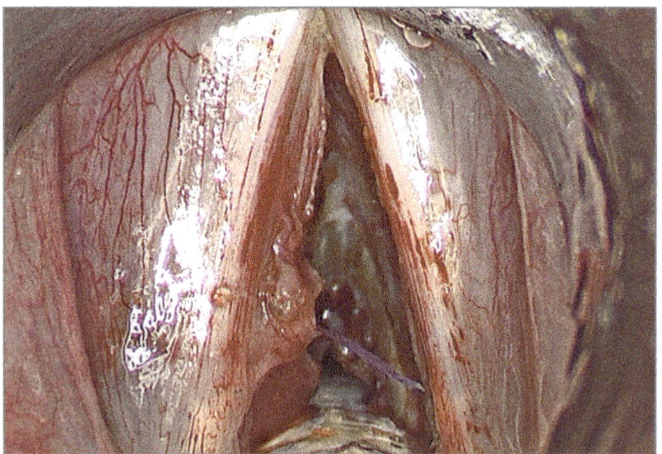

FIG. 10.39: The cartilage inner core was laserised to create an airway, fibrin glue was applied to encourage smooth reepithelization. The web undersurface was made raw and sutured to the left vocal fold infraglottic area

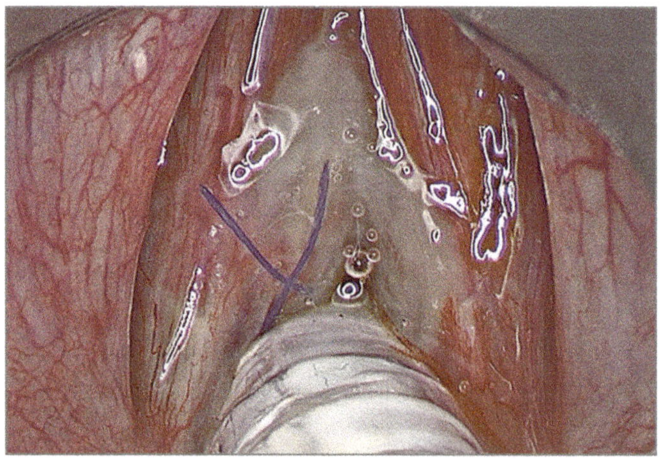

FIG. 10.40: Two weeks following the primary surgery the patient was taken up under anesthesia for slough clearance

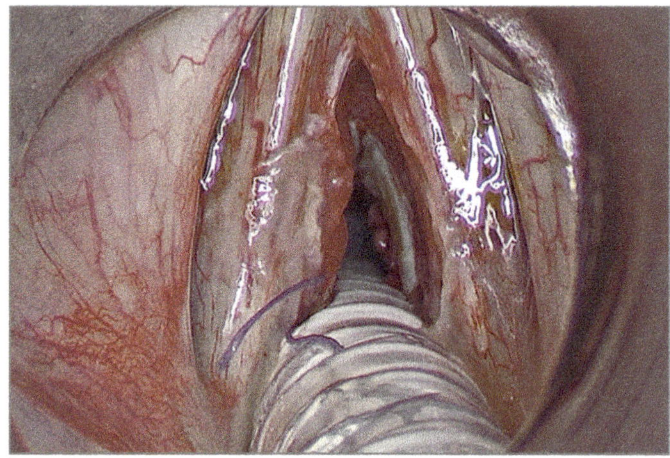

FIG. 10.41: Slough once cleared revealed a better subglottic airway

CASE 7

Anterior glottic webs can be deliberately and precisely created in patients who desire to increase the fundamental pitch of their voice. This surgery is commonly performed in patients who have undergone a male to female gender reassignment surgery.

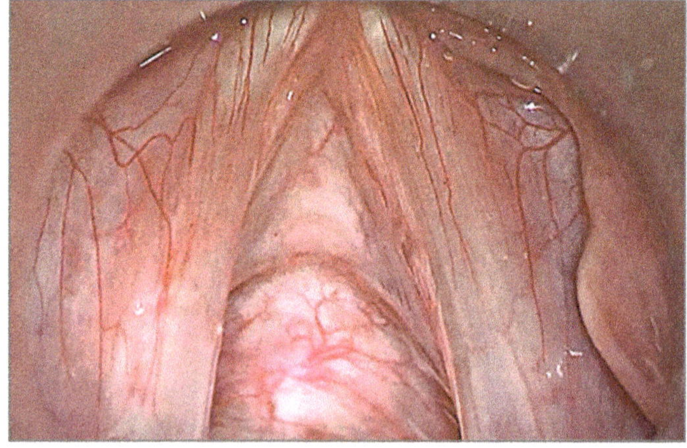

FIG. 10.42: Normal larynx in a patient who wants to increase her pitch following gender reassignment surgery

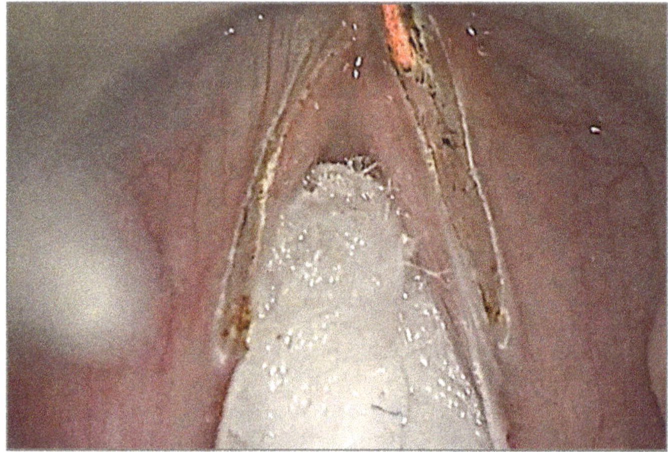

FIG. 10.43: CO_2 laser AcuBlade making the anterior half of the medial vibrating edge raw

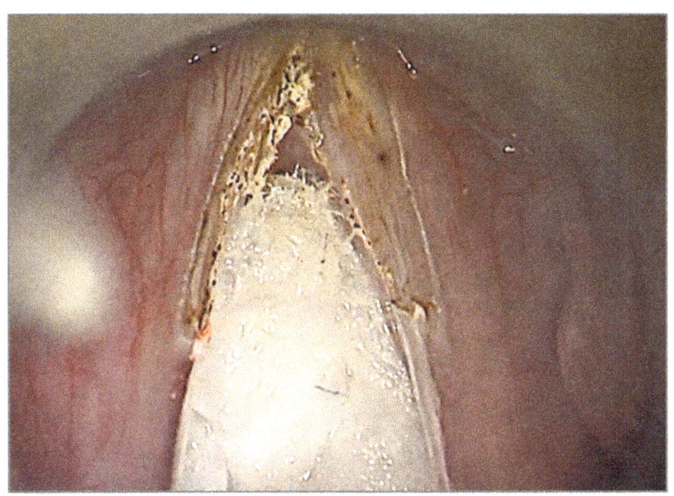

FIG. 10.44: CO_2 laser AcuBlade making the anterior half of the medial vibrating edge raw

Continued

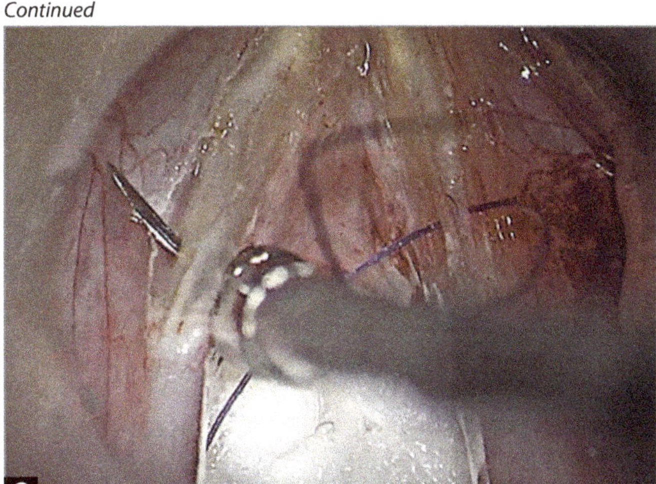

FIG. 10.45: 4-0 VICRYL suture being taken to suture the vocal folds to one another at the anterior commissure. The vocal ligament is taken in these sutures

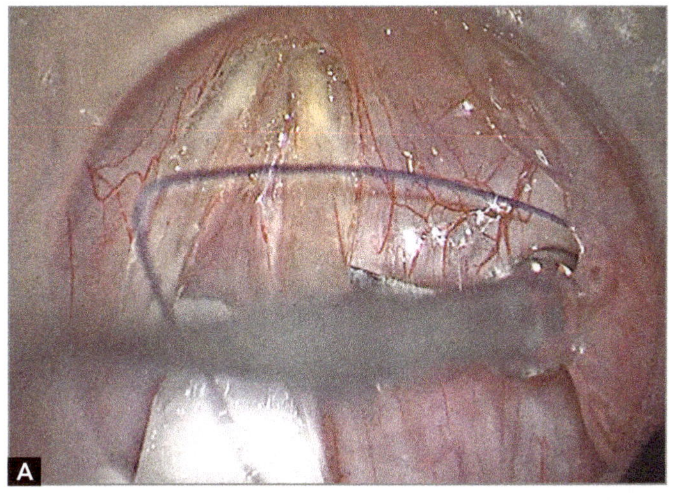

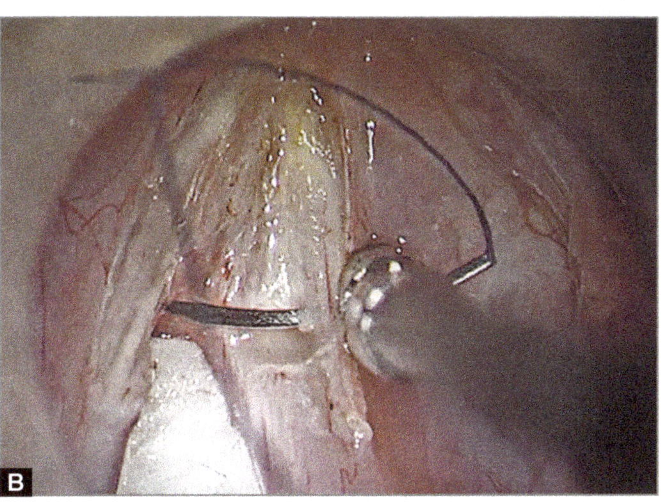

Continued

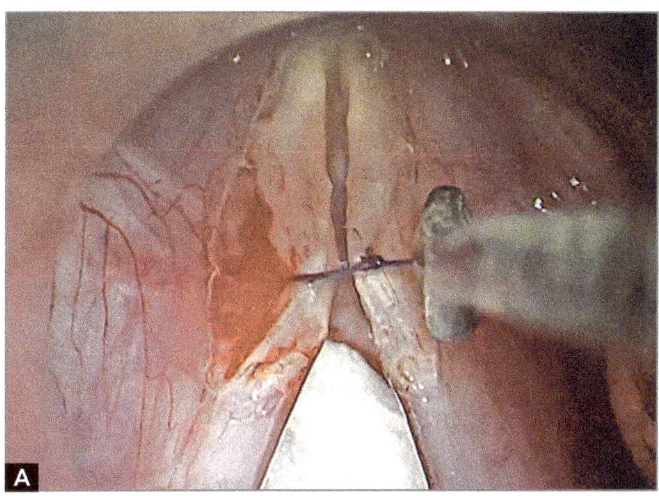

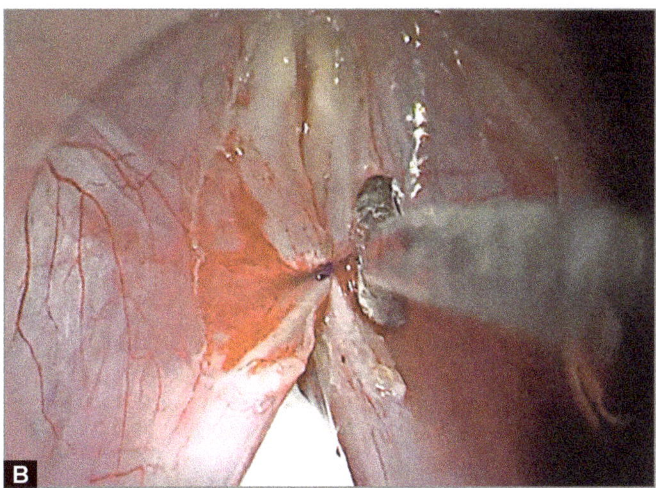

FIG. 10.46: The knot slider getting the knot in position

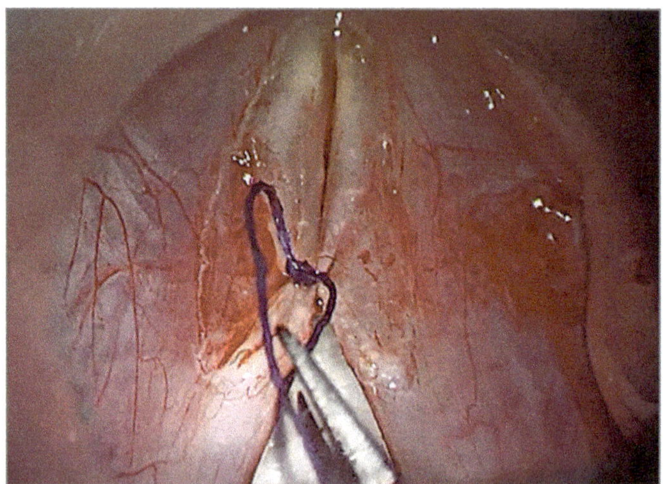

FIG. 10.47: Vicryl threads being cut once the knot has been taken

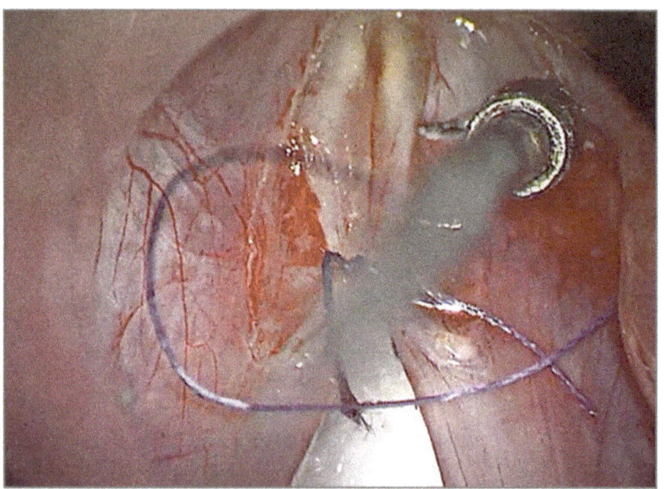

FIG. 10.48: Another knot being taken anterior to the previous one

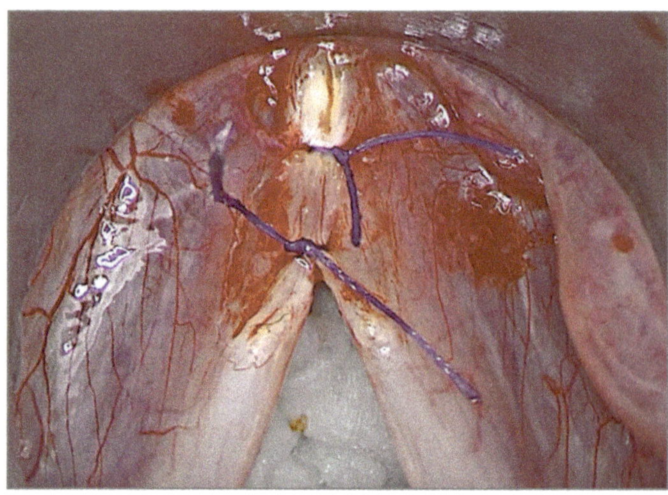

FIG. 10.49: Final postoperative image showing the creation of an anterior glottic web along half the membranous vocal fold

REFERENCES

1. Benmansour N, Remacle M, Matar N, et al. Endoscopic treatment of anterior glottic webs according to Lichtenberger technique and results on 18 patients. Eur Arch Otolaryngol. 2012;269 (9):2075-80.
2. Montgomery W. Management of glottic stenosis. Otolaryngol Clinics North Am. 1979;12:841-7.
3. McIlwain JC. A historical overview of the etiology and treatment of laryngeal stenosis. Arch Otolaryngol. 1989;246 (5):336-40.
4. Lahav Y, Shoffel-Havakuk H, Halperin D. Acquired glottic stenosis-the ongoing challenge: A review of etiology, pathogenesis and surgical management. J Voice. 2015;29(5);646.e1-e10.
5. Cohen SR. Congenital glottic webs in children. A retrospective review of 51 patients. Ann Otol Rhinol Laryngol Suppl. 1985;121:2-16.

CHAPTER 11

Keratosis

DEFINITION

White patches on the vocal folds, which are benign on histopathology, revealing multiple layers of keratin.

Keratosis may appear as a white-gray warty papillomatous lesion or may have a sharp, spiny, irregular surface.[1]

It is essential to rule out other causes of white patches (leukoplakia) such as fungal plaques, tuberculosis, and malignancy. Only once histopathology has confirmed keratosis may the term be accurately used.

PHILOSOPHY OF MANAGEMENT

Management of keratosis is not simple due to its propensity to recur often and its premalignant nature. The challenge in the management of keratosis is decision-making regarding surgical excision every time it appears. Excisional biopsy is always preferred to targeted biopsy so as not to miss the representative area. When the keratosis is diffuse, the anterior commissure needs to be respected to prevent postsurgical webbing and the excision of the keratosis may have to be staged.

When the recurrence is minimal, the decision to observe may be a tricky one.

A large study performed by the University of Wisconsin in 2008 [2] on leukoplakia revealed a 15% severe dysplasia rate in the biopsy samples with 18% of these patients subsequently developing squamous cell carcinoma. In their study 4% of patients with no dysplasia in the primary surgery had a malignant conversion.

In a study done by Gallo et al. there was no association found between human papillomavirus and malignant transformation of laryngeal keratosis. [3]

However, the presence of koilocytes along with keratin in some of the histopathology samples suggests the presence of viral infection.

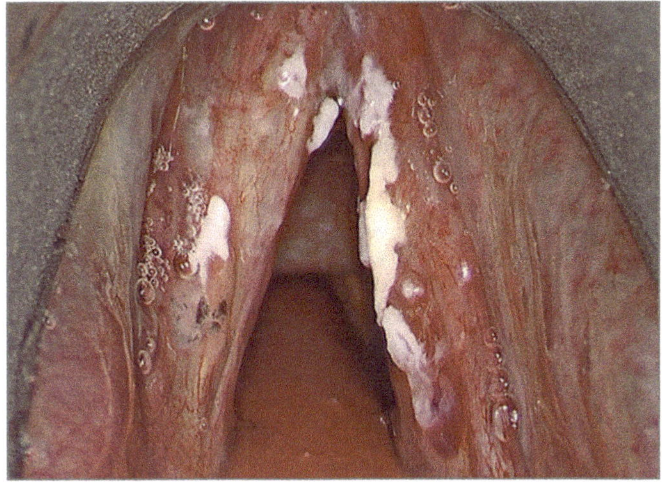

FIG. 11.1: Bilateral keratosis of the true vocal folds. (E-CC)

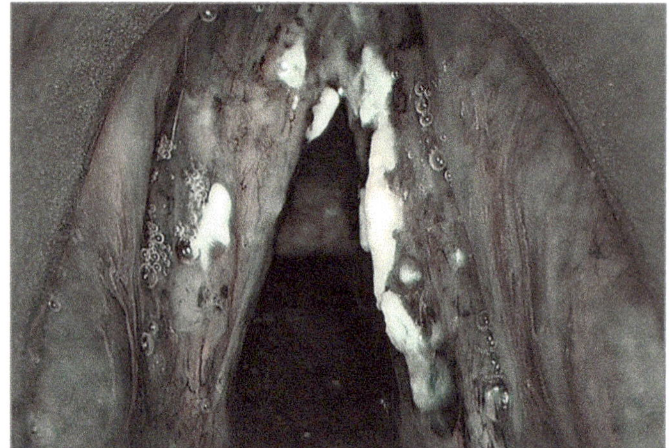

FIG. 11.2: Spectra A image of 11.1 (E-SA). The keratosis appears a brilliant white against a grey-blue background of the vocal folds in SA mode, and is a good tool to pick up early recurrence and to confirm excision points during surgery

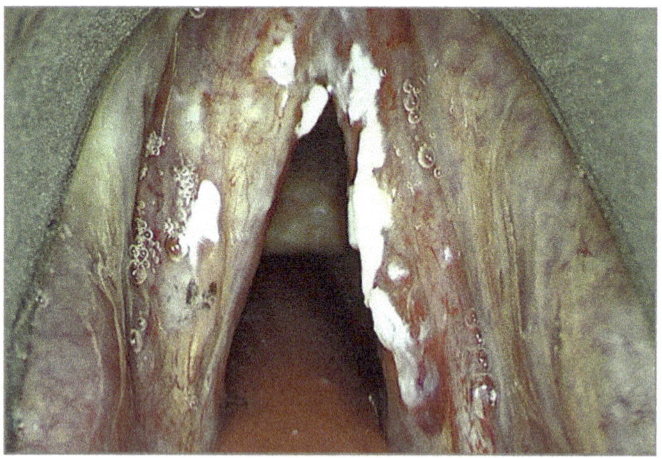

FIG. 11.3: Spectra B image of 11.1. The keratosis appears a brilliant white against a light pink background of the vocal folds; the blood vessels are a bright red in SA mode. (E-SB)

CASE 1

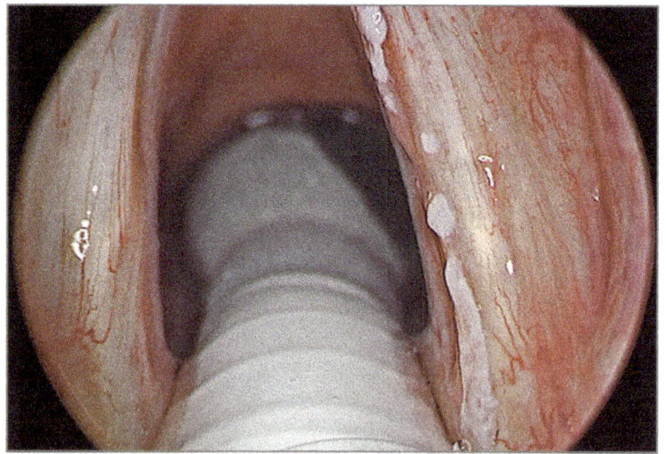

FIG. 11.4: An adult male patient was referred to our center following excision of right glottic keratosis and clinically seemed to have a recurrence. (E-CC)

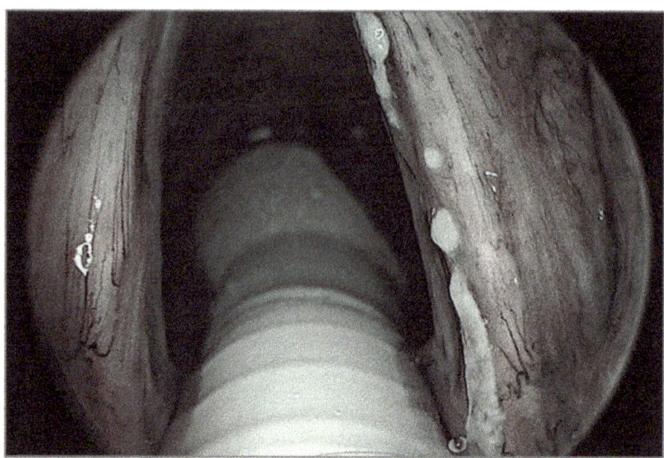

FIG. 11.5: Spectra A image of 11.4 with the keratosis clearly seen against a blue-gray backdrop. (E-SA)

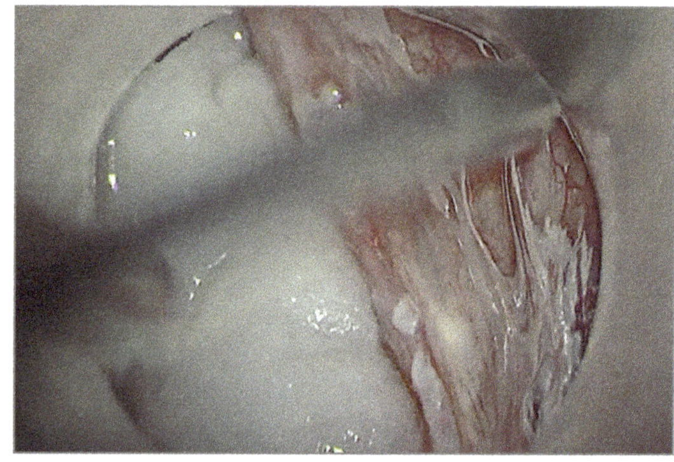

FIG. 11.6: Subepithelial infiltration technique being performed with a 27-gauge needle to bulk up the right vocal fold SLP prior to laser excision. A moist cotton pledget has been placed in the subglottis to protect the cuff of the endotracheal tube. (M-CC)

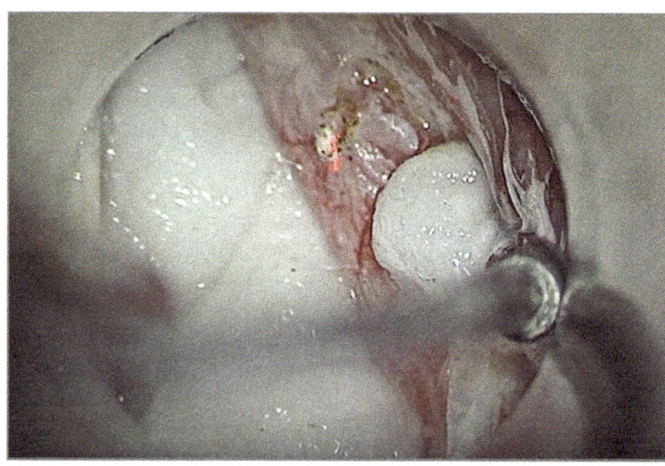

FIG. 11.7: A cotton ball being used to evert the vocal fold to aid in making the laser cut anterior to the keratosis. (M-CC)

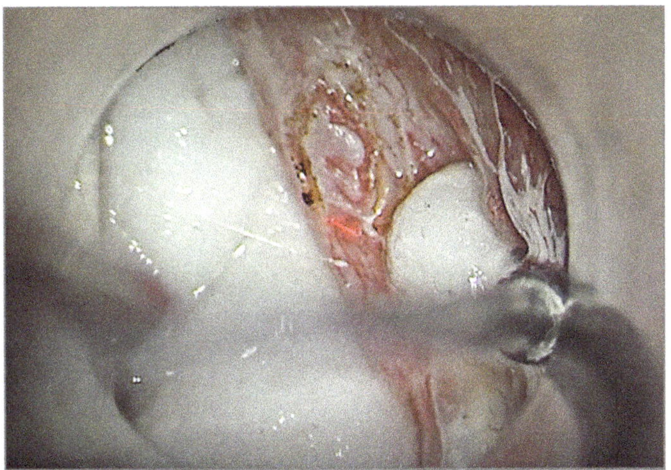

FIG. 11.8: The anterior keratosis being circumferentially excised with the CO_2 acuBlade. (M-CC)

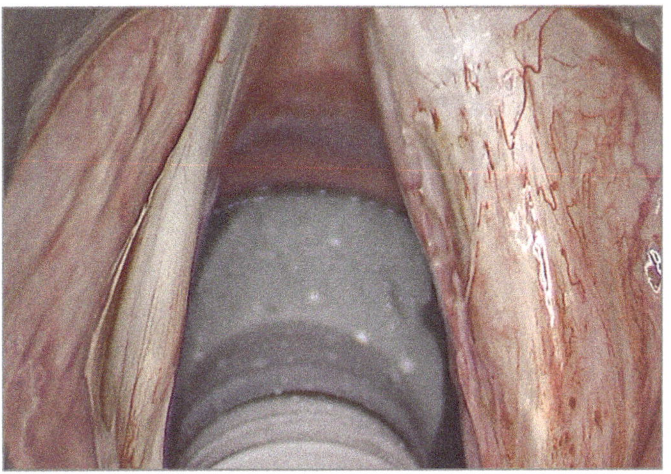

FIG. 11.9: The final postoperative image following excision of the entire right vocal fold keratosis. (E-CC)

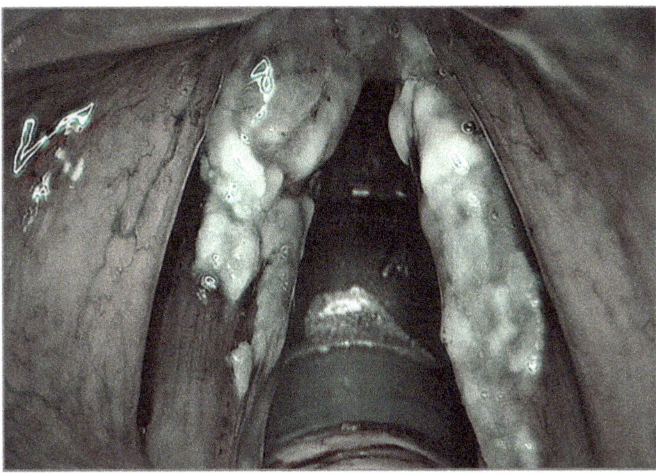

FIG. 11.11: Spectra A image of 11.10. The white keratosis is very marked against a gray-blue backdrop of the larynx. (E-SA)

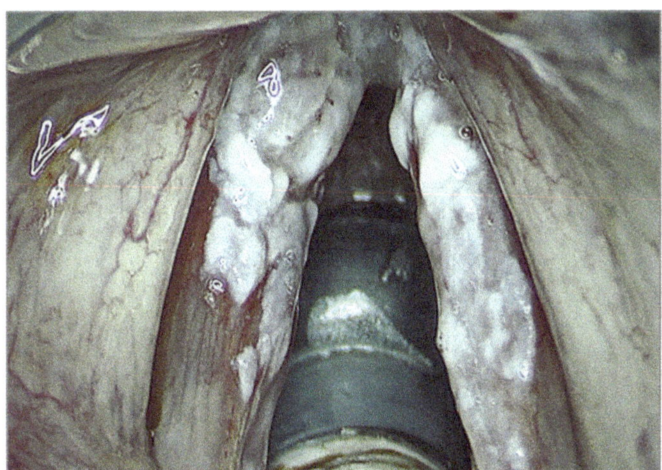

FIG. 11.12: Image in spectra B mode of 11.10. (E-SB)

CASE 2

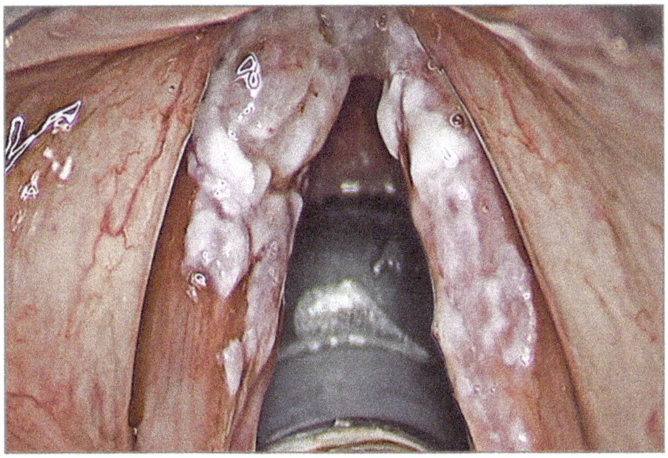

FIG. 11.10: An adult male patient with bilateral suspected keratosis with anterior commissure involvement. This diagnosis was confirmed with histopathology. (E-CC)

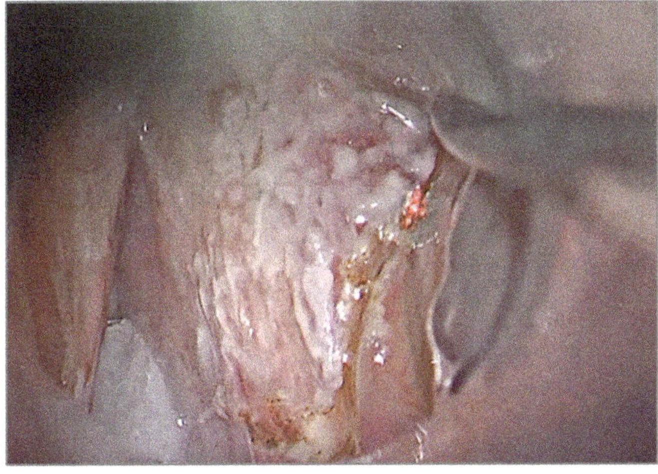

FIG. 11.13: CO_2 laser excision of the right keratosis following SEIT. The lateral extent of the keratosis is seen and can be excised after the right false vocal fold is retracted, in this case using a microflap elevator. (M-CC)

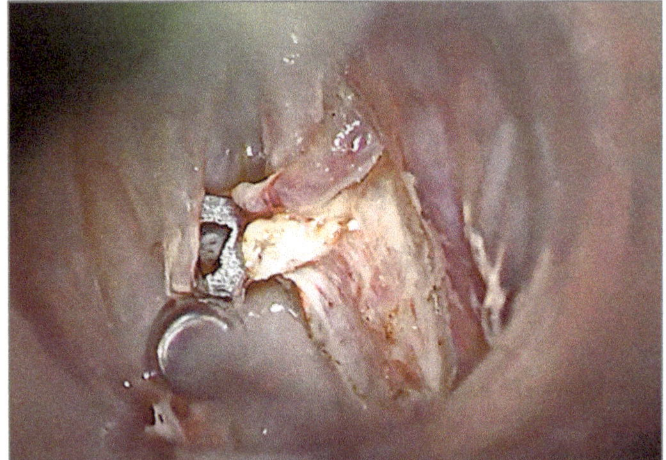

FIG. 11.14: Excision of the right posterior keratosis, maximally preserving the SLP

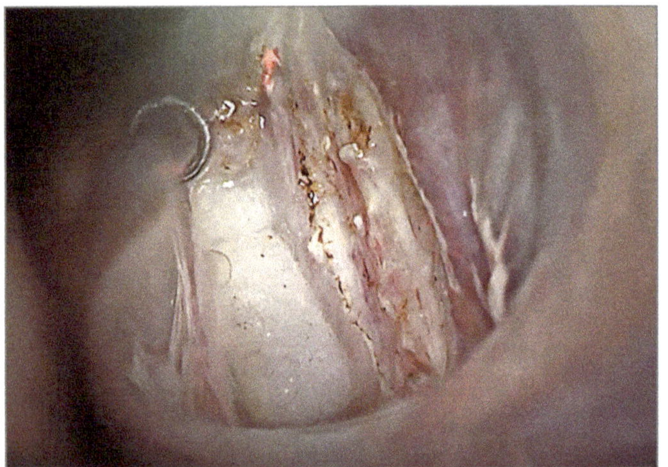

FIG. 11.15: Anterior extension of the excision. (M-CC)

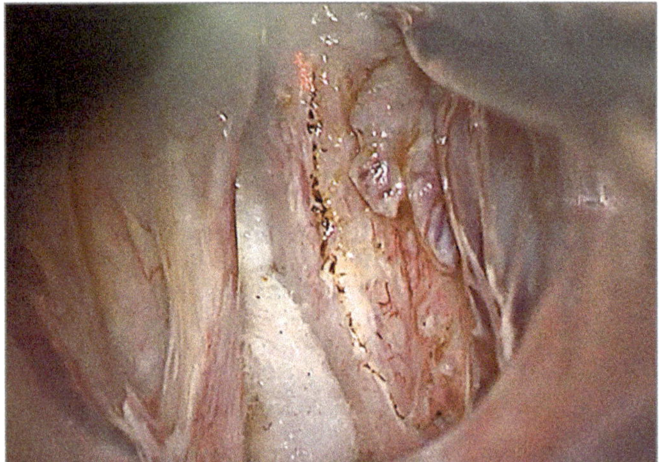

FIG. 11.16: Infraglottic cut being made anteriorly to complete the right glottic excision. The right vocal fold is everted laterally with the blunt microflap elevator to facilitate this step. (M-CC)

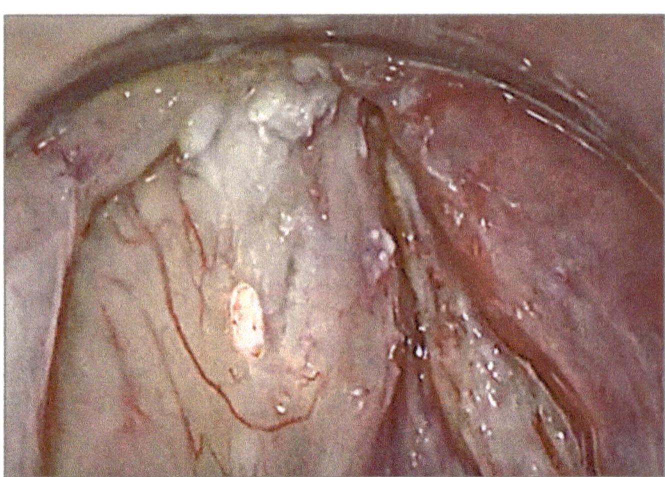

FIG. 11.17: The microlaryngoscope is repositioned to better expose the left vocal fold. (M-CC)

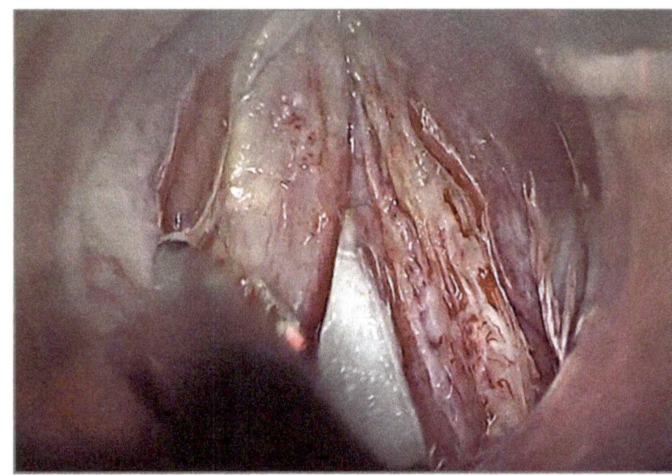

FIG. 11.18: The laser microflap excision on the left side is commenced from the posterior part of the vocal fold. (E-CC)

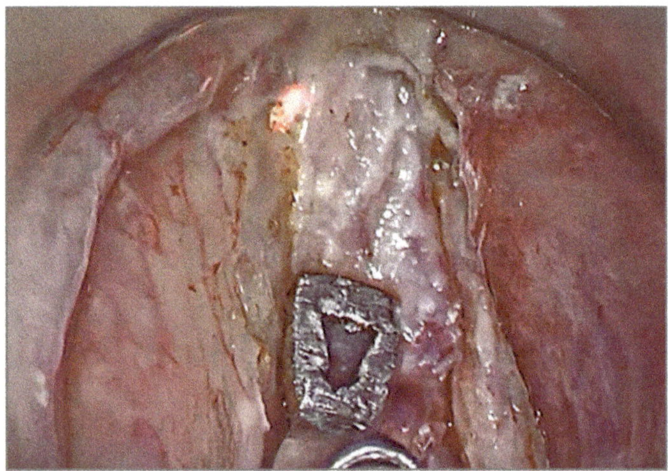

FIG. 11.19: The anterior cut is made such that some epithelium is left at the medial edge anteriorly to avoid a web formation. (M-CC)

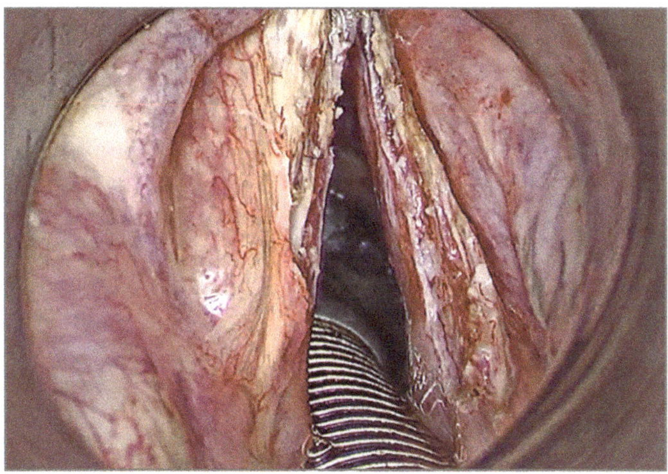

FIG. 11.20: Final postoperative image, a small amount of anterior keratosis of the left vocal fold is seen. (E-CC)

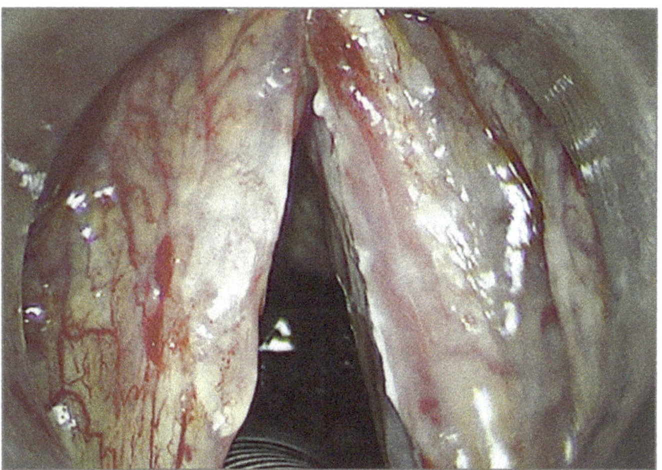

FIG. 11.23: Specta B mode of 11.21. The margins are distinct as compared to CC mode. The anterior commissure on the left seems to be free of disease. (E-SB)

CASE 3

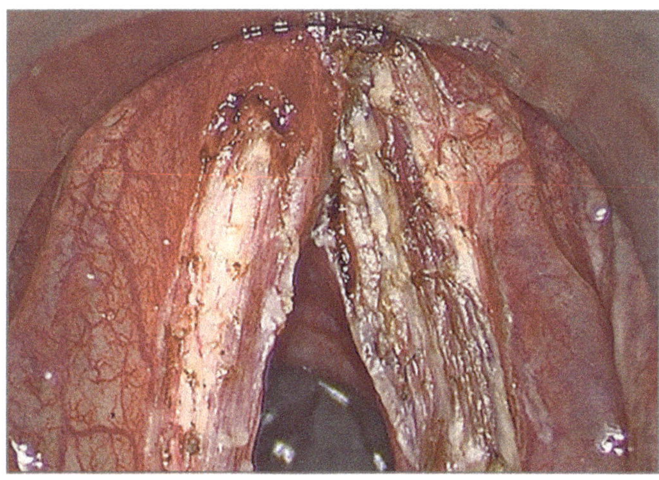

FIG. 11.24: Final postoperative image following excision. Uninvolved epithelium of the left anterior commissure will prevent a glottic web from developing. (E-CC)

FIG. 11.21: Thin layer of keratosis is clinically diagnosed on both the vocal folds. (E-CC)

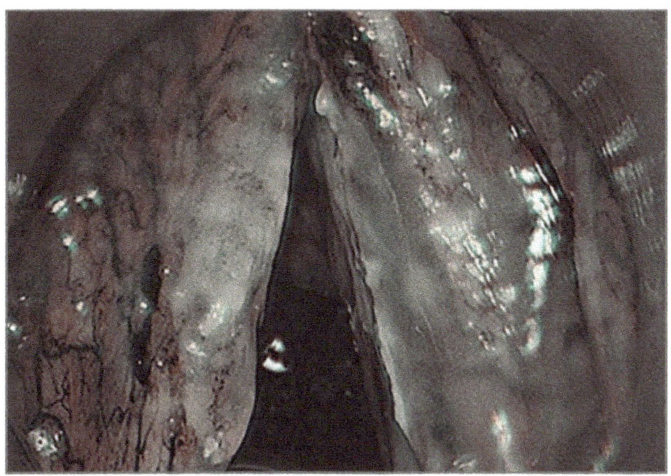

FIG. 11.22: Spectra A image of 10.21. The margins of the thin keratosis become more distinct and aid in planning the incisions for the surgical excision. (E-SA)

CASE 4

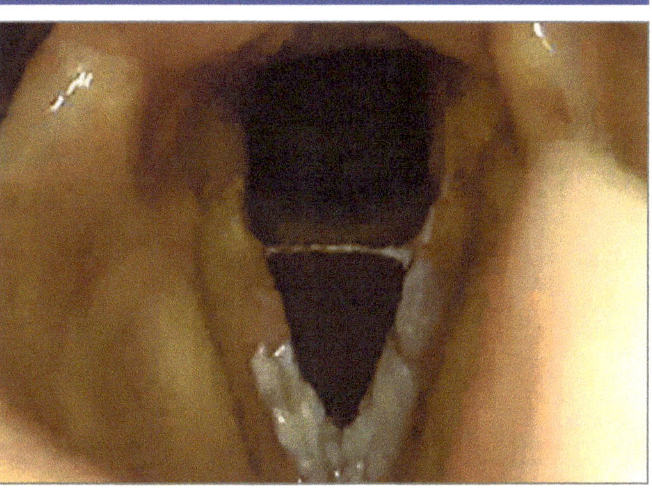

FIG. 11.25: Stroboscopic image of an adult male, nonsmoker, revealing anterior commissure suspected keratosis with extension posteriorly on the left vocal fold. (70 degree stroboscope)

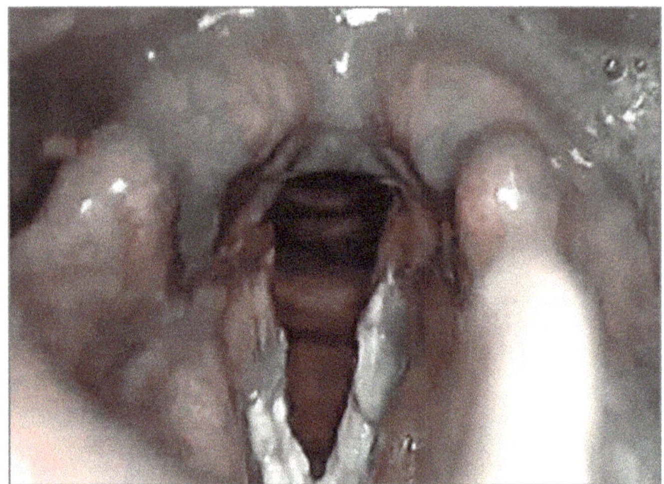

FIG. 11.26: Narrow band image of the same lesion. The keratosis and its margins are very distinct as a bright white against a gray-pink back drop. (70 degree laryngoscope with NBI)

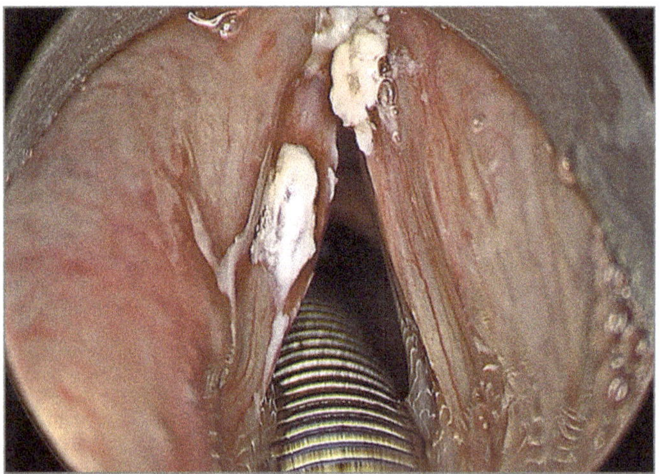

FIG. 11.27: The patient is taken up for laser excision with frozen histopathology planned. The keratosis on the left vocal fold is not a continuous sheet but in interrupted areas. (E-CC)

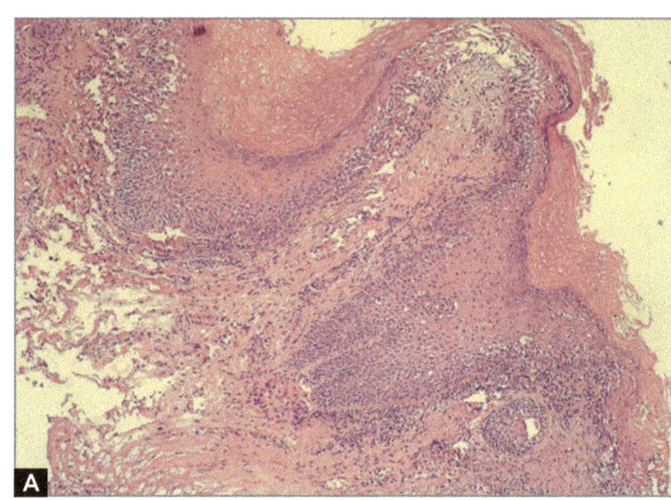

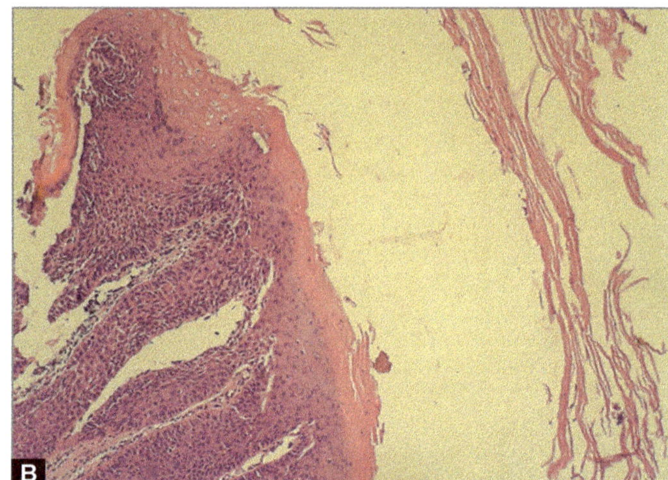

FIG. 11.29: The frozen histopathology of 11.25 revealing layers of keratin, confirming the clinical diagnosis of keratosis. (H&E staining)

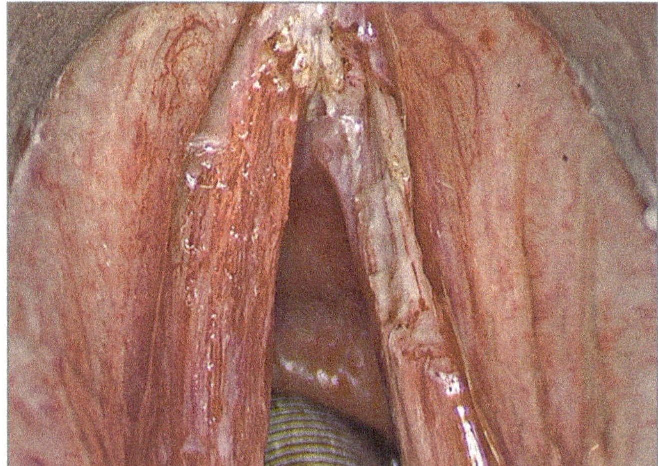

FIG. 11.28: The final postoperative image with minimal lesion left in situ at the anterior commissure to prevent webbing. (E-CC)

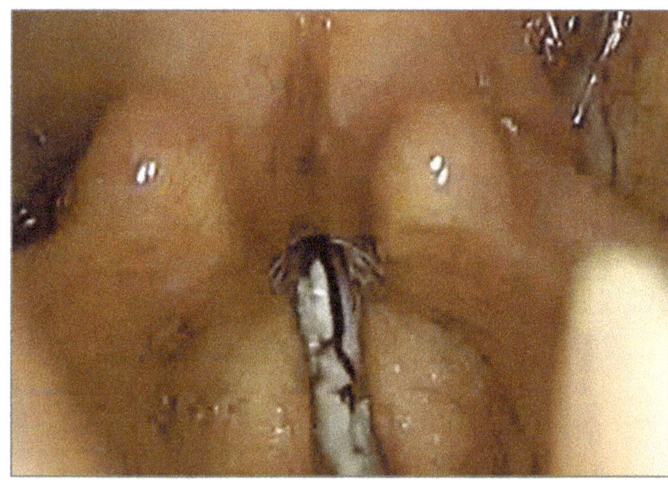

FIG. 11.30: Within 6 months, the patient had a complete recurrence of his keratosis with severe deterioration in voice quality. (70 degree stroboscopy)

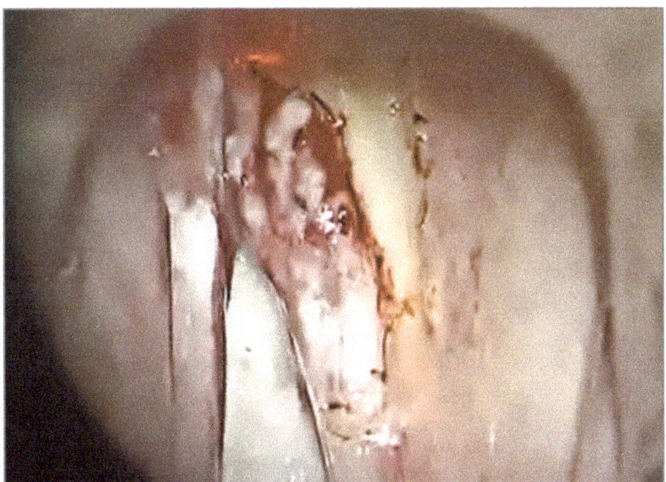

FIG. 11.31: The patient was taken up for surgical excision once again. The epithelial cordotomy on the right vocal fold revealed a healthy looking SLP. The ligament covered by the SLP can be seen on the right vocal fold. The CO_2 laser AcuBlade is seen making the anterior epithelial cut. (M-CC)

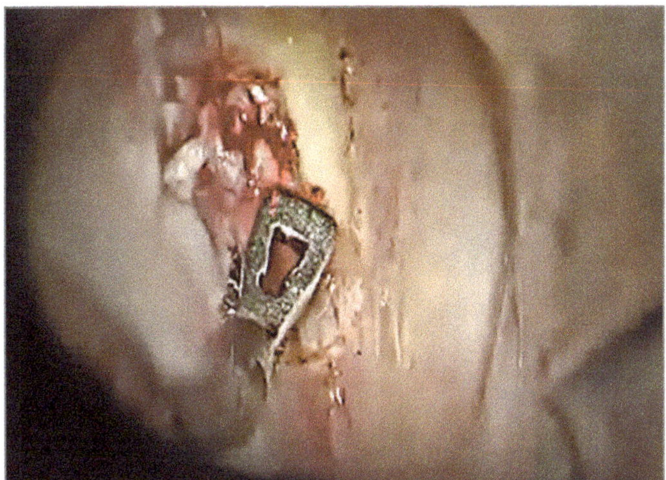

FIG. 11.32: An upward Bouchayer is holding the diseased epithelium to provide traction while performing the laser excision. (M-CC)

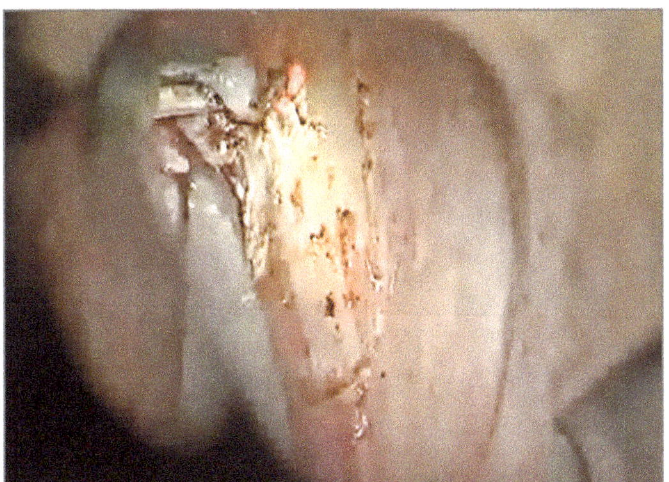

FIG. 11.33: Final anterior excision being performed. (M-CC)

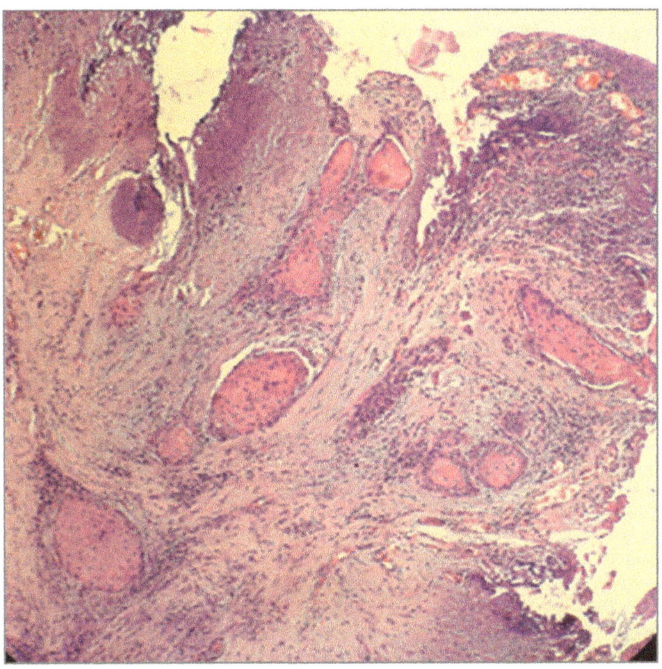

FIG. 11.34: The histopathology was squamous invasive carcinoma. This was unexpected as the SLP was very healthy looking under the microscope. This case highlights the importance of tissue testing at every recurrence as well as the importance of excising and sending the entire tissue sample for histopathology and not small selected pieces. (H&E)

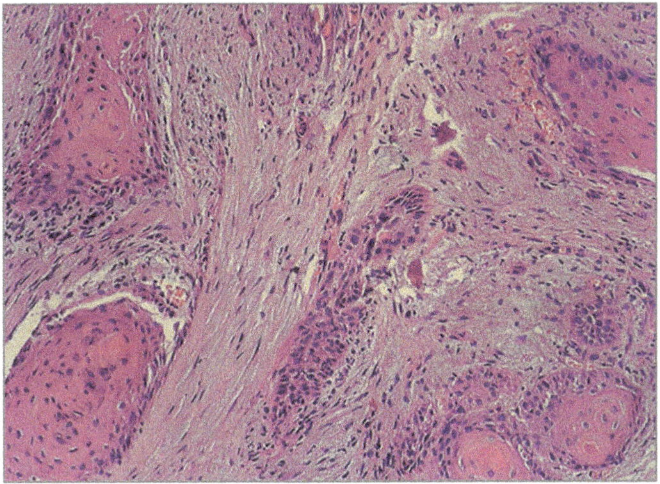

FIG. 11.35: Zoomed image of 11.34

CASE 5

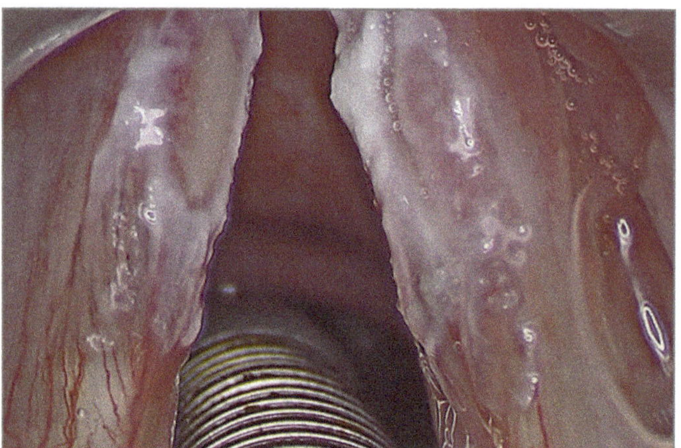

FIG. 11.36: Patient gives a history of long standing hoarseness with microscopic examination revealing left striking zone ulceration surrounded by possible keratosis and right vocal fold possible keratosis extending to the anterior commissure. (E-CC)

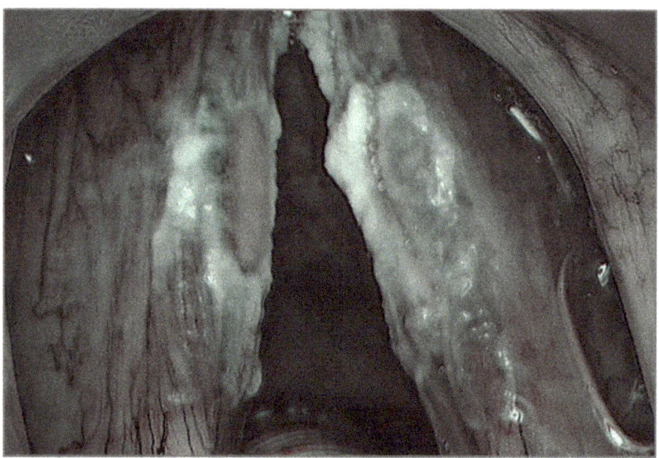

FIG. 11.37: SA mode of case 5 clearly demarcating the edges of the left vocal fold ulcer from the surrounding suspected keratosis. The anterior extent of the keratosis can be clearly appreciated. (E-SA)

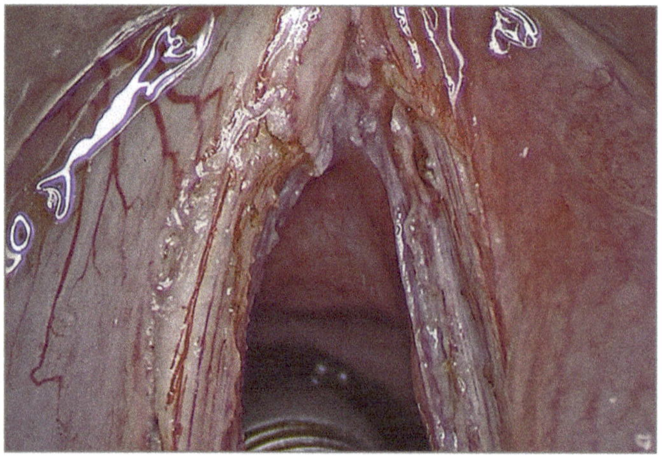

FIG. 11.38: Final postoperative image revealing left anterior commissure intact mucosa. (E-CC)

CASE 6

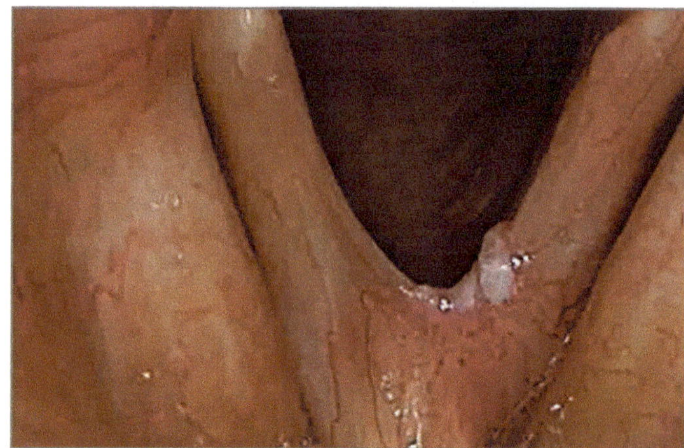

FIG. 11.39: Patient referred with history of keratosis excision performed 2 months back from the left vocal fold. The patient has an anterior glottic web with a recurrence of keratosis at the anterior commissure, more towards the left side with increased anterior vascularity as seen on WL laryngoscopy. (70 degree laryngoscopy)

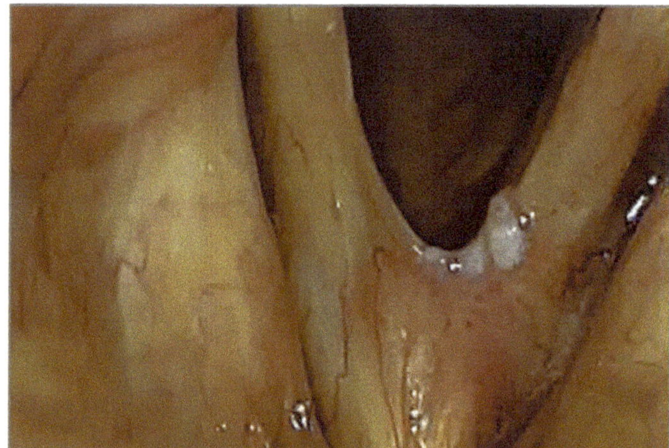

FIG. 11.40: Stroboscopic image of the same patient

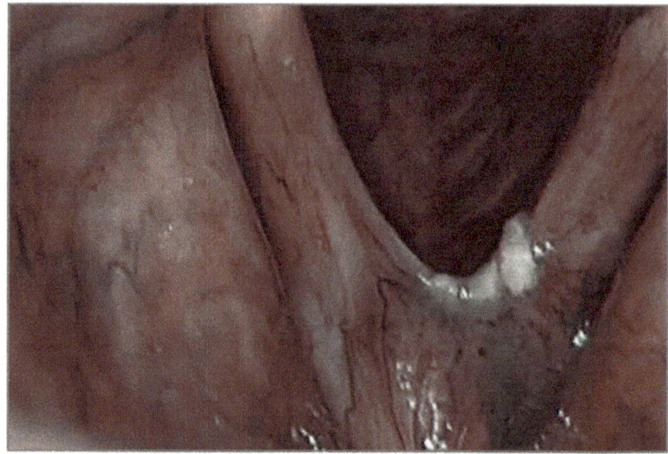

FIG. 11.41: Narrow band image of the same patient with a few scattered brown dots along with a Ni type 1 pattern. As keratosis often hides the underlying vascular pattern and only the peripheral vascular pattern can be studied, a decision to excise the lesion was taken

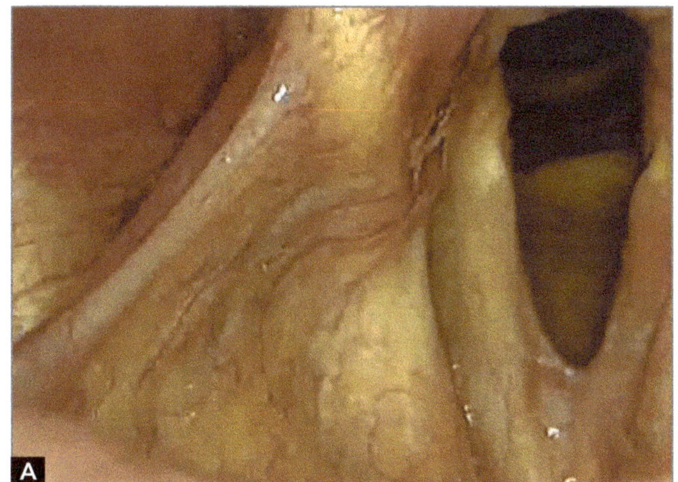

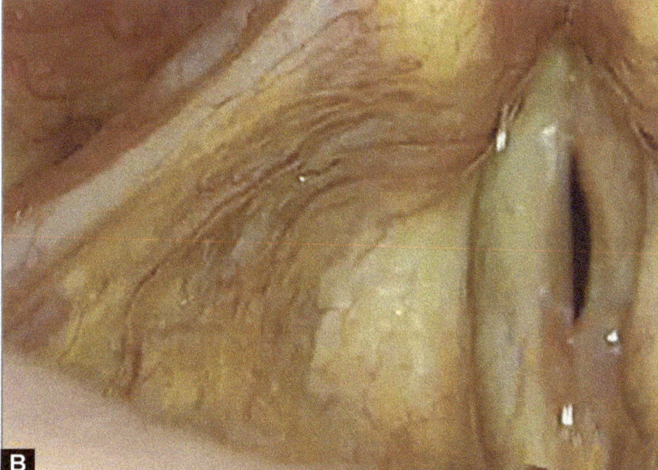

FIG. 11.42: Postoperative stroboscopy images in **A,** abduction and **B,** adduction. The histopathology was keratosis with no dysplasia. Web surgery was planned for a later date once the keratosis stops recurring

REFERENCES

1. Arthur JC. Hyperkeratosis of the larynx. AMA Arch Otolaryngol. 1959;70(3): 287-91.
2. Jason SI, Daniel LC, Seth HD. Institutional and comprehensive review of laryngeal leukoplakia. 2008 (Online). Available from: http://journals.sagepub.com/doi/10.1177/000348940811700114.
3. Gallo O, Bianchi S, Giannini A, et al. Lack of detection of human papillomavirus (HPV) in transformed laryngeal keratoses by in situ hybridization (ISH) technique. Acta Otolaryngol. 1994;114(2):213-7.

CHAPTER 12

Contact Granuloma

DEFINITION

A contact granuloma in the larynx is a polypoidal lesion attached to the arytenoid cartilage, typically the vocal process.

Granulomas of the larynx may be specific (tuberculosis, syphilis)[1] or nonspecific granulomas.

Chevalier Jackson first identified contact ulcers in 1928.[2] He collected 127 case reports dating to 1888. In 1935, Jackson and Jackson suggested a mechanical cause related to the hammer and anvil effect of the vocal processes colliding against each other, leading to superficial mucosal ulceration (the contact ulcer) and focal granulation tissue response.[3]

The mucosa covering the vocal processes of the arytenoid cartilage is a thin layer of stratified squamous epithelium. This thin layer of mucosa is susceptible to being crushed between any unyielding object (i.e., an endotracheal tube, the opposite arytenoid) and the firm cartilage beneath the mucosa.[4]

Histologically, nonspecific granulomas resemble pyogenic granulomas consisting of chronic inflammatory infiltration with neovascularization and fibrosis covered by squamous epithelium.

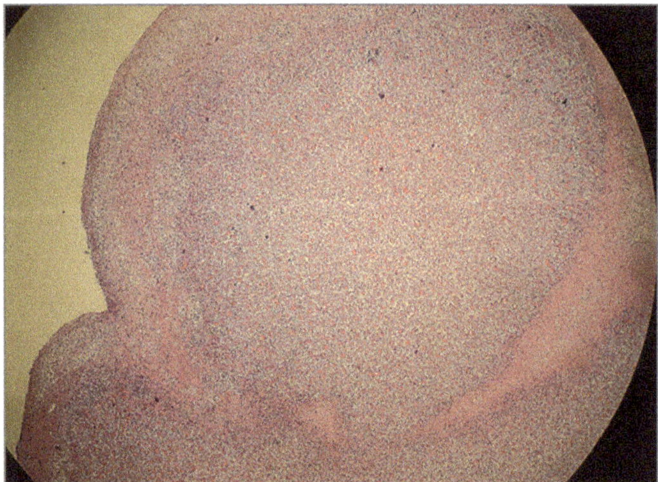

FIG. 12.1A: H&E staining of a nonspecific pyogenic granuloma consisting of chronic inflammatory infiltration with neovascularization and fibrosis covered by squamous epithelium

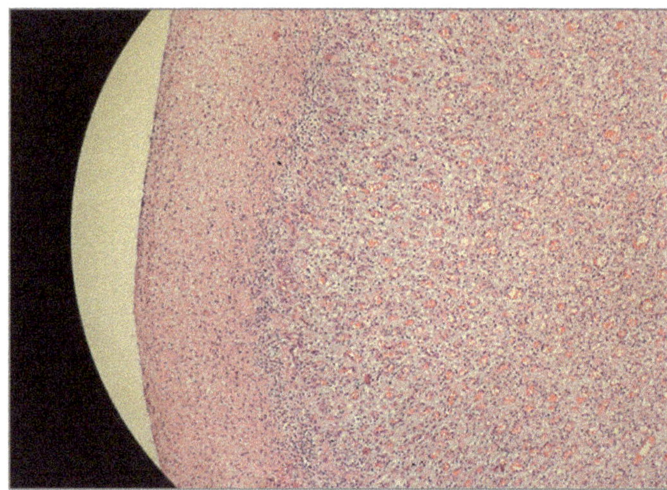

FIG. 12.1B: High power image of Fig. 12.1A

RISK FACTORS

The risk factors responsible for the development of a contact granuloma are laryngopharyngeal reflux, vocal abuse, and severe cough. When the granuloma develops following trauma to the arytenoid due to intubation, it is called an intubation granuloma.

FARWELL CLASSIFICATION OF CONTACT GRANULOMAS[5]

- Grade 1: Sessile, nonulcerative granuloma limited to vocal process
- Grade 2: Pedunculated or ulcerated granuloma limited to vocal process
- Grade 3: Granuloma extending past vocal process but not crossing midline of airway in fully abducted position
- Grade 4: Granuloma extending past vocal process and past the midline of the airway in the fully abducted position.

The granulomas were additionally graded A if unilateral and B if bilateral.

AUTHOR'S PHILOSOPHY OF MANAGEMENT

Contact granulomas that are Farwell grade 1 and 2 but asymptomatic and incidentally picked up are treated with proton pump inhibitor (PPI) and lifestyle changes. Botulinum toxin is injected into the adductor muscle group, under laryngeal electromyography control, for the symptomatic Farwell grade 1 and 2.

Contact granulomas that are Farwell grade 3 and 4 are excised, leaving behind a stump, and the thyroarytenoid muscle injected with botulinum toxin at the time of surgery. They also receive PPI twice a day along with lifestyle modifications to curb reflux.

If a recurrence is seen after surgery, a repeat botulinum injection of a greater dose is advocated along with steroid inhalation.

PHILOSOPHY OF SURGERY

Historically, contact granulomas are surgically excised only when symptomatic, due to the high rate of recurrence associated with this procedure (35–50%).[4] The reasons postulated for the recurrence are an exposed and infected perichondrium of the vocal process facing constant phonotraumatic injury from the contralateral vocal process, in an acidic environment caused by laryngopharyngeal reflux.

In order to decrease the chances of recurrence, the following options may be considered:

- Injection of botulinum toxin in the thyroarytenoid (adductor) muscle of the ipsilateral vocal fold. The paresis caused by this does not permit contact of the contralateral vocal process with the operated site, during phonation, cough, or swallowing, thus allowing for good healing. The dose injected may vary from 3.75 mouse unit (MU) to 10 MU depending on the patient response. The author initially injects 5 MU
- Steroid inhalation once or twice a day to promote healing. The steroid inhalation is followed by steam inhalation in order to prevent fungal laryngitis
- Proton pump inhibitors twice a day along with alginate and lifestyle modifications to decrease reflux
- The surgical excision is performed such that a stump of the granuloma is retained, so as to not create an unnecessary raw area on the vocal process. This stump settles in time with the other medical measures being advised.

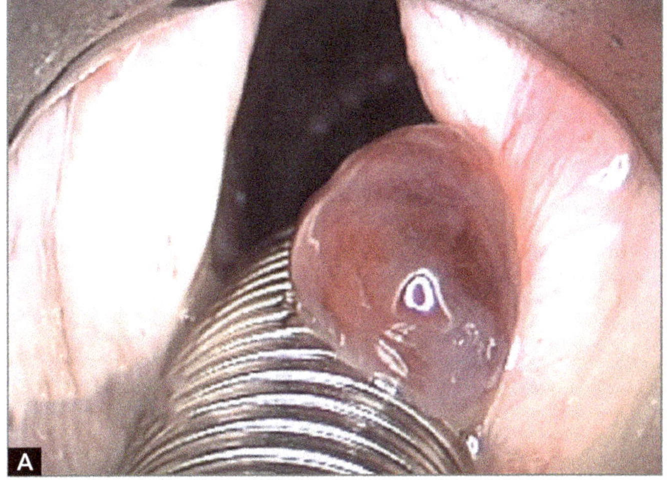

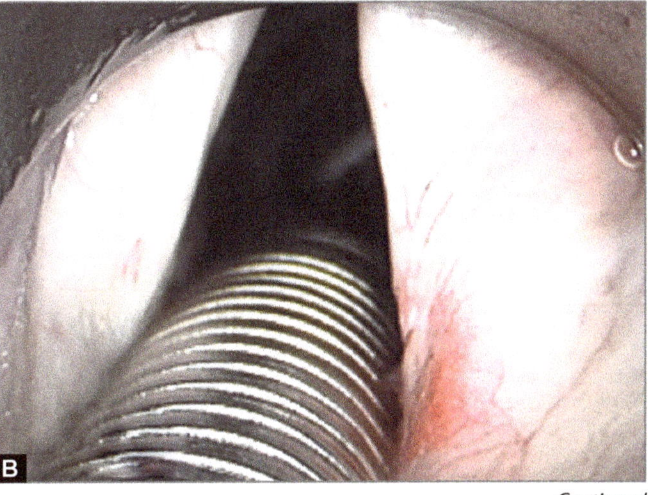

Continued

Continued

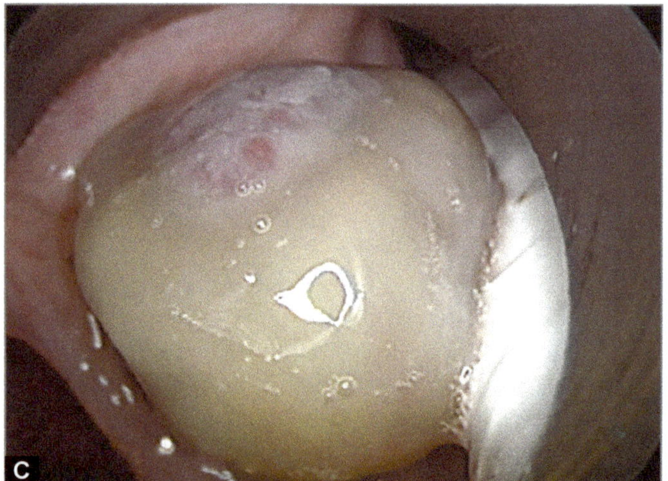

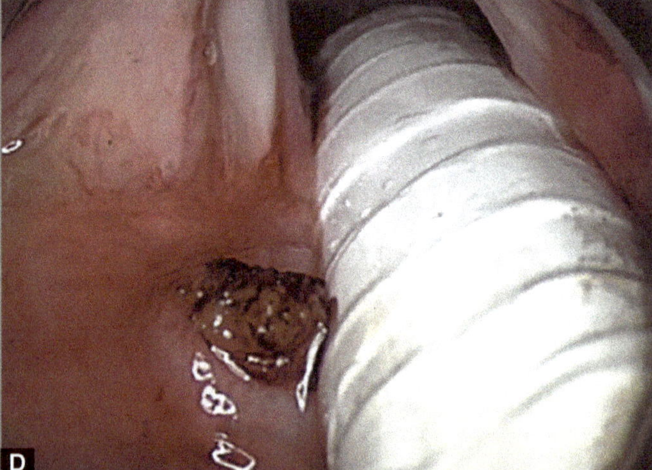

FIG. 12.2: A Farwell grade 3 (**A**) and grade 4 (**C**) contact granuloma prior to surgical excision and following surgery (**B** and **D**).

CASE 1

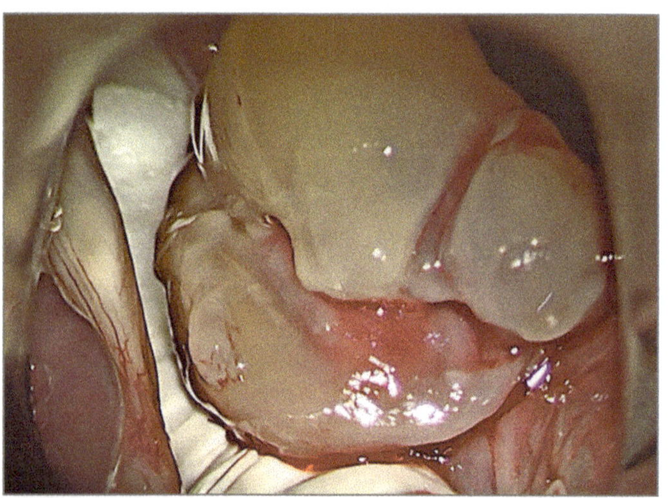

FIG. 12.3: Multilobulated massive contact granuloma of the right vocal fold

FIG. 12.4: The granuloma is retracted medially and the attachment of the granuloma is seen to be the vocal process

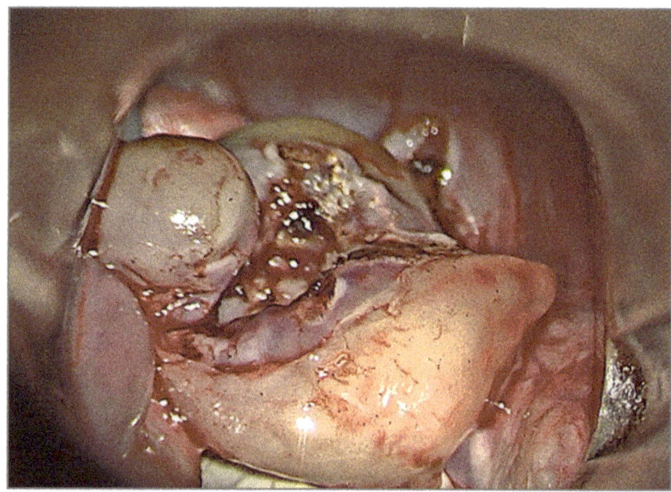

FIG. 12.5: Laser excision of the pedicle of the granuloma with a CO_2 AcuBlade

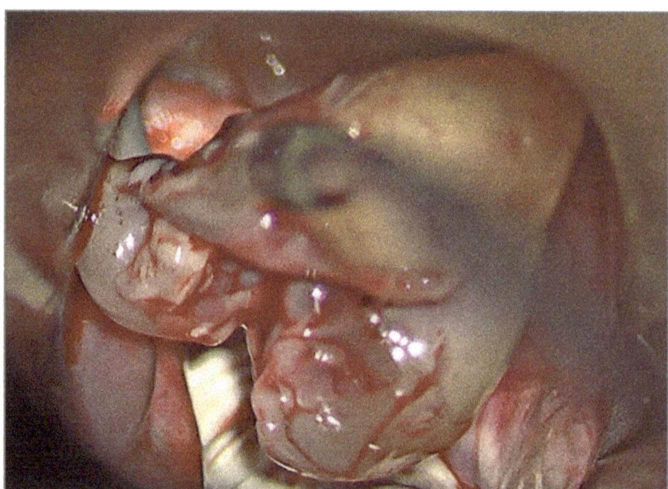

FIG. 12.6: The granuloma is being excised in toto

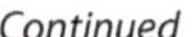

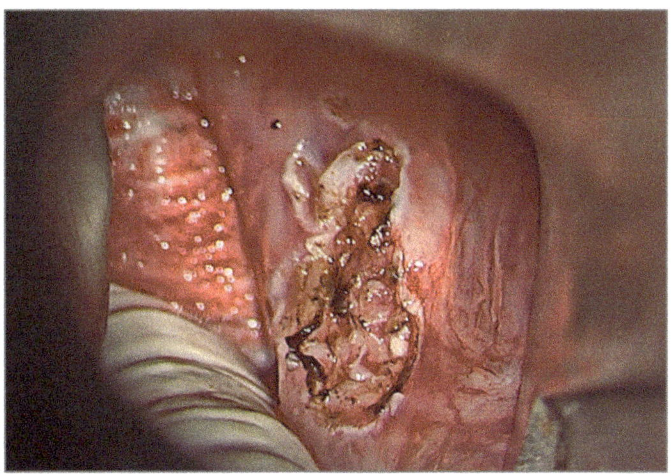

FIG. 12.7: The surgical site reveals a perichondrial cover to the vocal process

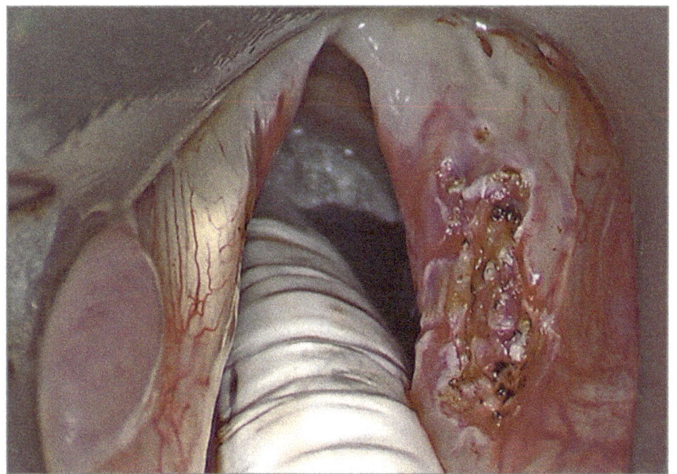

FIG. 12.8: Final postoperative image

CASE 2

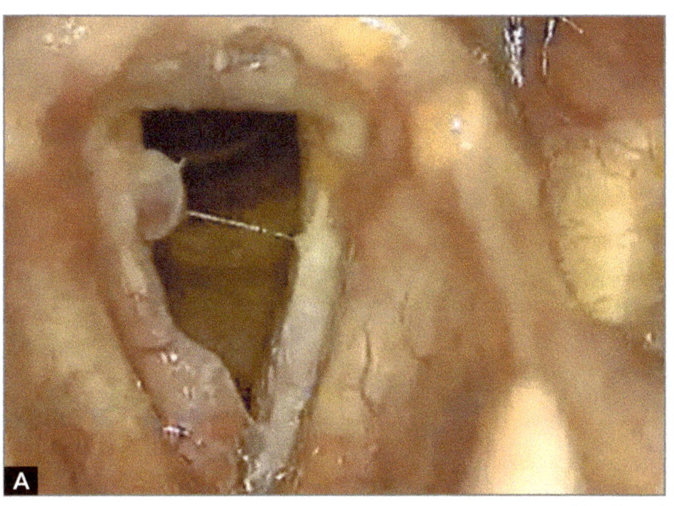

Continued

Continued

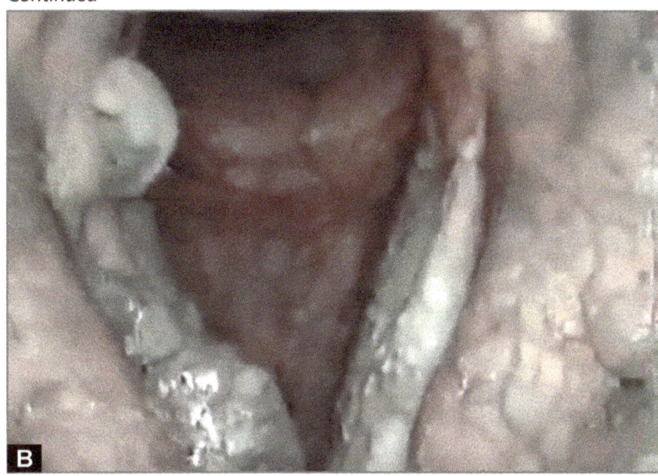

FIG. 12.9: An adult male smoker was referred to our hospital with a diagnosis of a right vocal fold polyp. Stroboscopy at the institute revealed two lesions of the right vocal fold. A posterior contact granuloma and an anterior growth (**A**), possibly with dysplastic features on narrow band imaging (**B**)

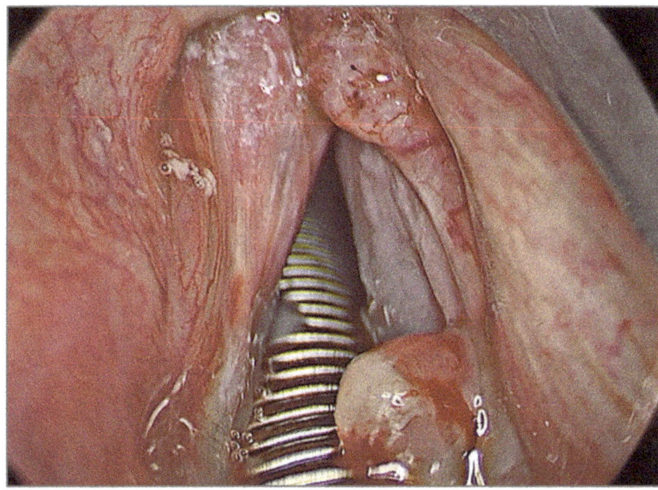

FIG. 12.10: Image under anesthesia confirming two separate lesions. (E-CC)

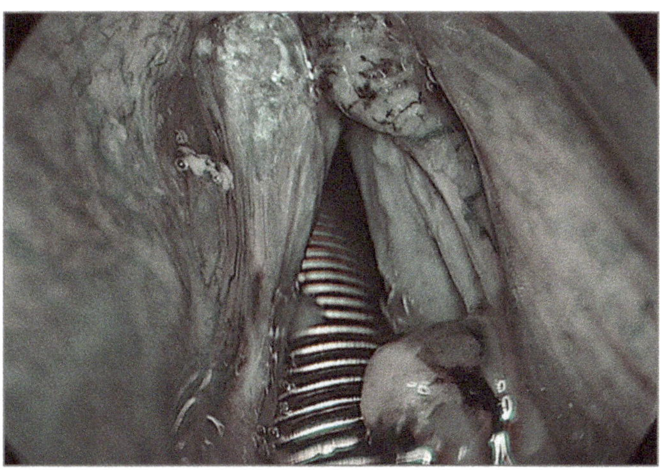

FIG. 12.11: The Spectra A image revealing a type 5b pattern of the right anterior lesion suggesting malignancy. Histopathology confirmed invasive carcinoma of the right anterior lesion. (E-SA)

CASE 3

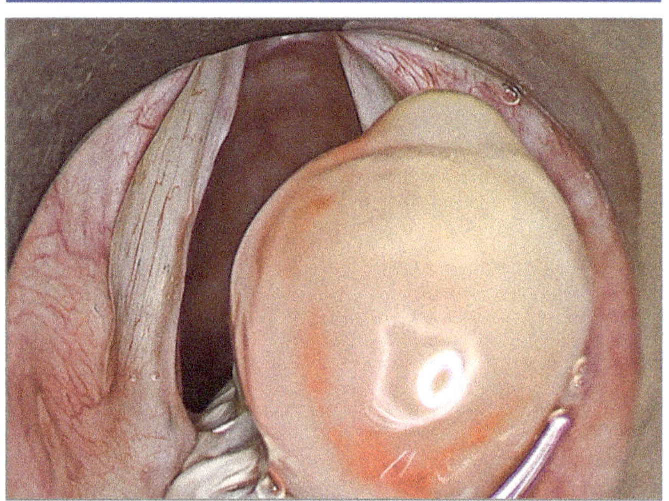

FIG. 12.12: A large contact granuloma of the right vocal fold. (E-CC)

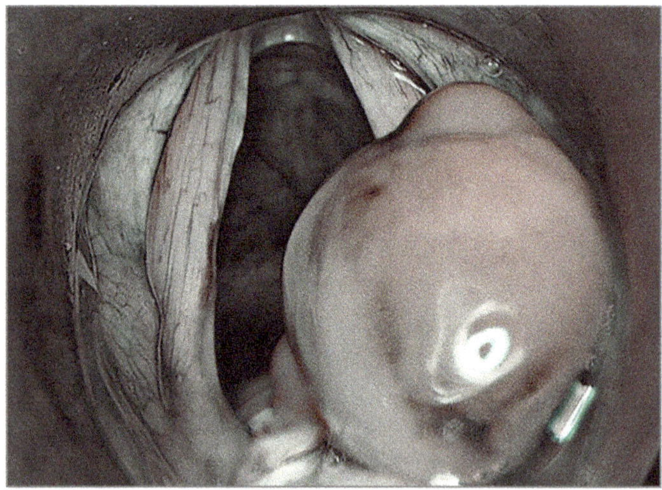

FIG. 12.13: Spectra image of 12.12. (E-SA)

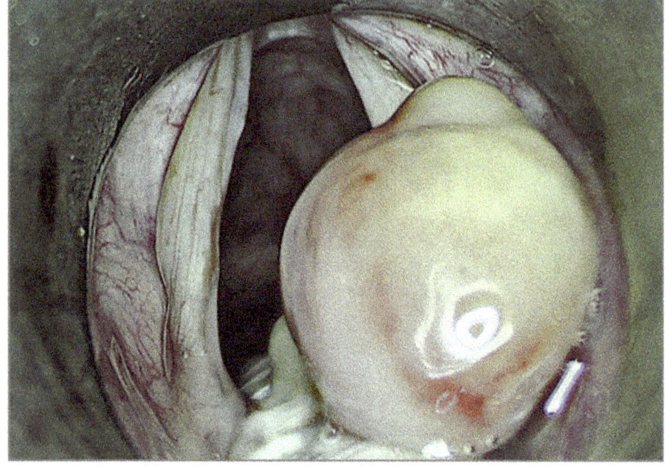

FIG. 12.14: Spectra B image of 12.12. (E-SB)

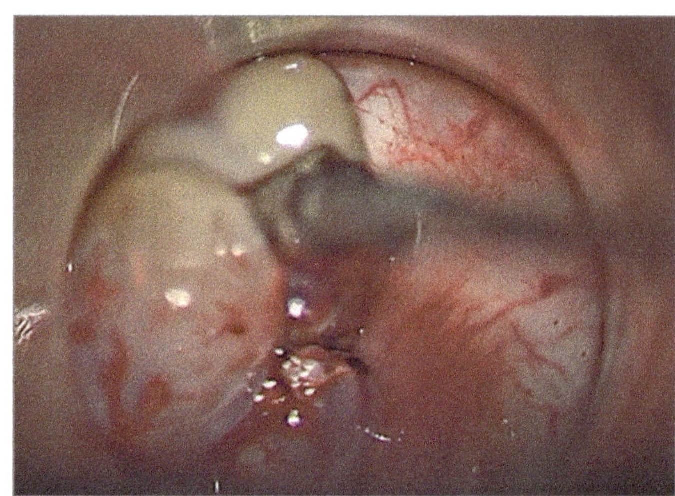

FIG. 12.15: Medial retraction of the granuloma reveals its attachment to the vocal process of the right arytenoid. This attachment is being excised with the CO_2 AcuBlade. (M-CC)

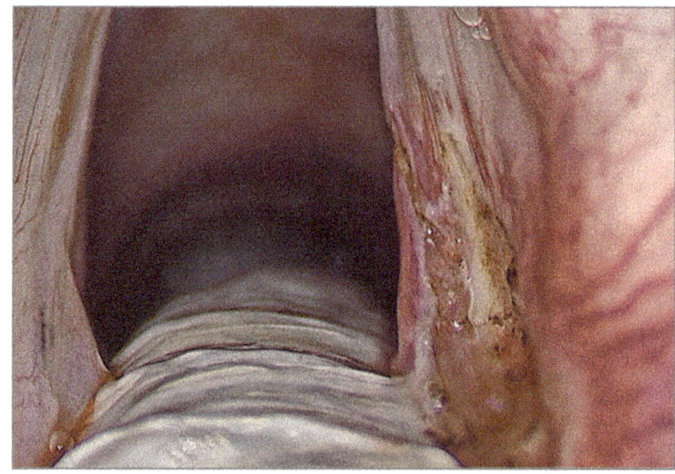

FIG. 12.16: Final postoperative image of the patient following complete excision of the granuloma.

CASE 4

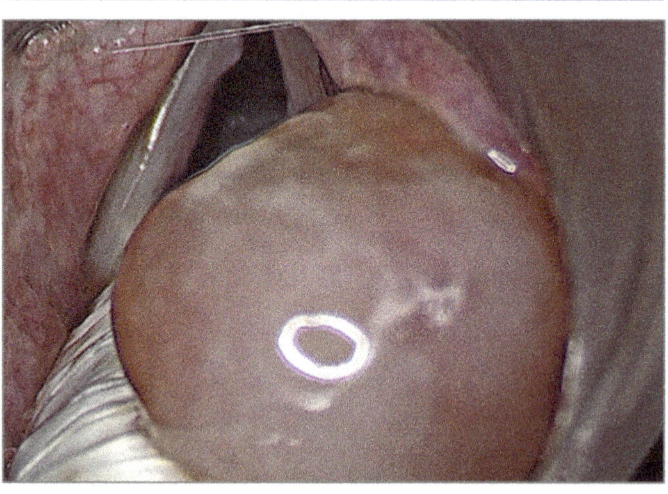

FIG. 12.17: Large contact granuloma of the right vocal fold. (E-CC)

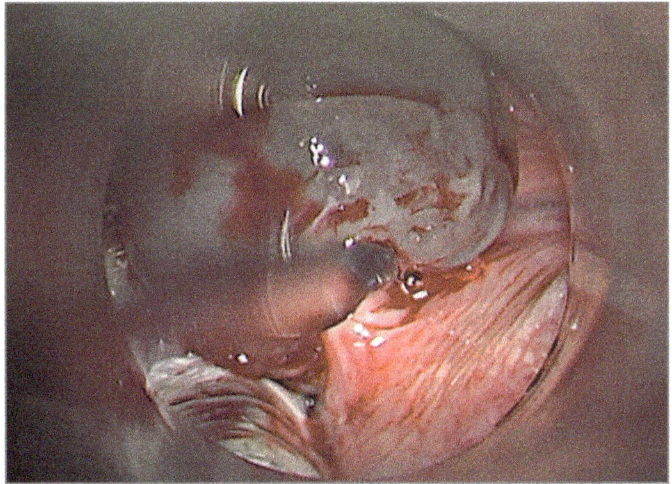

FIG. 12.18: Retraction of the granuloma to reveal the attachment of the pedicle to the arytenoid. (M-CC)

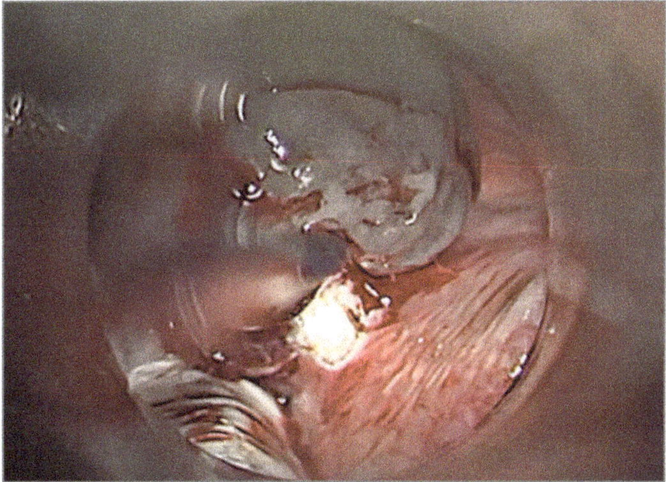

FIG. 12.18: CO_2 laser AcuBlade excision of the pedicle of the contact granuloma. (M-CC)

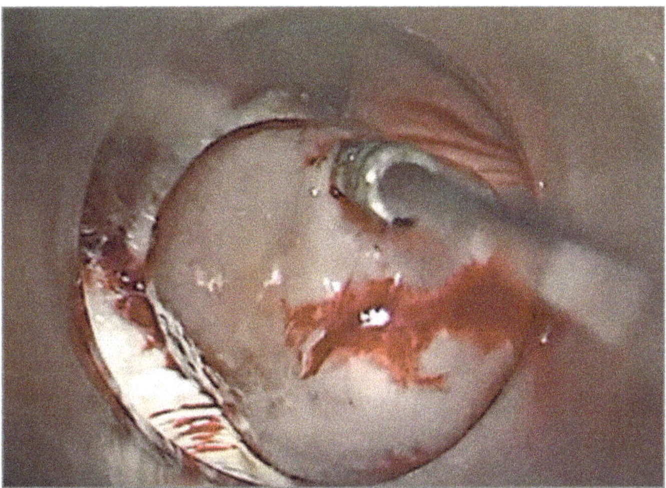

FIG. 12.19: In toto removal of the granuloma. (M-CC)

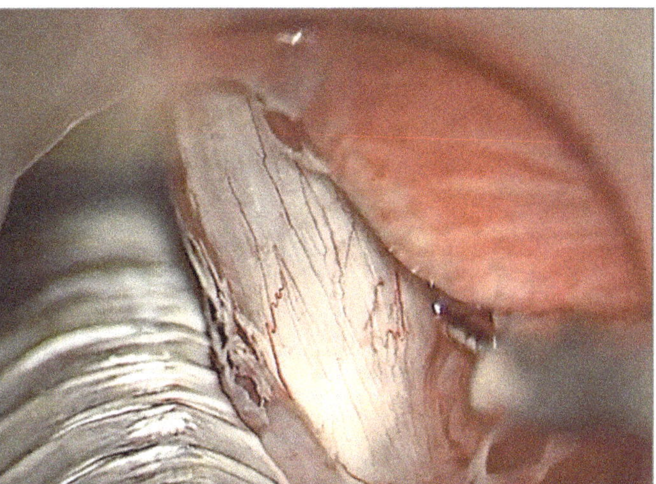

FIG. 12.20: Injection of 5 MU of botulinum toxin into the thyroarytenoid muscle of the right vocal fold

REFERENCES

1. Beham AW, Puellmann K, Laird R, et al. A TNF-regulated recombinatorial macrophage immune receptor implicated in granuloma formation in tuberculosis. PLoS Pathog. 2011 Nov. 7(11):e1002375.
2. Jackson C. Contact ulcer of the larynx. Ann Otol Rhinol Laryngol. 1928;37:227-30.
3. Jackson C, Jackson CL. Contact ulcer of the larynx. Arch Otolaryngol. 1935;22:1-15.
4. Garnett JD, Meyers AD. Contact granulomas. Online. Available from: http://emedicine.medscape.com/article/865924-overview
5. Farwell DG, Belafsky PC, Rees CJ. An endoscopic grading system for vocal process granuloma, J Laryngol Otol. 2008;122(10):1092-5.

CHAPTER 13

Lipoma of the Larynx

DEFINITION

Lipomas in the head and neck region are rare, and its presentation in the larynx is even more unusual, constituting only 0.6% of all benign laryngeal tumors.[1]

Laryngeal lipomas mostly remain asymptomatic, but with a gradual increase in size can give rise to pressure symptoms, such as progressive hoarseness, dysphagia, and dyspnea.[2]

Laryngoscopic evaluation usually reveals a submucosal bulge and computed tomography (CT) of the area is diagnostic. The common differential diagnosis of lipoma is a laryngocele, which can be easily ruled out in the CT scan. Till today, no case of a lipoma of the true vocal folds has been documented.[3,4]

The management of symptomatic laryngeal lipomas is, as complete an excision as possible. Lipomas may be partly or totally encapsulated. In most cases, a microlaryngeal CO_2 laser excision is performed, however, large lipomas may occasionally warrant an external neck surgery.

CASE 1

A 59-year-old female patient presented with progressive hoarseness and vocal fatigue since the last 3 years. A left supraglottic smooth bulge was observed on laryngoscopy, which was resulting in a phonatory gap with ventricular pattern of speech.

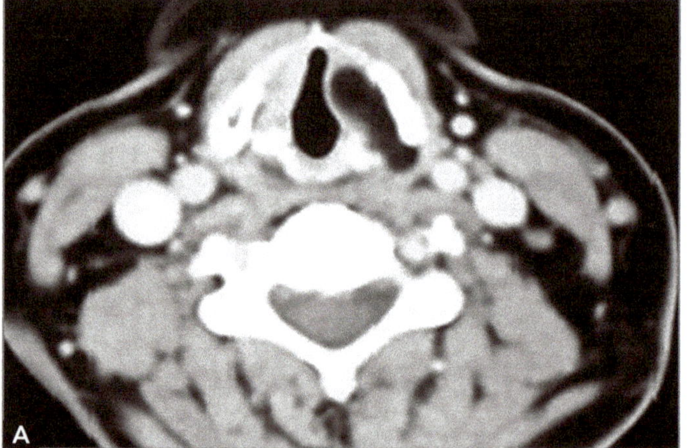

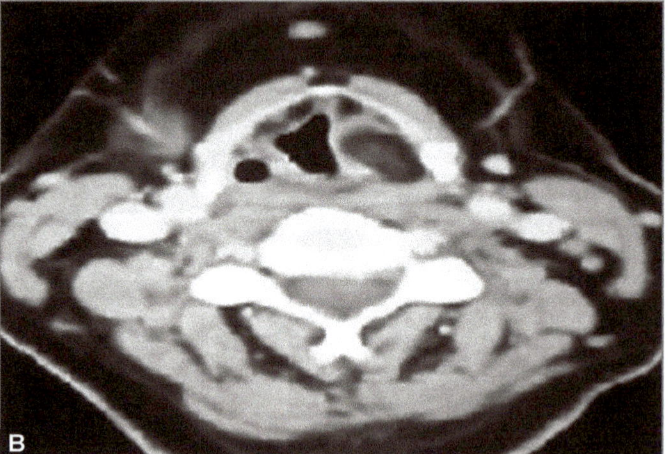

Continued

Continued

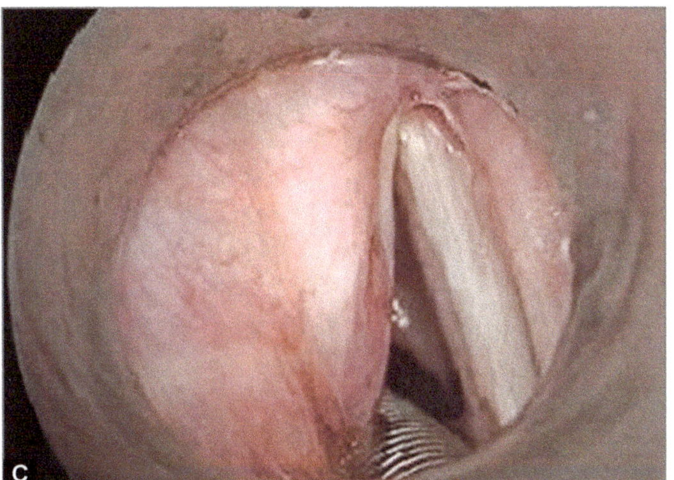

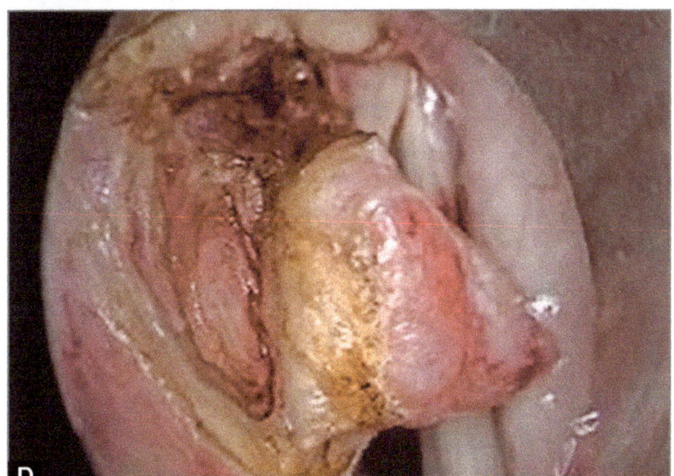

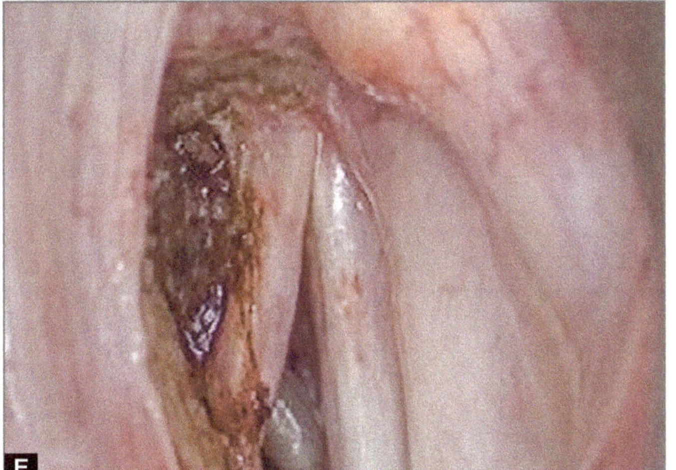

Continued

Continued

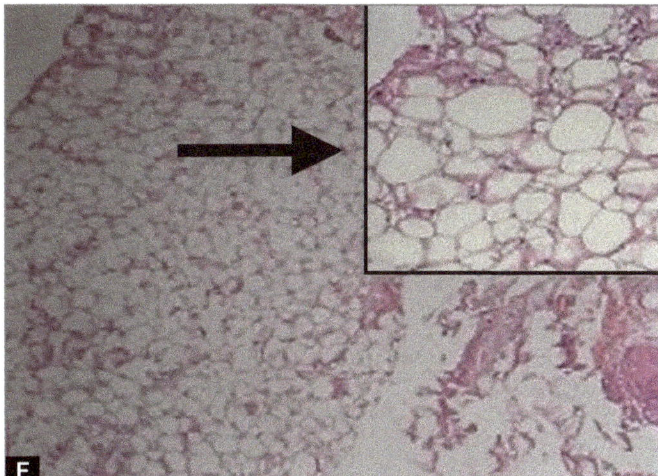

FIG. 13.1: A and **B,** Contrast-enhanced CT scan of neck (axial view) showing fat containing soft tissue lesion on the left side. The lesion measures approximately 2.8 × 0.9 × 2.1 cm in maximum CC × TR × AP dimensions, extending cranially into aryepiglottic fold and inferiority almost up to the inferior margin of cricoid cartilage. The lesion is displacing the left vocal fold medially and is in very close approximation to the internal carotid artery laterally. **C,** Preoperative picture showing left-sided false vocal fold bulge obscuring the view of left true vocal fold. **D,** Intraoperative picture showing CO_2 laser excision of the lipoma. **E,** Postoperative picture showing excision site and the left vocal fold. **F,** Histopathology slide (low power, H&E stain) showing a nodular fragment of mature adipose tissue with lobules of mucous glands and skeletal muscle at the periphery, confirming our clinical diagnosis of lipoma. Mature adipocytes seen in high power (inset)

CASE 2

An adult male patient was referred with a foreign body sensation and throat pain of a short duration. On laryngoscopy, a left ventricular bulge was seen anteriorly. A CT scan confirmed this bulge to be a lipoma. As the patient had no hoarseness and the presenting pain sensation settled conservatively, the lipoma is under observation only.

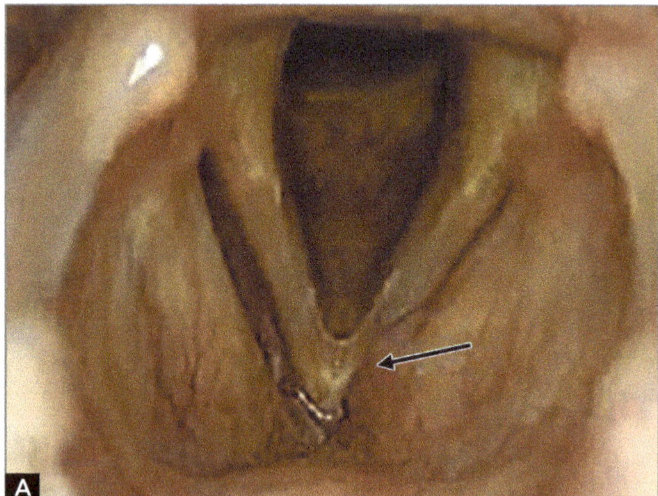

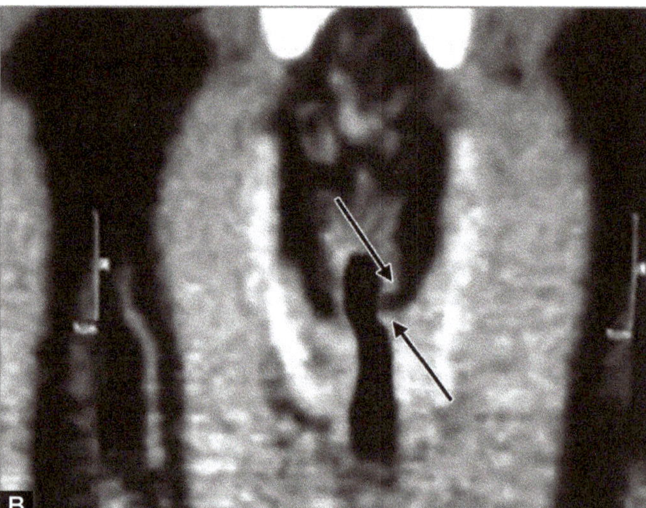

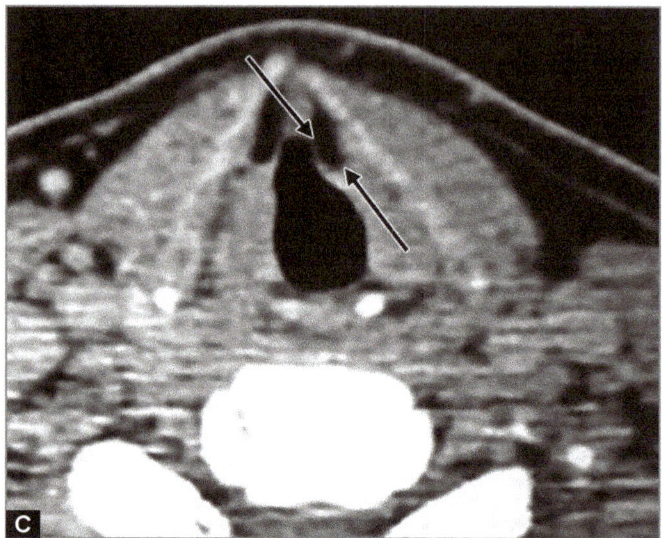

FIG. 13.2: Laryngostroboscopy. **A,** A very small left-sided ventricular bulge (arrow) seen. **B** and **C,** The same bulge can be corroborated with CT scan on coronal and axial views

CASE 3

An adult female presented with longstanding hoarseness and a history of a recent laryngeal biopsy revealing a lipoma. The CT scan image revealed a large lipoma but the patient was not willing for excision.

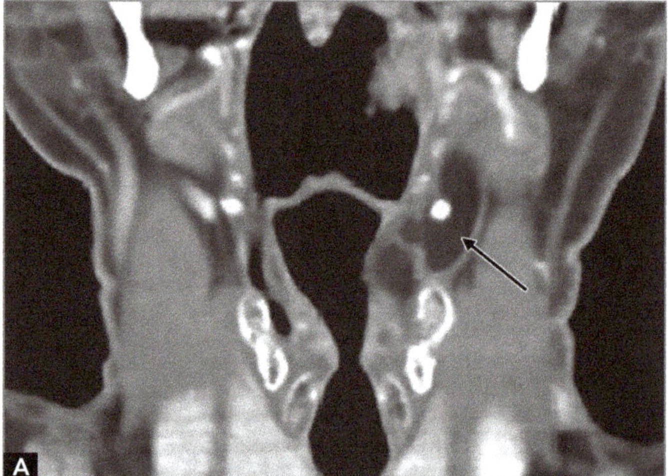

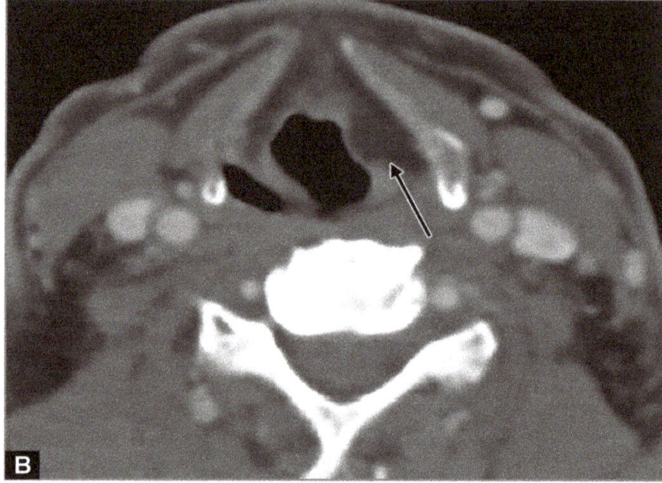

FIG. 13.3: Contrast-enhanced CT scan of neck (coronal and axial view, respectively) showing left supraglottic homogenous hypodense fat density mass (lipoma) extending superionty from above the level of hyoid bone to inferionty up to the thyriod cartilage (arrow)

REFERENCES

1. Khorsandi Ashtiani MT, Yazdani N, Saeedi M, et al. Large lipoma of the larynx: A case report. Acta Med Iran 2010;48(5):353-6.
2. Nerurkar NK, Jain AA, Desai BH. Lipoma of the Larynx: Our experience. Int J Phonosurg Laryngol. 2016;6(2):89-92.
3. Oguz G, Murath A, Barutcu O, et al. The case of laryngeal lipoma. J Otol Rhinol. 2013;2:2.
4. Bildirici K, Kecik C, Peker B, et al. Lipoma of the Larynx: A case report. Cerrahpasa J Med. 2001;32:112-4.

CHAPTER 14

Laryngeal Manifestations of Rheumatoid Arthritis

Rheumatoid arthritis (RA) is a destructive autoimmune disease that affects 3% of the adult population. It is characterized by the formation of both articular and extra-articular lesions with a predilection for small joints.[1] The prevalence of laryngeal manifestations of rheumatoid arthritis has been on the rise. In a report by Lawry et al. in 1960, the prevalence of laryngeal symptoms was up to 31%.[2] Towards the end of the century, the prevalence increased to seventy-five percent.[1]

When present, the laryngeal manifestations span an array of findings ranging from cricoarytenoid joint (CAJ), fixation and neuropathy of the recurrent laryngeal nerve, to myositis and presence of laryngeal nodules.[3-5]

FIXATION OF THE CRICOARYTENOID JOINT

Laryngeal electromyography can differentiate between vocal fold paralysis and CAJ fixation. Palpation of the CAJ under general anesthesia can confirm the presence of joint fixation and rule out any possible posterior glottic stenosis. High-resolution computerized tomography is also helpful for early detection of CAJ arthritis. The most common findings are increased density of the joint, narrowing of the joint space, ankylosis, and vocal fold thickening. Steroids may be injected into the effected CAJ.[1]

BAMBOO NODES OF THE TRUE VOCAL FOLDS

Other laryngoscopic findings include the presence of inflammatory masses or rheumatoid nodules in the larynx and pharynx. Bamboo nodes may be seen in patients of rheumatoid arthritis.

Bamboo nodes were initially described by Hosako et al. in a female patient with lupus erythematous. Endoscopic visualization shows transversally arranged cystic yellowish bamboo nodes in the submucosal space of the middle portion of the vocal folds. Similar to other laryngeal lesions in patients with rheumatoid arthritis, these nodes are more often seen in patients with active disease rather than inactive and correlates with antibody deposits.[6] Voice therapy is initially advised for hoarseness due to bamboo nodes and surgical excision of the nodes with steroid administration locally is reserved for the recalcitrant cases.

CASE 1

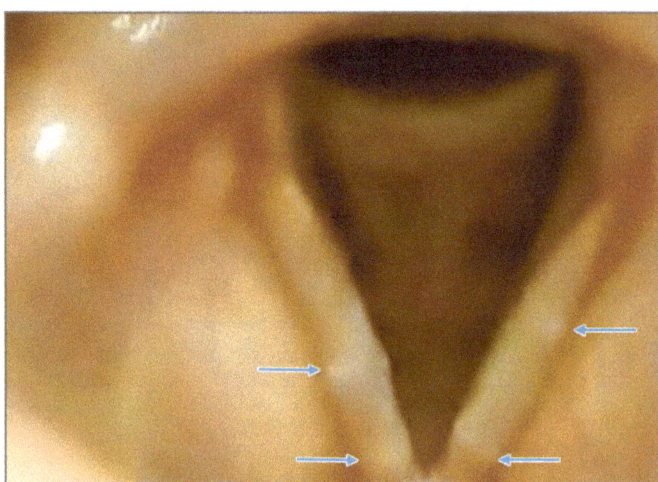

FIG. 14.1: Bilateral, multiple, bamboo nodes (blue arrows) are seen on the vocal folds in a patient recently diagnosed with rheumatoid arthritis. This patient gave history of 5–6 months of hoarseness. Patient has been advised voice therapy

REFERENCES

1. Hamdan AL, Sarieddine D. Laryngeal manifestations of rheumatoid arthritis. Autoimmune Dis. 2013;2013:103081.
2. Lawry GV, Finerman ML, Hanafee WN, et al. Laryngeal involvement in rheumatoid arthritis. A clinical, laryngoscopic, and computerized tomographic study. Arthritis Rheum. 1984;27(8):873-82.
3. Mikkelson WM, Duff IF, Robinson WD. Unusual manifestation of rheumatoid nodules; report of three cases. J Mich State Med Soc. 1955;54(3):292-7.
4. Murano E, Tayama N, Miyaji M, et al. Bamboo Node: Primary Vocal Fold Lesion as Evidence of Autoimmune Disease. J of Voice. 15(3):441-50.
5. Voulgari PV, Papazisi D, Bai M, et al. Laryngeal involvement in rheumatoid arthritis. Rheumatology International. 2005;25(5):321-25.
6. Hosako Y, Nakamura M, Tayama N, et al. Laryngeal involvements in systemic lupus erythematosus: a case report. Larynx. 1993;5(2):171-5.

CHAPTER 15

Recurrent Respiratory Papilloma

DEFINITION

Recurrent respiratory papilloma (RRP) is a disease of human papillomavirus (HPV) induced epithelial proliferation affecting the respiratory tract.

TYPES

When the onset of RRP is at a younger age, typically under 5 years but prior to adolescence, it is classified as juvenile-onset recurrent respiratory papillomatosis (JORRP). The commonest laryngeal tumor in children is JORRP. An adult onset of RRP, typically between 20 and 40 years of age, is classified as adult onset recurrent respiratory papillomatosis (AORRP).

Besides the peak of RRP in childhood and between 20 and 40 years, there is a third possible peak at 64 years.[1]

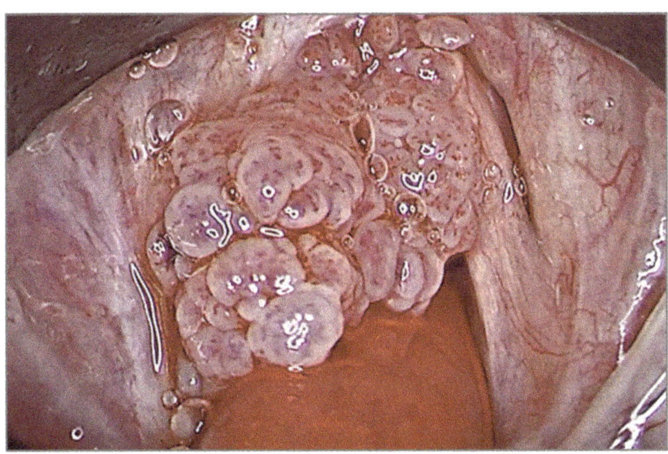

FIG. 15.1: JORRP in a 3-year-old child revealing multiple fronds of left sided papilloma. (E-CC)

Juvenile-onset recurrent respiratory papillomatosis typically behaves more aggressive than AORRP, possibly due to the presence of an immature immune system in children.

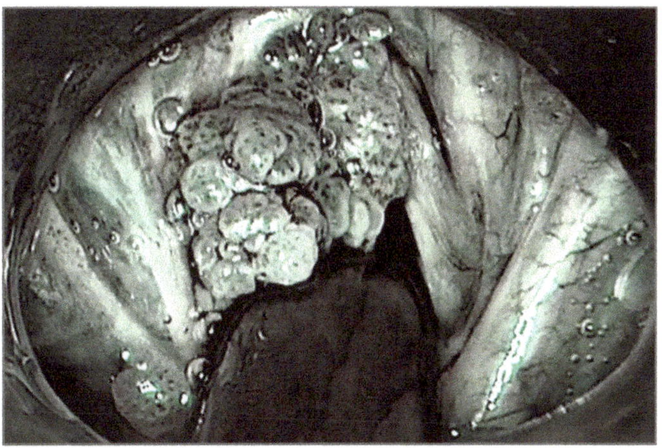

FIG. 15.2: Image 15.1 in SA mode

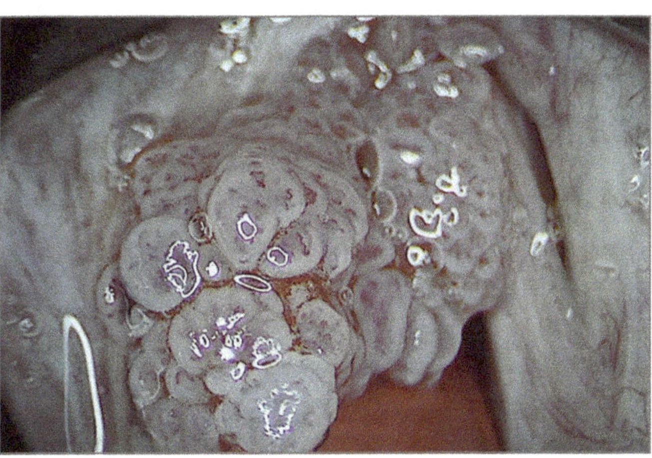

FIG. 15.3: Image 15.1 in SB mode

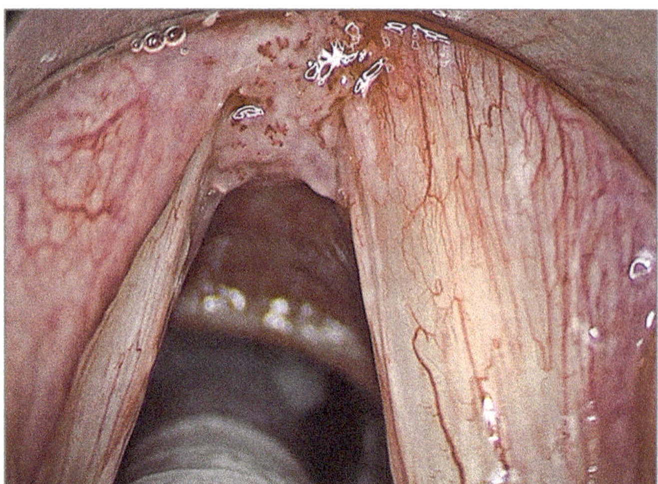

FIG. 15.4: AORRP showing disease limited to the anterior commissure. (E-CC)

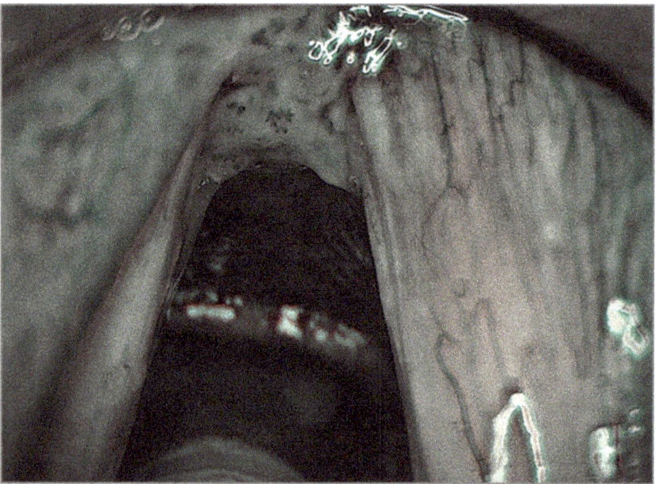

FIG. 15.5: Image 15.4 in SA mode

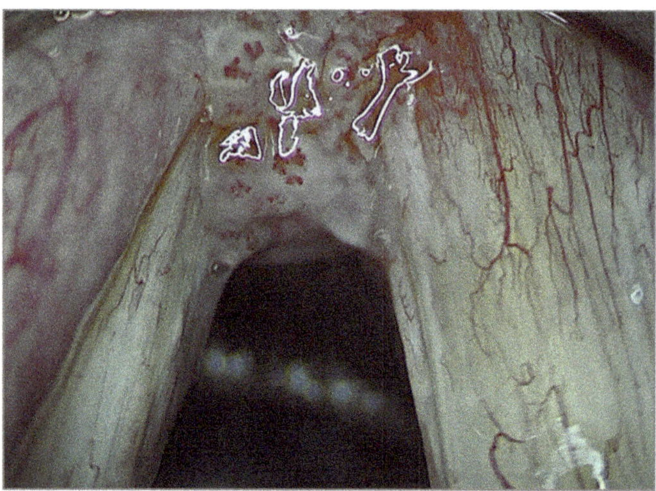

FIG. 15.6: Image 15.4 in SB mode

HUMAN PAPILLOMAVIRUS AND ITS TRANSMISSION

Human papillomavirus 6 and 11 are typically responsible for RRP while HPV 16 and 18, though uncommon, are more frequently associated with malignant changes. An absence of any HPV being detected (no type) is not necessarily a good thing in RRP as a higher association with malignant change has been suggested in these cases.[2,3]

Between HPV 6 and 11, HPV 11 has been found to be more aggressive in children and HPV 6 more aggressive in adults.[4,5]

Though the transmission of the virus in JORRP is thought to be a vertical peripartum transmission of the virus from infected mother, a C-section is not found to be completely protective. Furthermore, one out of several hundred children born to HPV positive women develops JORRP. It is possible that the viral transmission may take place via the cord blood.

Kashima et al. postulated the triad of a first borne, vaginally delivered child of a teenage mother being likely to develop JORRP.[6]

The transmission of the virus is thought to be horizontal in the case of AORRP, with sexual transmission as one route of infection. It may, however, be possible that AORRP is simply an activation of quiescent HPV infection of the basement membrane of the respiratory tract, present since childhood. The mode of transmission in AORRP is also possible via inhalation of the infected laser plumes during surgery being performed for RRP.

The HPV has an affinity for the basement membrane of the epithelium. As only the basal epithelial cells can proliferate, the virus infects this cell layer. Human papillomavirus DNA integrates in the basal epithelial layer within the epithelial transition zones of the body where stratified squamous epithelium meets ciliated columnar epithelium, such as true vocal folds and site of tracheostomy. Human papillomavirus also has an affinity for traumatized epithelium as found subsequent to a tracheostomy.

Recurrence following surgical excision is common as the virus also resides in the epithelium that appears normal.

HISTOPATHOLOGY

Hemotoxylin and eosin (H&E) staining reveals exophytic projections of keratinized stratified squamous epithelium overlying a fibrovascular core. Occasionally, vacuolated cells with clear cytoplasmic inclusion are found (koilocytes) which signal the presence of viral infection. The histopathology in children does not differ from that in adults.

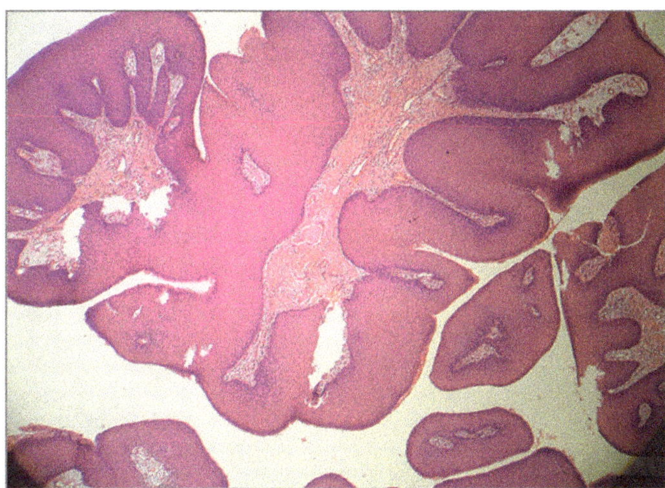

FIG. 15.7: H&E staining in an adult RRP patient revealing keratinized stratified squamous epithelium overlying a fibrovascular core

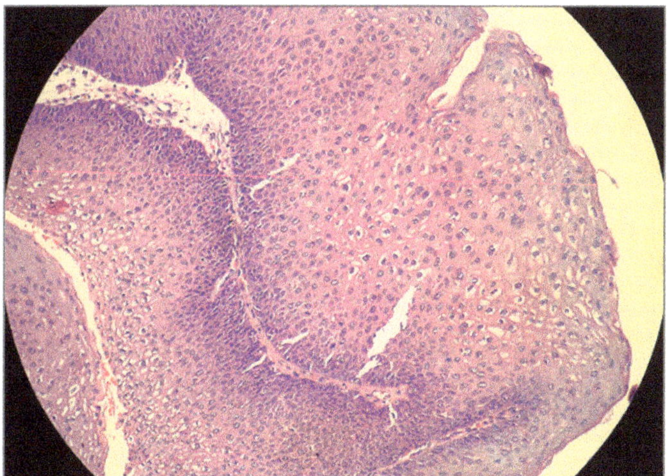

FIG. 15.8: H&E staining in a pediatric RRP revealing a magnified single papilloma. The HP in children does not differ in any way from that in adults

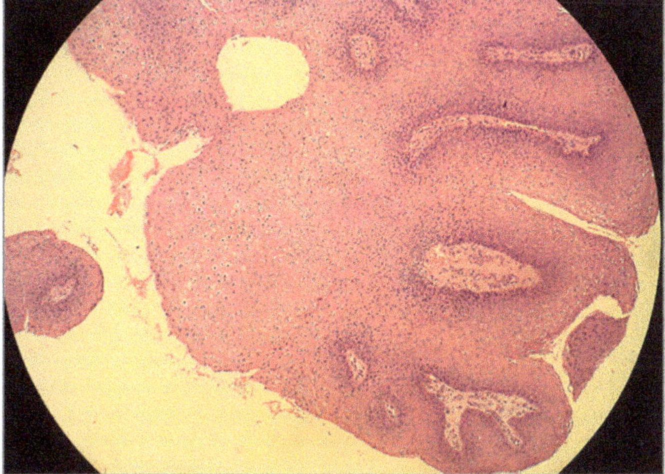

FIG. 15.9: Vacuolated cells with clear cytoplasmic inclusion (koilocytes) found within the papilloma suggest viral presence

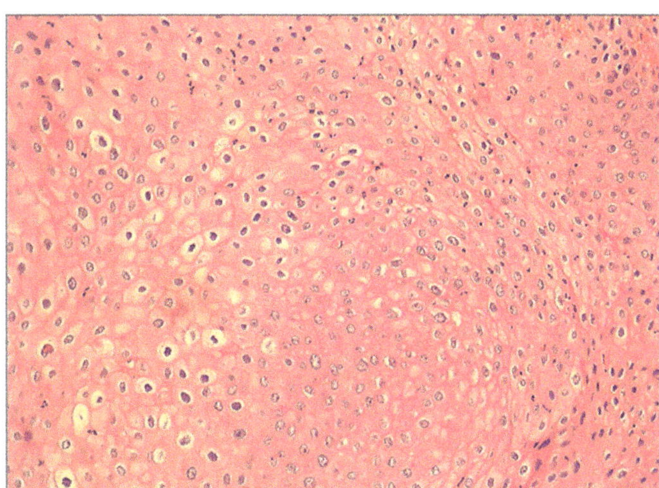

FIG. 15.10: Magnified image of 15.3 clearly showing the koilocytes

TABLE 15.1: Common characteristics of of JORRP and AORRP

JORRP	AORRP
Onset < adolecence	20–40 years; 60 years
Male = female	Male preponderence
Firstborn, teenage mother, vaginal delivery	Orogenital route or activation of virus, laser plumes, instruments
Aggressive	Less aggressive
HPV 11 more aggressive	HPV 6 more aggressive
Try to avoid a tracheostomy	Microflap excision when possible
Anterior commissure to be respected in all RRP	Try office laser procedures under local anesthesia if frequent recurrences

Presentation and diagnosis in children

The AORRP is picked up early, as the patient's complaint of hoarseness, and the laryngoscopy is not a challenge. In the case of children, this does not hold true. The child may not complain of hoarseness and the caretakers may not identify a problem till the hoarseness is severe or accompanied by stridor. Children are best evaluated without anesthesia with a pediatric flexible laryngoscope by bundling up the child in a sheet. A preprocedure oxygen saturation (SpO_2) should guide if the flexible laryngoscopy may be performed in the operation theater or as an office procedure. A single puff of 4% lignocaine spray in one nostril suffices for the procedure with no sedation.

Laryngoscopy reveals typical warty growths or a mottled appearance of lesions which are often found typically in multifocal fronds.

Staging of Recurrent Respiratory Papilloma

There are various staging systems that may be utilized for RRP.

Derkay-Coltrera Staging System[7]

This provides a uniform staging worksheet for assessment of RRP and the Derkay grading describes the amount of RRP by clinical parameters (voice, stridor, urgency, distress) and anatomical parameters (25 subsites). The scores predict intervals between surgery.

Dikkers Staging System[8]

Dikkers grading (3 grades) is beneficial for predicting surgical need.

1. Grade 1: Sessile growth unifocal or multifocal
2. Grade 2: Exophytic RRP unifocal
3. Grade 3: Exophytic RRP multifocal.

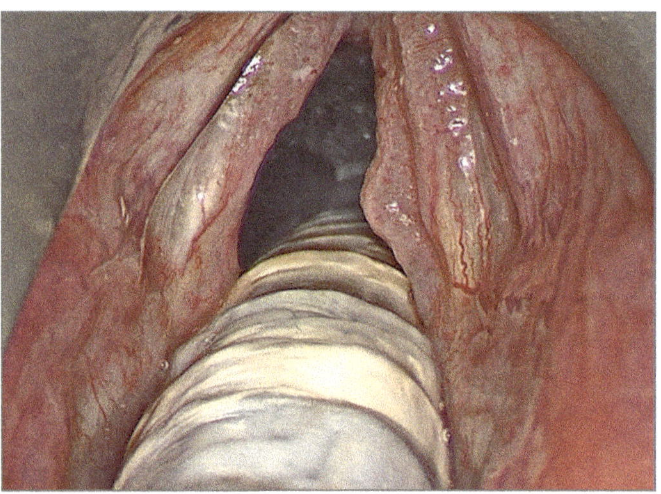

FIG. 15.11: Dikkers grade 1

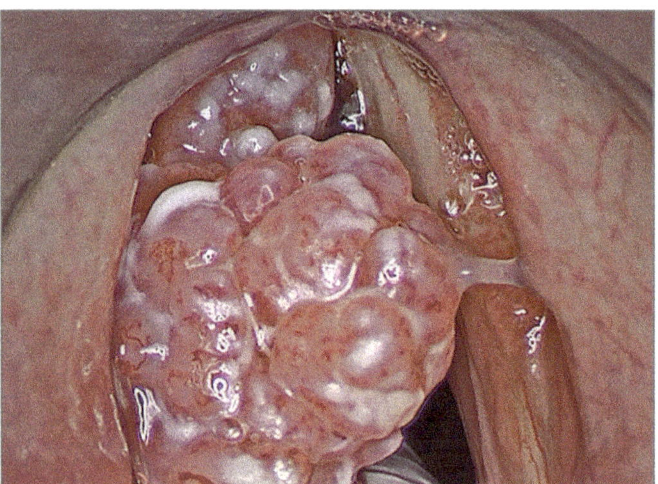

FIG. 15.12: Dikkers grade 2

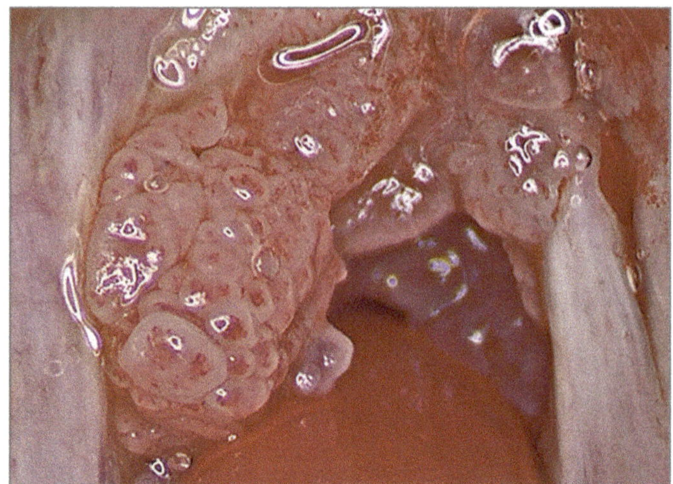

FIG. 15.13: Dikkers grade 3

PHILOSOPHY OF MANAGEMENT

Evaluation of the entire airway, preferably with documentation is advisable. This should be an atraumatic evaluation to prevent seedling deposition. Interval biopsies to confirm the histopathology are important as occasionally the RRP may have undergone a malignant conversion.

Human papillomavirus subtyping is recommended once in order to ascertain the aggressiveness of the disease.

For bulky lesions, debulking using a tricut followed by a skimmer laryngeal microdebrider system is preferred. The author prefers microflap laser excision in case of small isolated fronds.

Complete removal of the epithelium along with the basement membrane (which harbors the virus) without making an incision on the ligament or traumatizing the normal mucosa is important to prevent new seedling deposits of disease.

CONCERNS

Tracheostomy

Since tracheostomy is associated with a 50% chance of tracheal disease,[9] it should be avoided as far as possible. If a tracheostomy has been performed, early decannulation should be planned. A study by Derkay in 1995 suggests the need of tracheostomy in 14% of JORRP patients.[10]

The overall chances of tracheal spread in JORRP is 17–26%[11] and bronchopulmonary spread less than 5%.[12]

Anterior Commissure

Multiple surgeries and disease in the anterior commissure are the primary reasons for the formation of an anterior glottic web in RRP patients. Staging the disease is the best way to avoid this complication.

Malignant Transformation (3–5%)

Typically described in children with tracheobronchial pulmonary involvement as compared to AORPP where laryngeal transformation is seen. Malignant conversion is seen more often in patients with no HPV type detected.[2,3]

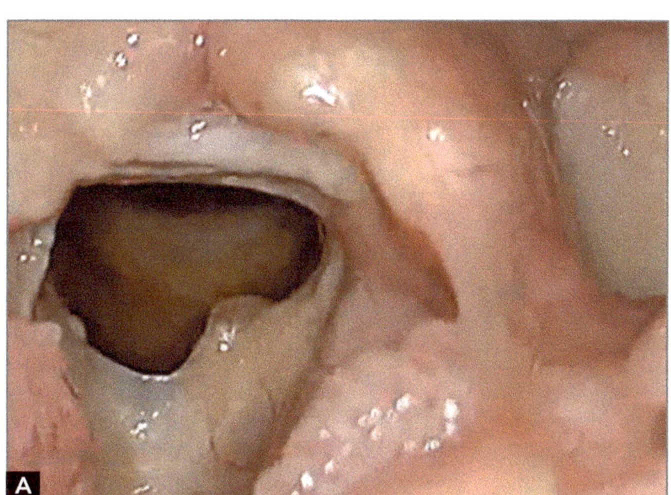

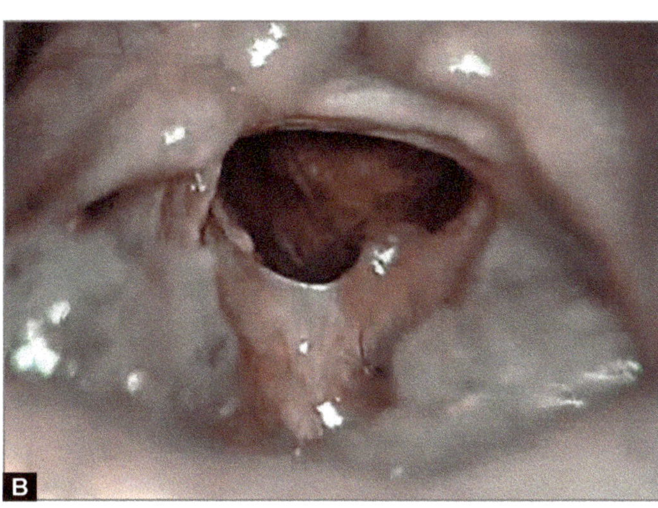

FIG. 15.14: An iatrogenic anterior glottic web is seen in a patient with active RRP in **A,** WL laryngoscopy and **B,** NBI light

REMISSION AND PUBERTY

Many reports suggest spontaneous regression of JORRP in adolescence. An alteration of the immune system at puberty may play a role. However, some patients progress to extensive disease involving the lower airways.

In the author's experience as well, the occurrence of remission is variable and often not at puberty.

Human papillomavirus vaccination is widely prevalent today and must be encouraged in both boys and girls. Vaccines in principle are not therapeutic agents, however, an increased number of antibodies against HPV post-Gardasil vaccine (quadrivalent HPV 6,11,16, and 18) may prevent new papilloma formation.[13]

CASE 1

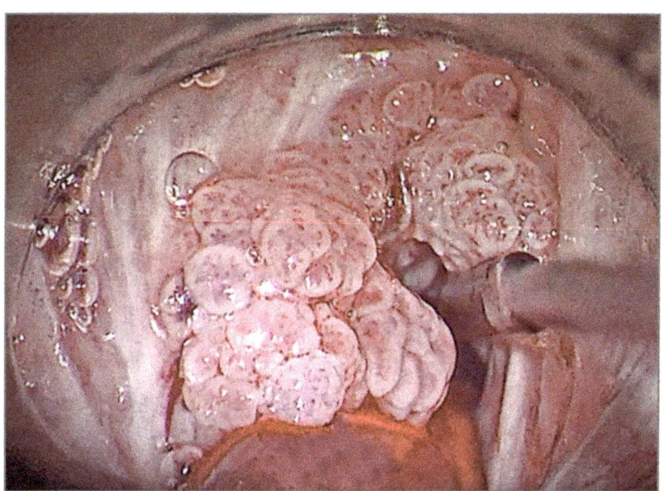

FIG. 15.15: A 3-year-old girl with grade 3 (Dikkers) JORRP with a retractor being used to evaluate the attachments of the papilloma fronds. (M-CC)

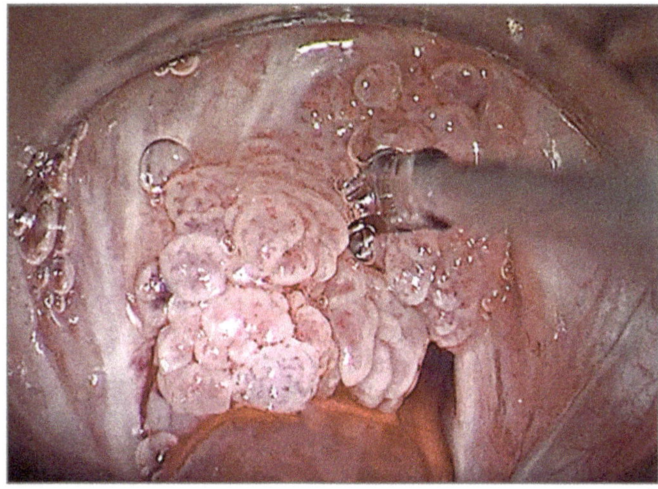

FIG. 15.16: A conventional biopsy being taken for histopathological confirmation as well as viral typing. (M-CC)

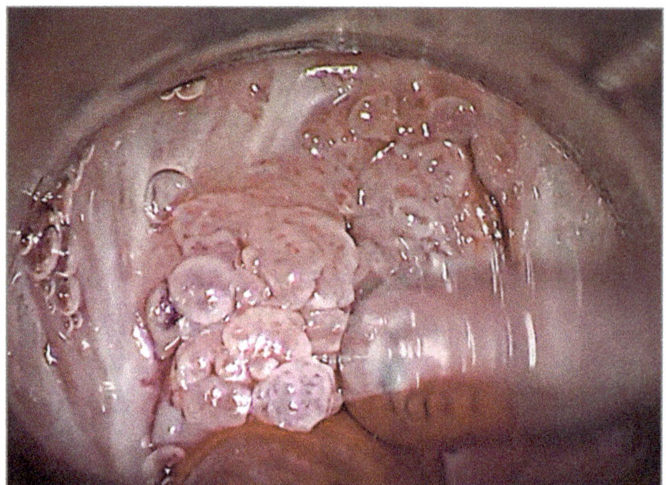

FIG. 15.17: Tricut laryngeal microdebrider being used to debulk the papillomas. (M-CC)

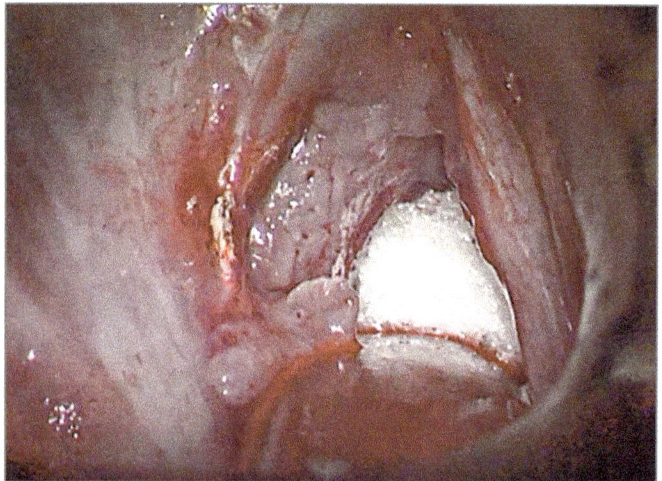

FIG. 15.18: Image following debulking with the microdebrider. Fronds seen in the Anterior commissure and posteriorly on the left vocal fold. (M-CC)

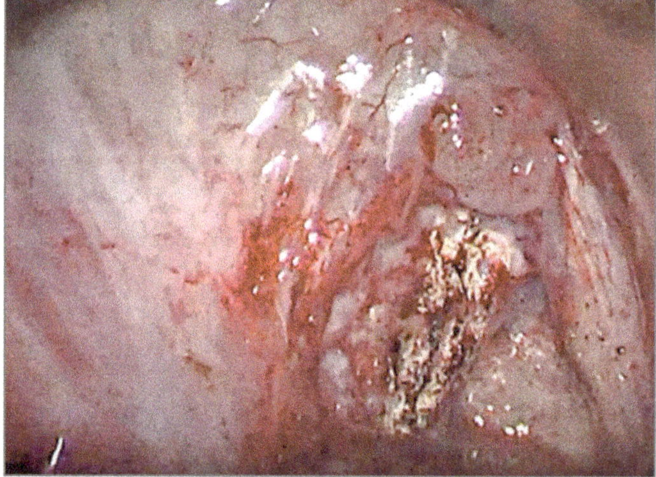

FIG. 15.19: Laser ablation of the carpet of papillomas on the left vocal fold and the left posterior frond

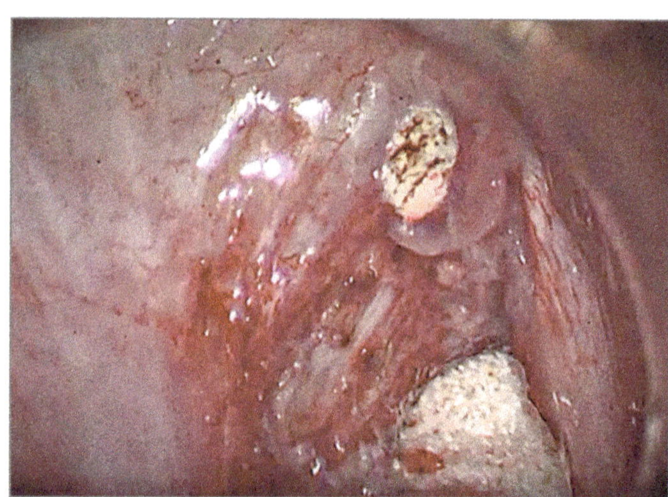

FIG. 15.20: Laser ablation of anterior commissure disease from the left lateral aspect. (M-CC)

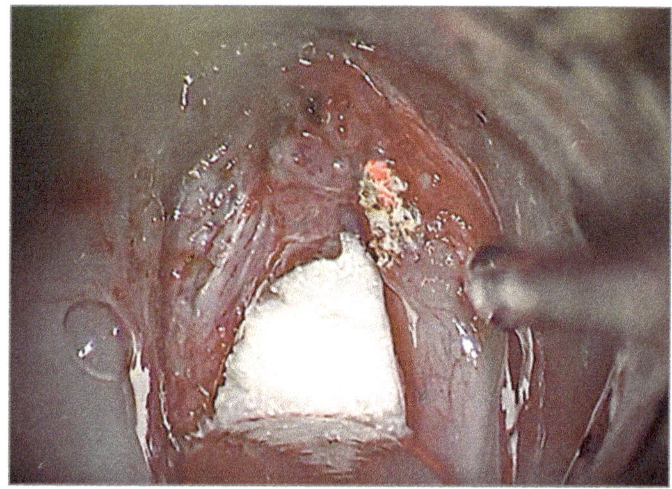

FIG. 15.21: Laser ablation of right anterior commissure disease. (M-CC)

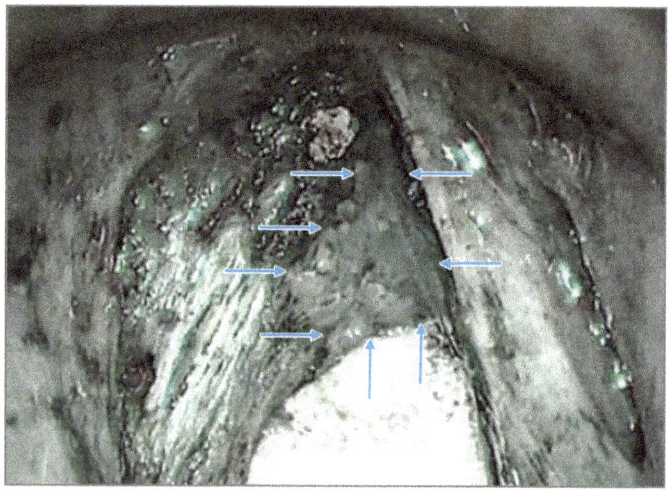

FIG. 15.22: Spectra A image to delineate the anterior commissure disease left intentionally to prevent webbing (in arrows). (M-SA)

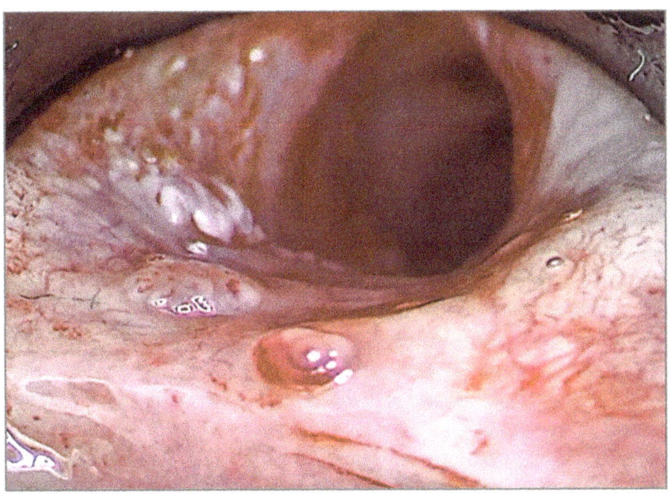

FIG. 15.23: Left posterior commissure disease seen clearly after removal of the endotracheal tube and apnea technique being used. (M-CC)

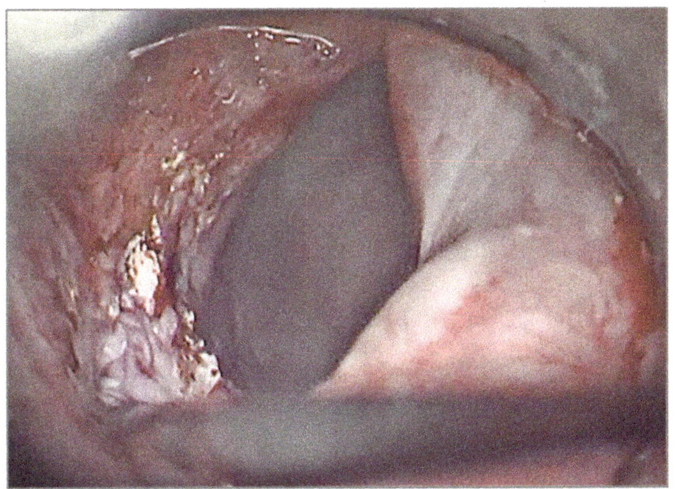

FIG. 15.24: Laser ablation of the posterior RRP. (M-CC)

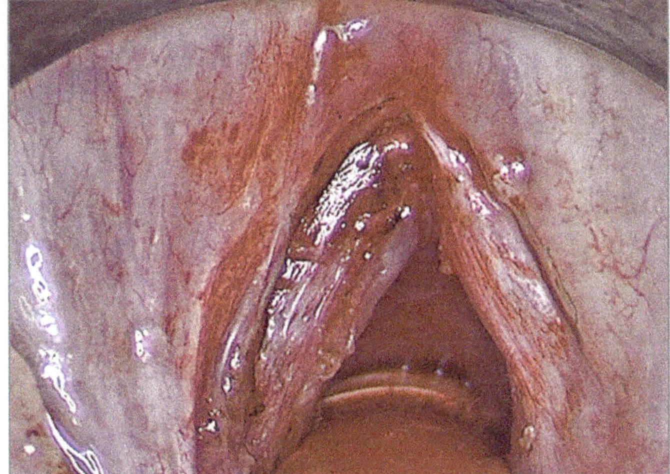

FIG. 15.25: Final postoperative image with staging of anterior commissure disease on the left side in order to prevent webbing. (M-CC)

CASE 2

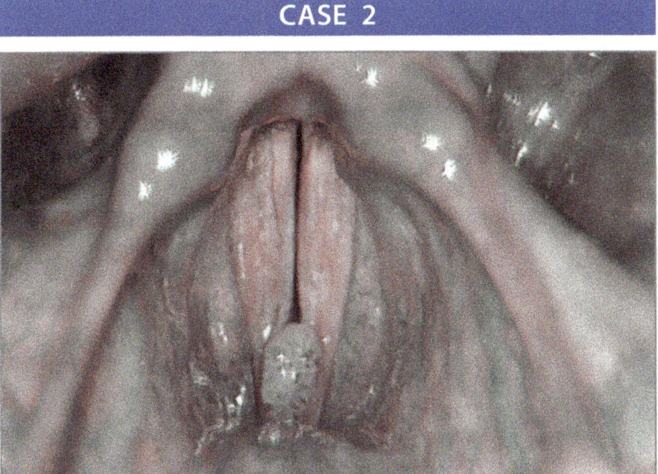

FIG. 15.26: RRP frond seen at the anterior commissure in an adult male patient with the NBI light. (RL-NBI)

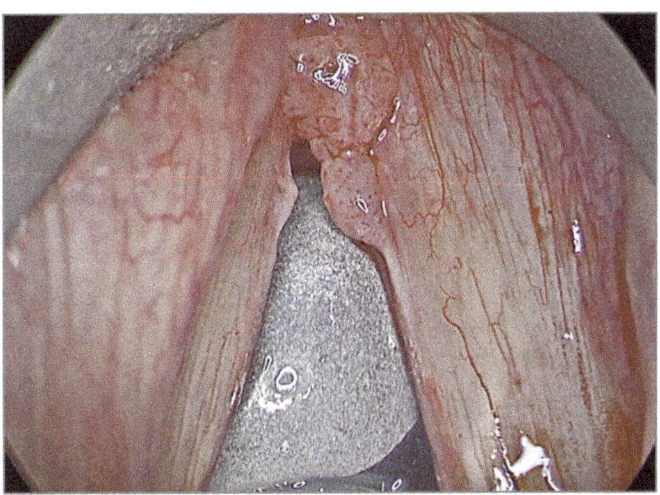

FIG. 15.27: Image after taking patient under anesthesia revealing the anterior commissure growth based primarily on the right side. (E-CC)

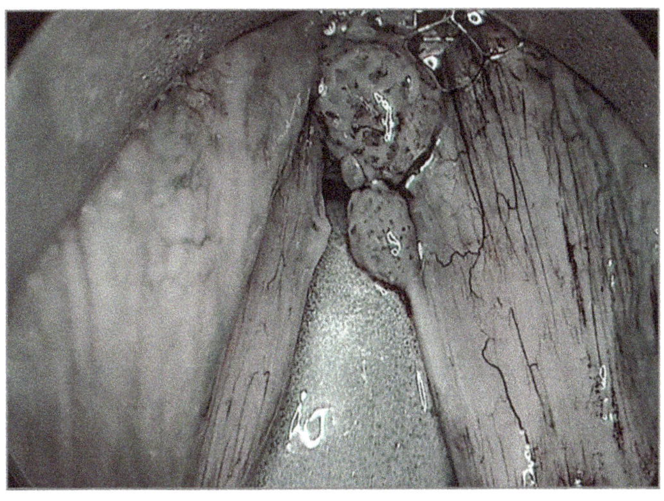

FIG. 15.28: Image 15.27 in SB mode. (E-SB)

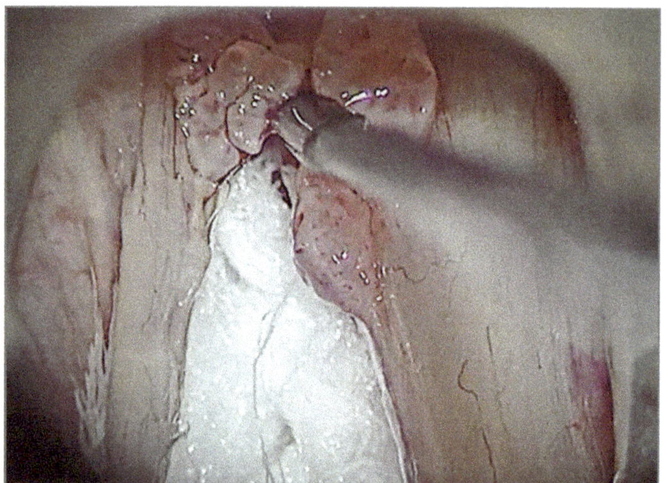

FIG. 15.29: Microflap elevator being used to retract and study the pedicles of the papilloma fronds. Cuff being protected by a moist cotton pledglet. (M-CC)

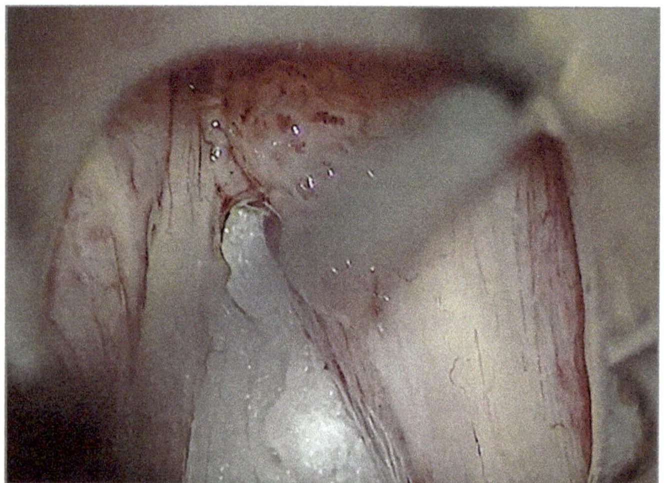

FIG. 15.30: SEIT being used, 27 gauge needle being used to inject 1–2 cc of 1:10,000 saline adrenaline. (M-CC)

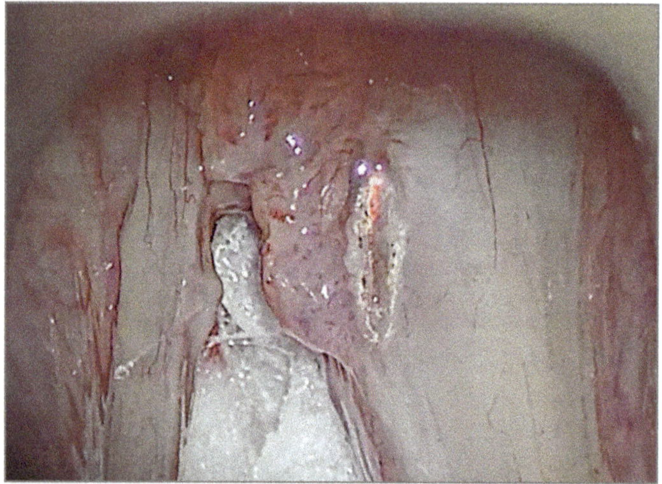

FIG. 15.31: Acublade CO_2 laser epithelial cordotomy being made just lateral to the papilloma fronds of the right vocal fold. (M-CC)

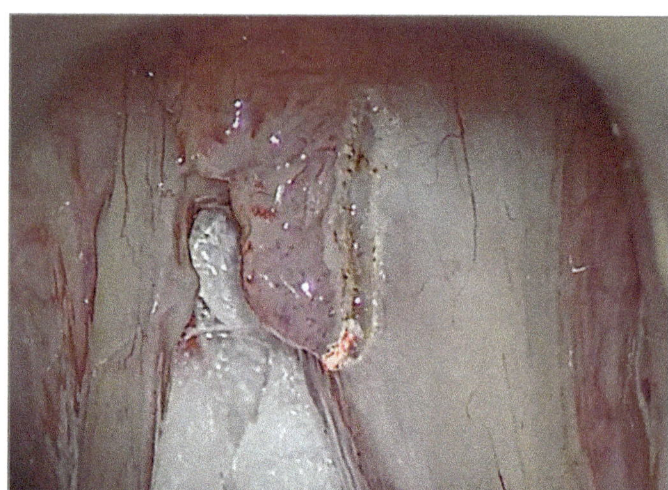

FIG. 15.32: Extension of the incision. (M-CC)

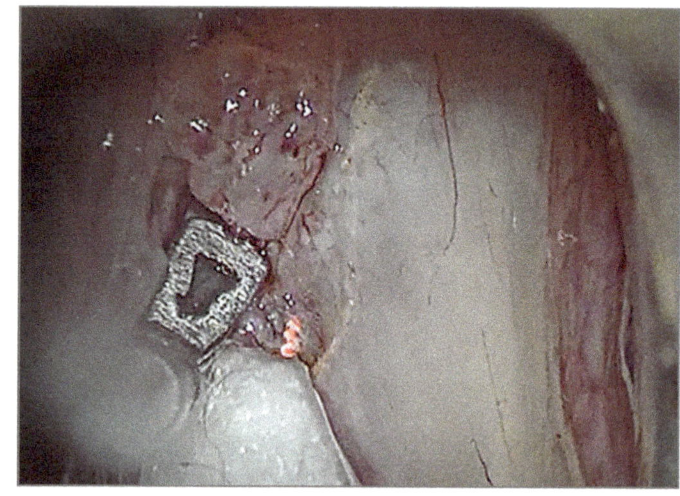

FIG. 15.33: Upward Bouchayer holding and gently retracting the papillomas medially for easier laser excision

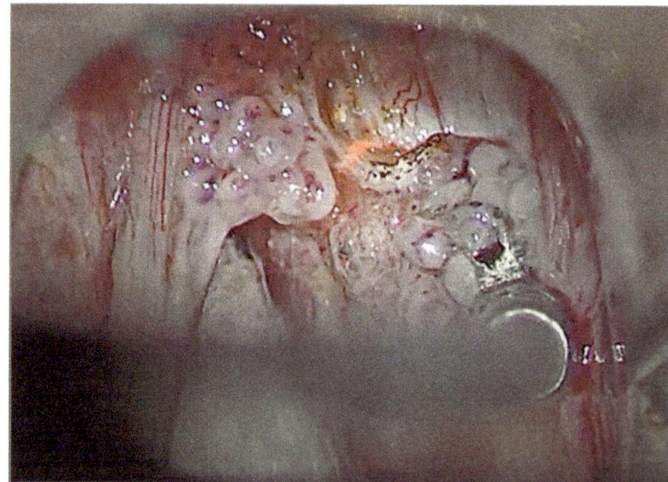

FIG. 15.34: Anterior cut being made to release the last attachments. (M-CC)

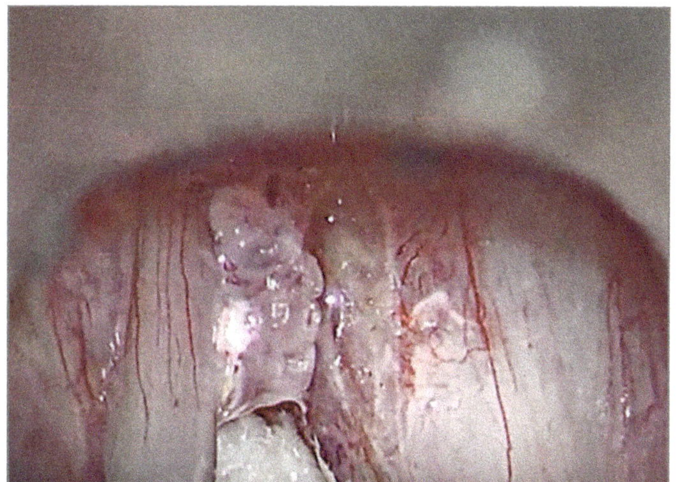

FIG. 15.35: Decision made to partially excise the papilloma's on the left vocal fold at the anterior commissure

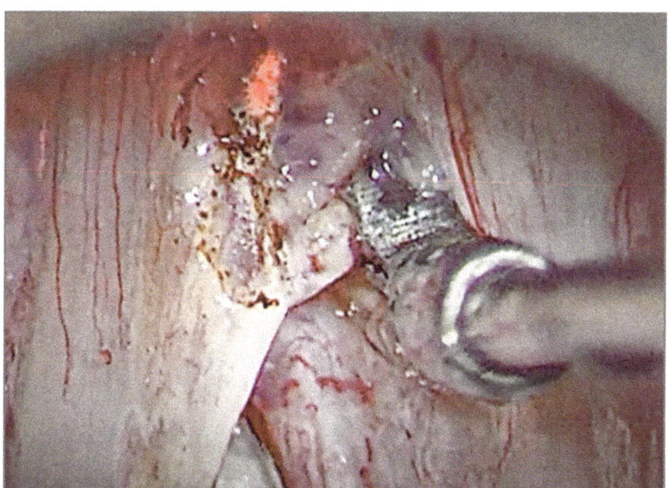

FIG. 15.36: Laser excision of the left RRP. (M-CC)

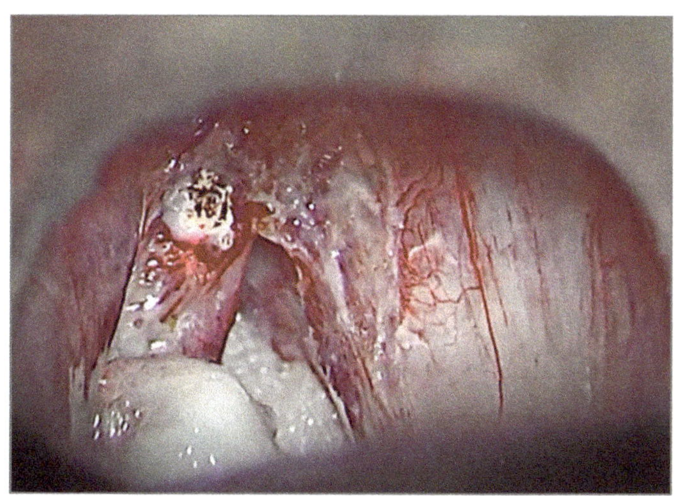

FIG. 15.37: Laser ablation of the left anterior commissure, laterally. (M-CC)

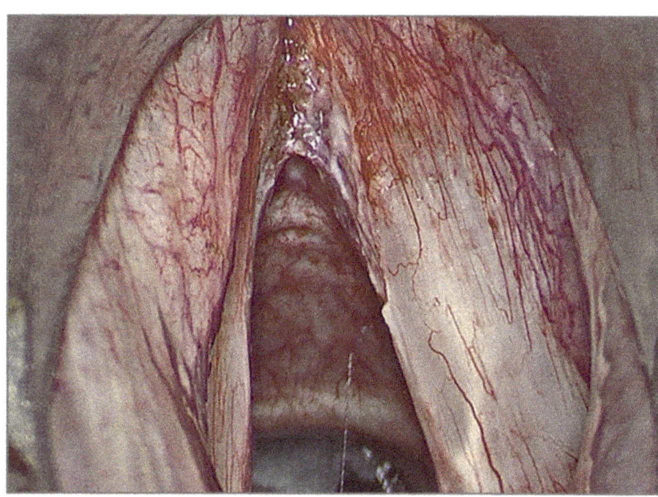

FIG. 15.38: Final postoperative image of the patient revealing few papillomas at the anterior commissure. (E-CC)

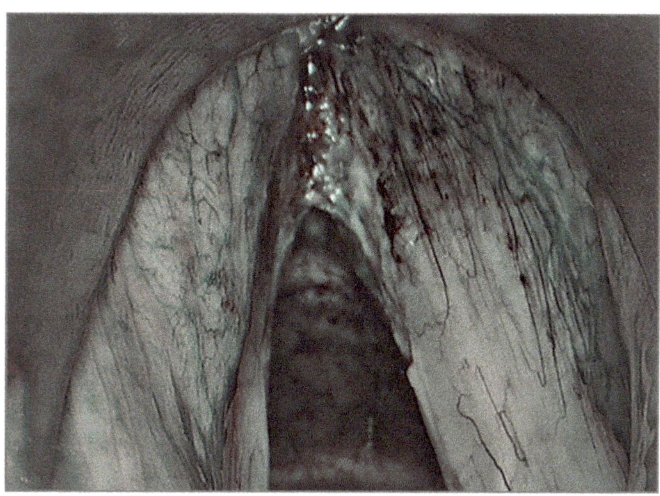

FIG. 15.39: Image 15.38 in SA. (E-SA)

CASE 4

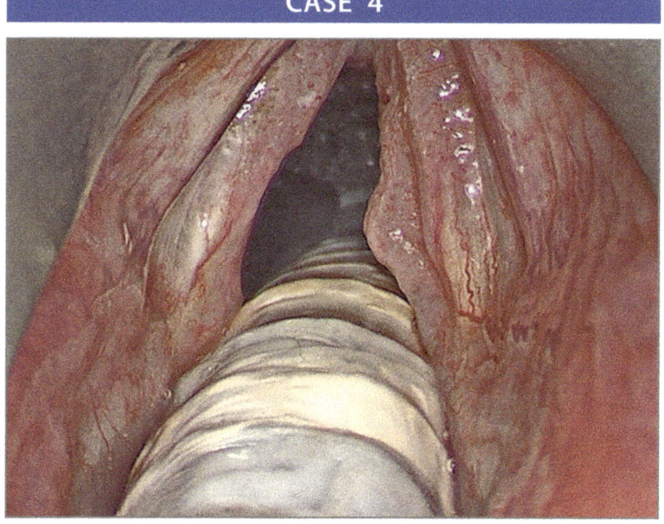

FIG. 15.39: AORRP with Dikkers grade 1 for planned staged surgery. (E-CC)

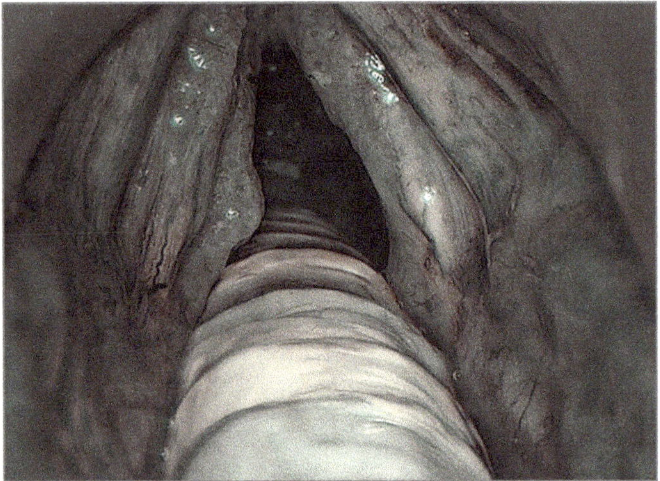

FIG. 15.40: Image 15.39 in SA mode

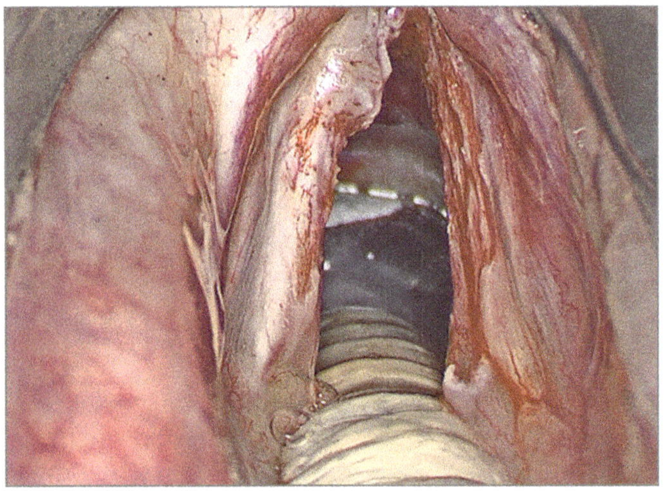

FIG. 15.41: Immediate postoperative image revealing right vocal fold complete excision with left anterior commissure residual disease left behind for subsequent excision at 4–6 weeks. (E-CC)

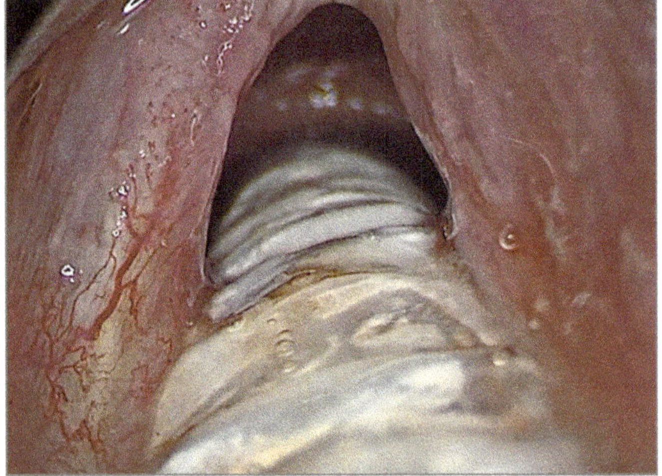

FIG. 15.42: Six weeks later. Good epithelial healing with a left vocal fold carpet of residual RRP

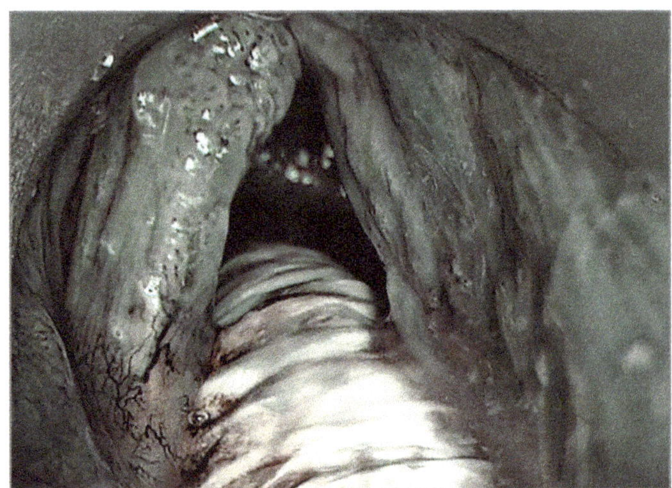

FIG. 15.43: Image 15.42 in SA mode. (E-SA)

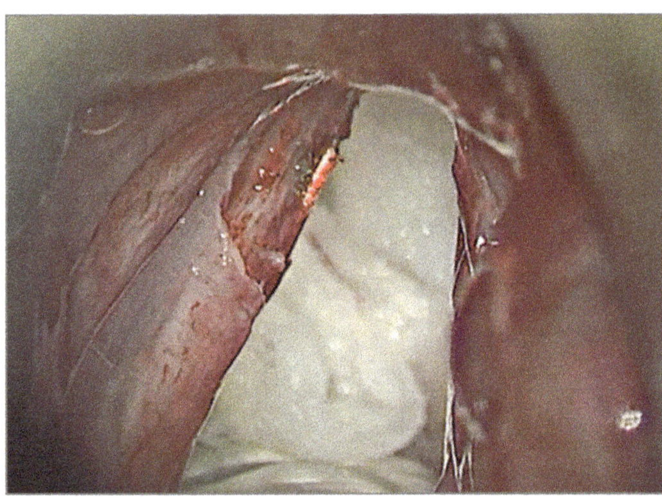

FIG. 15.44: The localized left anterior commissure disease can be relatively easily removed by elevating a flap or laser ablation. (E-CC)

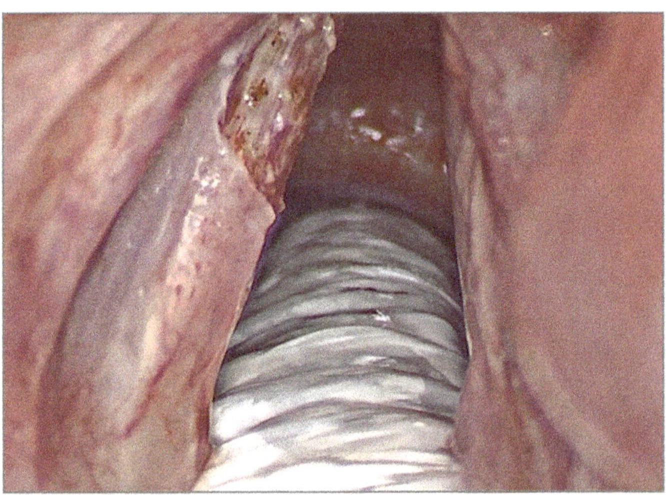

FIG. 15.45: Final postoperative image. (E-CC)

CASE 5

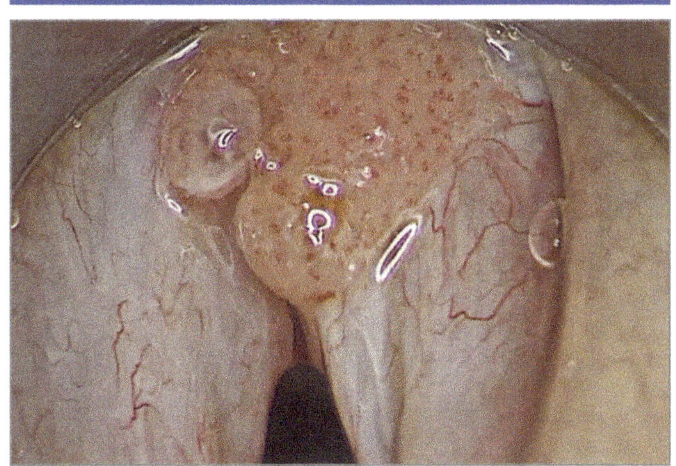

FIG. 15.46: Horseshoe RRP excised in one stage with clean up planned after 2 weeks. (E-CC)

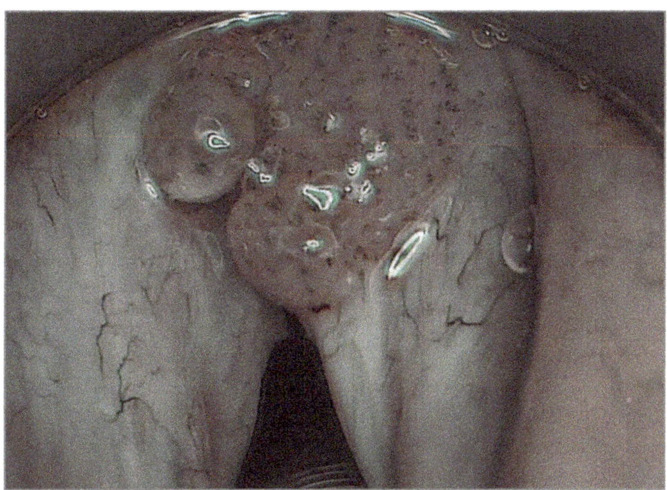

FIG. 15.47: Image 15.45 in SB mode. (E-SA)

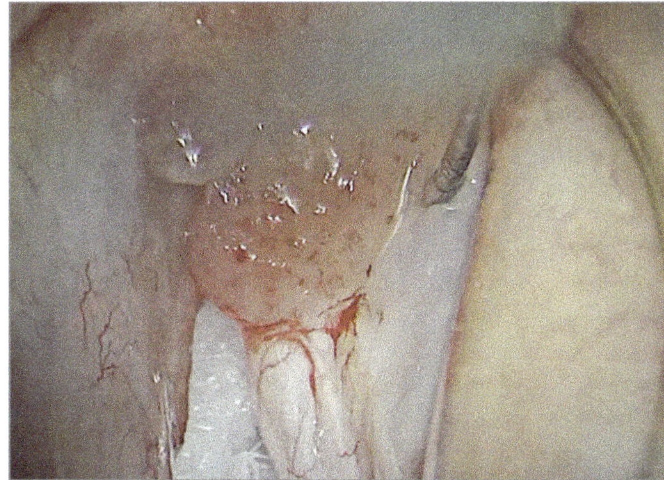

FIG. 15.48: SEIT, blanching of right vocal fold due to infiltration. (M-CC)

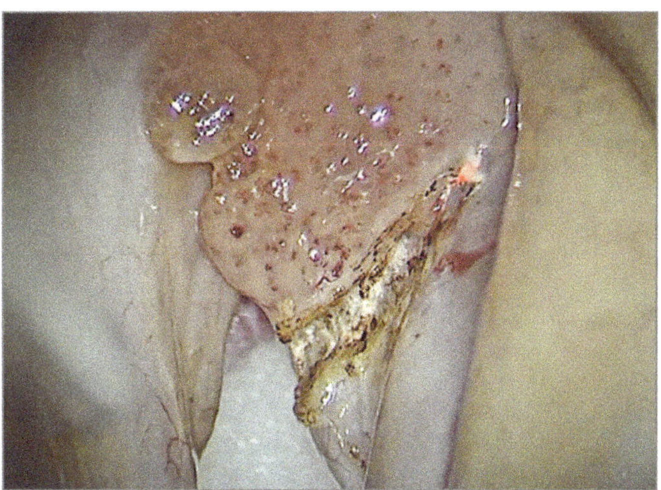

FIG. 15.49: CO_2 laser excsion using the acublade is performed. The epithelial cordotomy is made lateral to the lesion from a posterior to anterior direction in this case. (M-CC)

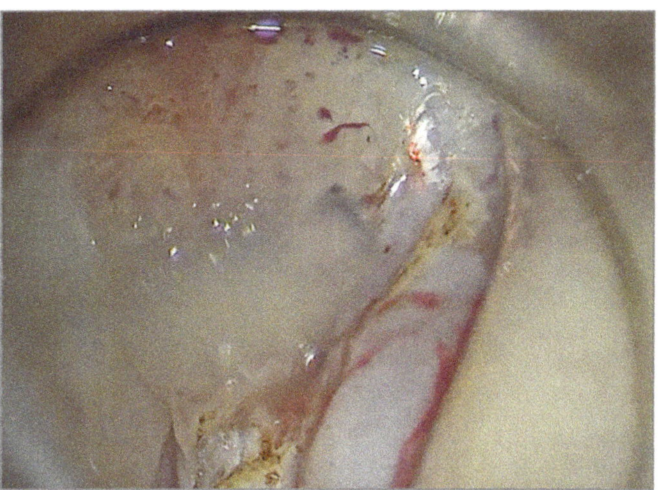

FIG. 15.50: Retraction of the lesion medially, with a blunt microflap elevator, permits anterior dissection. (M-CC)

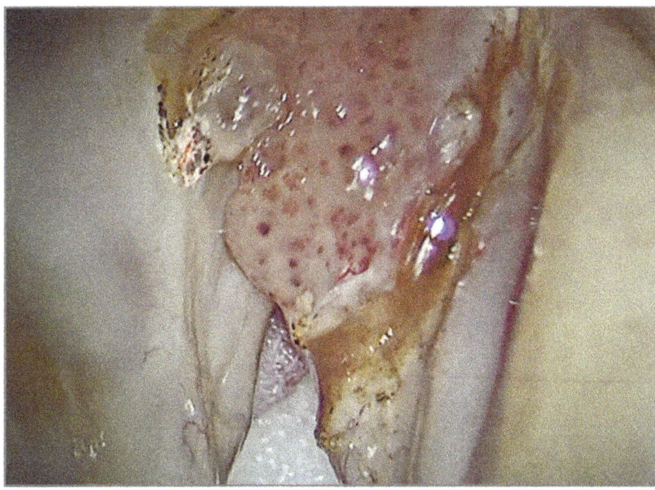

FIG. 15.51: The incision is now carried forward onto the left vocal fold, lateral to the anterior commissure lesion on the left side. Thus a horseshoe excision of the entire lesion is performed. (M-CC)

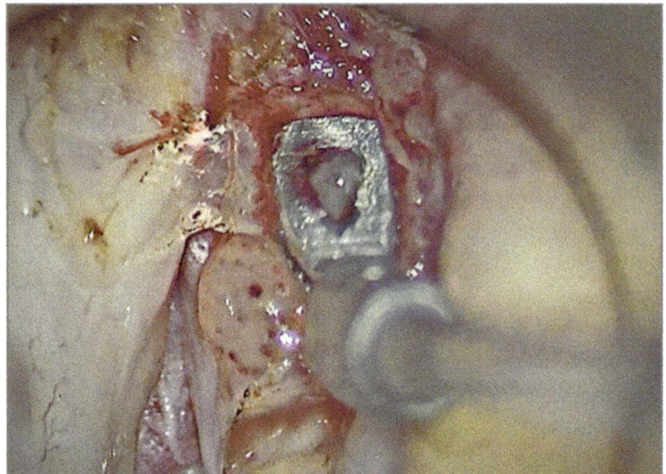

FIG. 15.52: Medial retraction of the lesion at the anterior commissure aids in the final excision. (M-CC)

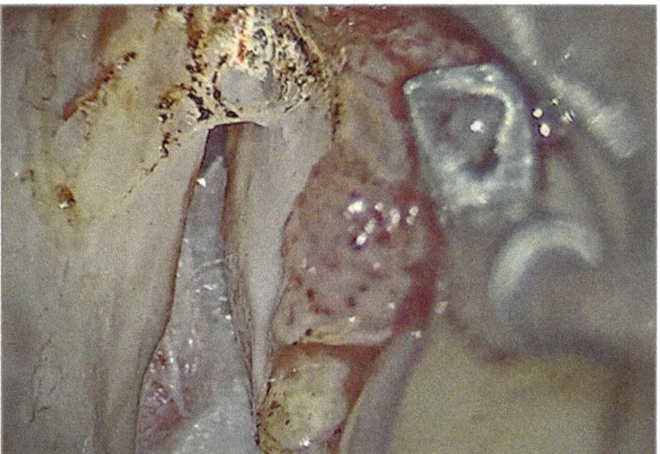

FIG. 15.53: The raw area created at the anterior commisure would result in a postoperative web, thus the patient has been counseled that a clean up procedure shall be performed in 7–10 days time. The slough is cleaned up at that time, minimising the web formation. (M-CC)

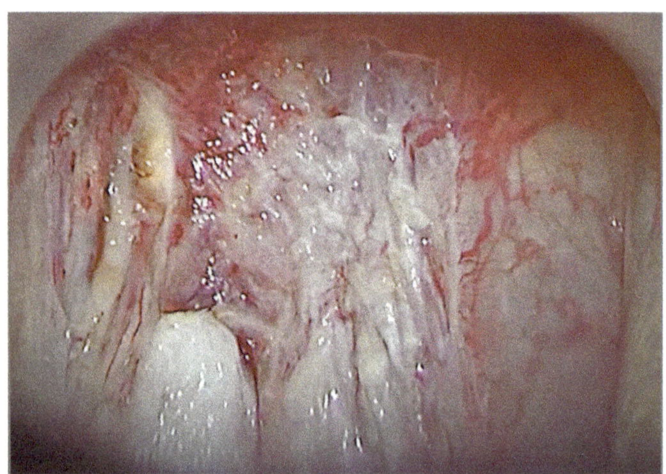

FIG. 15.54: Final postoperative image. (M-CC)

CASE 6

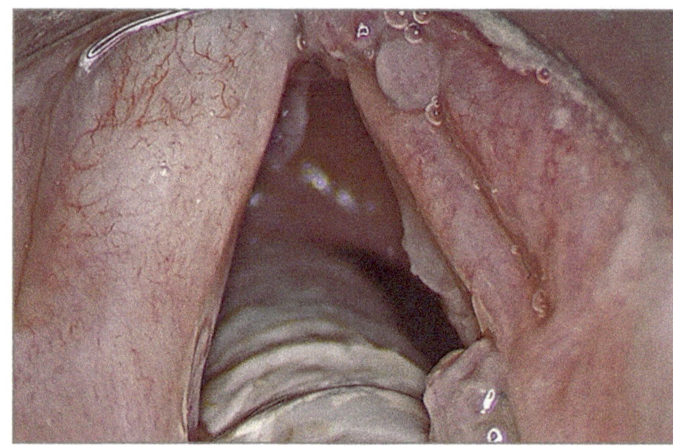

FIG. 15.55: AORRP in an adult male patient, with fronds of papilloma at the right ventricle, right infraglottic surface, and over the vocal process area of the right vocal fold. An area of fibrosis is seen near the left posterior ventricle due to the previous surgeries. (E-CC)

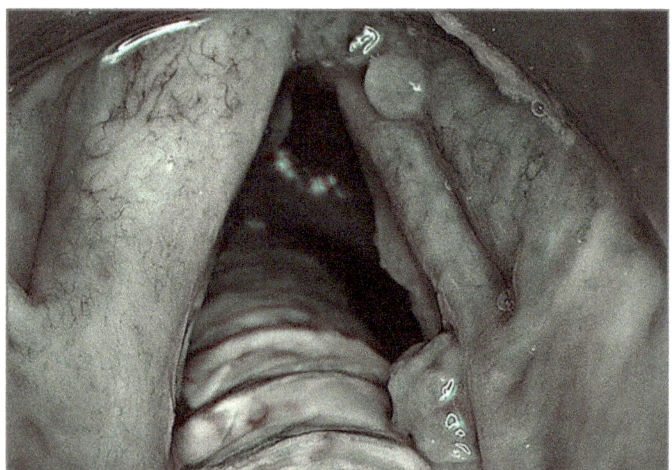

FIG. 15.56: Image 15.55 in SA mode. (E-SA)

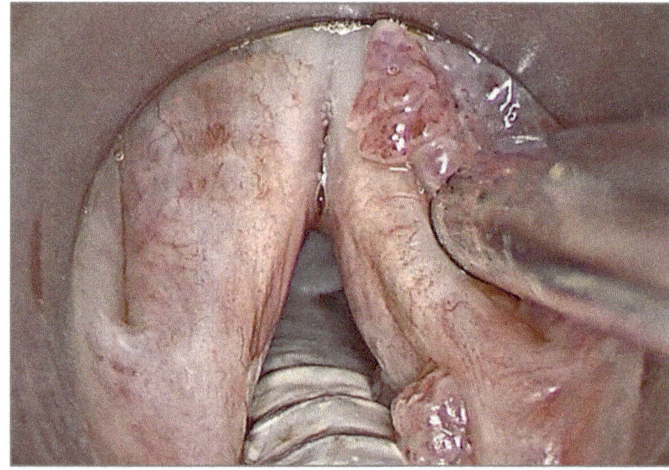

FIG. 15.57: Tricut laryngeal microdebrider, 3.5 mm, being used to excise the right anterior papillomas. This entire case is managed with a 0 degree bronchoscopic telescope and microdebrider. (M-CC)

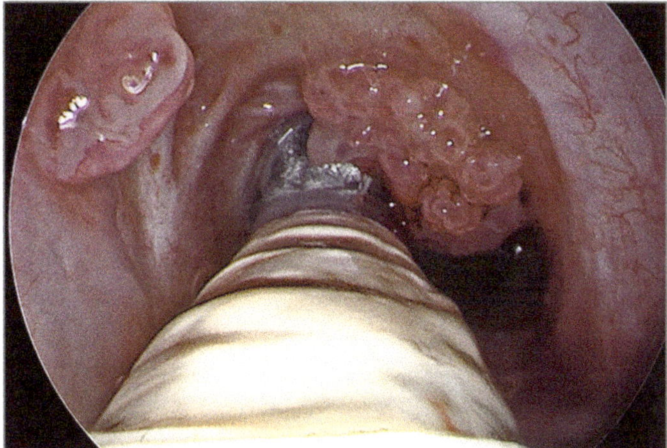

FIG. 15.58: This patient has subglottic and tracheal papillomas seen by the side of a 5 number laser endotracheal tube. (E-CC)

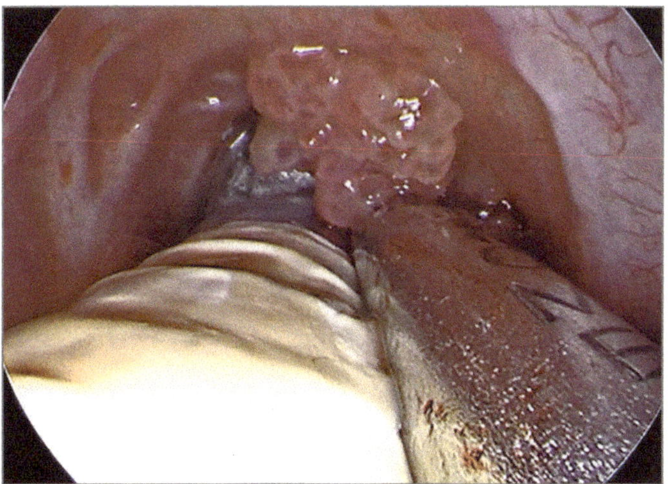

FIG. 15.59: Tracheal papillomas being debulked with a 3.5 tricut microdebrider blade. (E-CC)

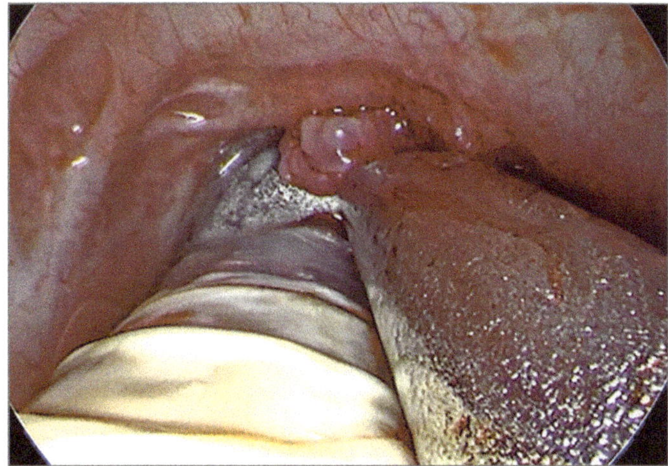

FIG. 15.60: As the debridement is currently above the inflated cuff of the endotracheal tube, the patients airway is protected. (E-CC)

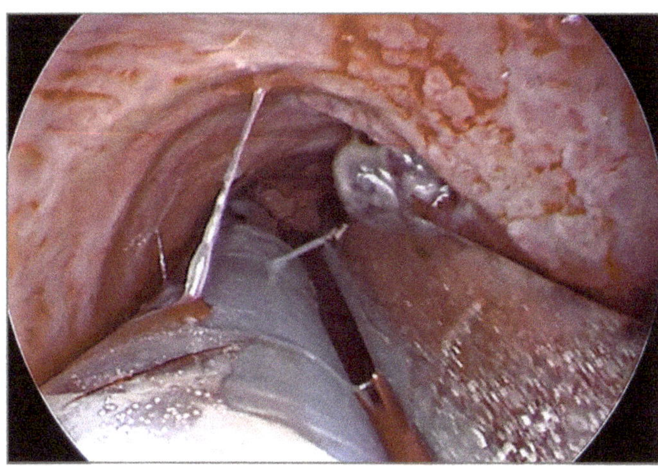

FIG. 15.61: In order to access the distal tracheal papillomas, the cuff is deflated and debulking performed by the side of this deflated cuff. Suctioning is performed as needed to protect the distal airway. (E-CC)

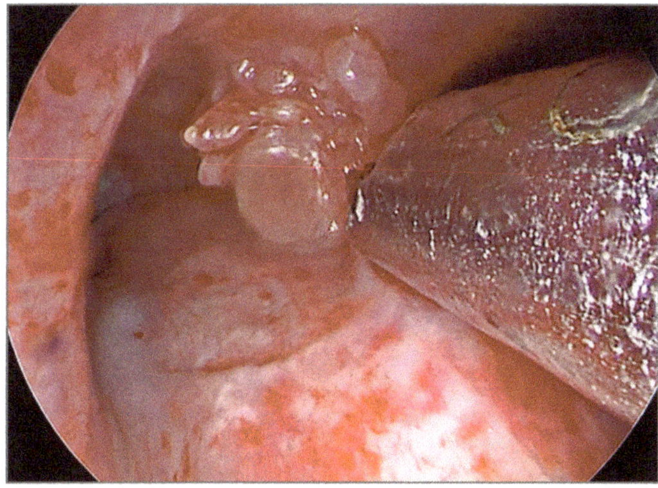

FIG. 15.62: The patient also has carinal papillomas and a tracheal blade (longer length than laryngeal blade) is used for debulking of disease at this point. (E-CC)

CASE 7

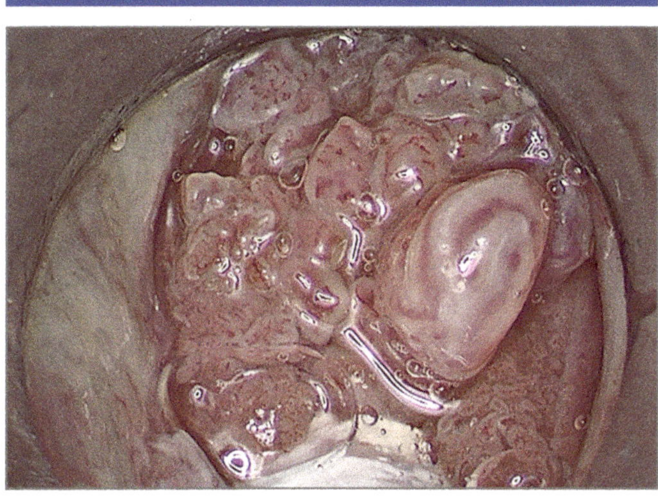

FIG. 15.63: JORRP in a 4-year-old patient, Dickers grade 3. (E-CC)

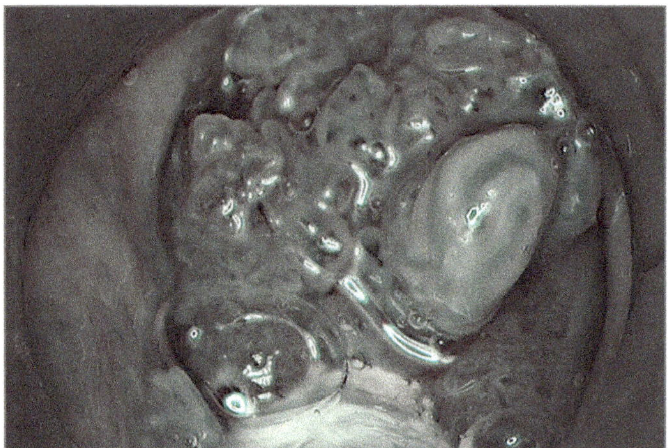

FIG. 15.64: Image 15.63 in SA mode. (E-SA)

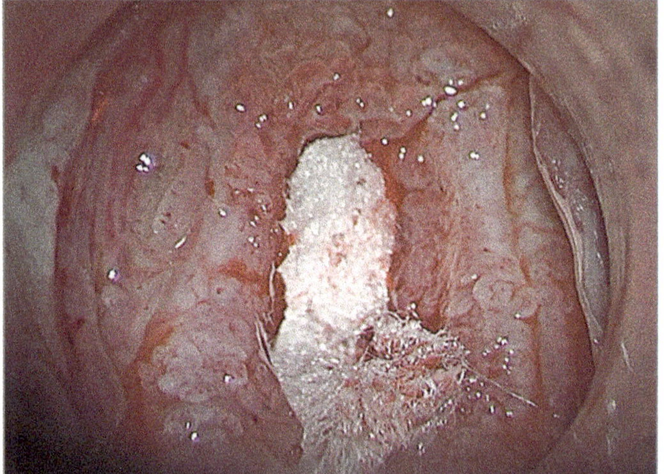

FIG. 15.65: Microdebrider debulking with a resultant oval airway. Subglottic cotton pledget is seen. (M-CC)

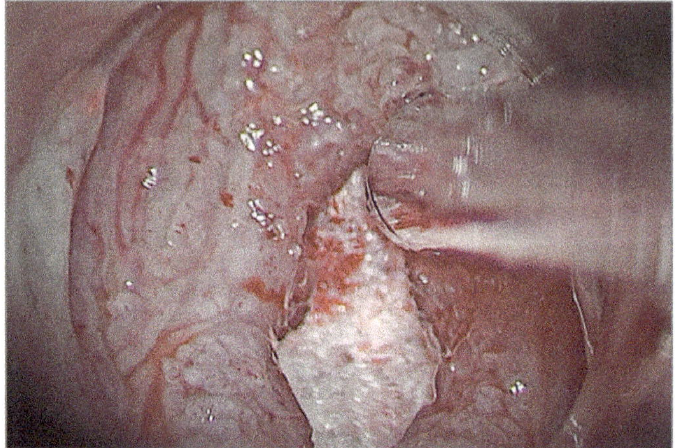

FIG. 15.66: Debulking of the right anterior commissure. (M-CC)

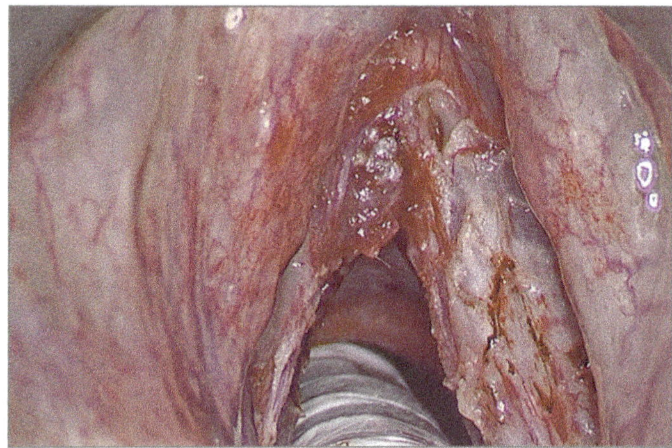

FIG. 15.67: Final postoperative image , disease intentionally left behind at the left anterior commissure in order to prevent webbing. (E-CC)

CASE 8

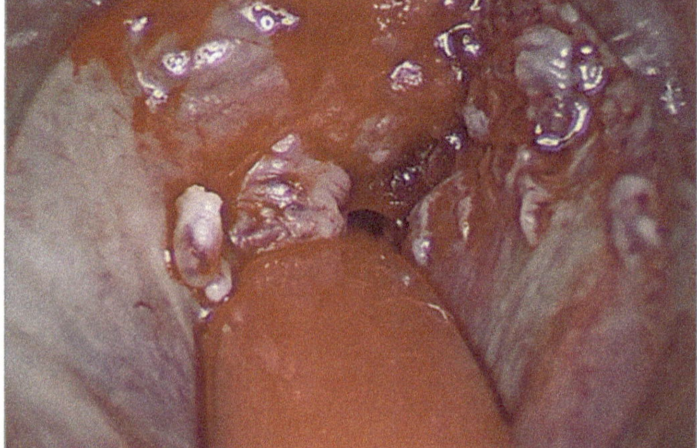

FIG. 15.68: A 19-year-old female patient was referred to our center for management of her airway. She had been operated at the age of 17 and 18 years prior to this referral, but with no definite histopathology available. The patient presented with diffuse papillomatous growths over her larynx and a right immobile vocal fold. There was a bilateral subepithelial supraglottic bulge. The histopathology of the first four surgeries was RRP, however, at the time of the 5th surgery, the disease appeared more invasive and the histopathology was invasive squamous cell carcinoma. (M-CC)

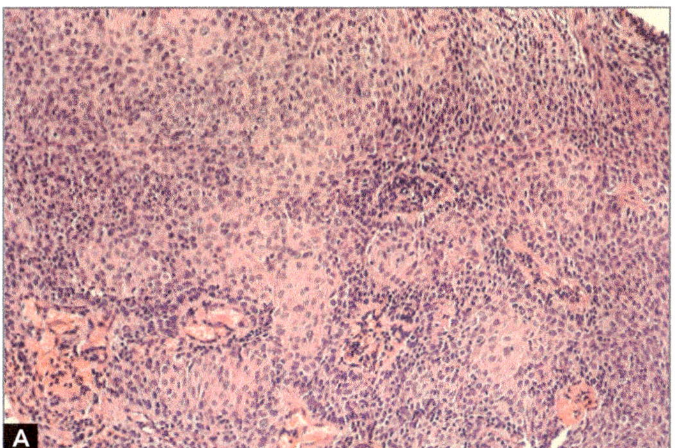

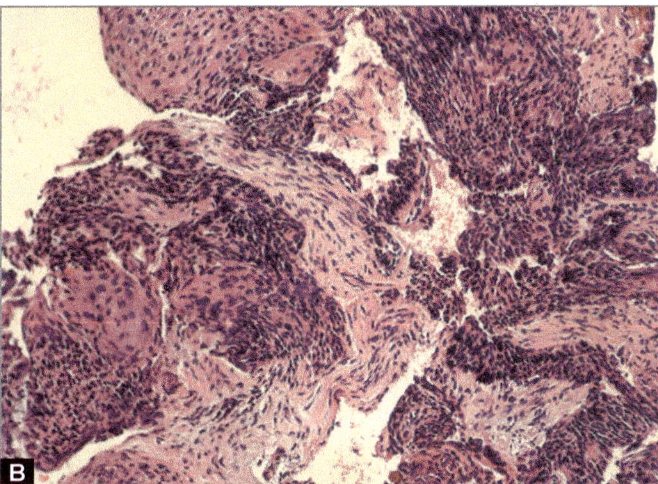

FIG. 15.69: The histopathology of the 5th surgery revealed invasive squamous cell carcinoma. She has undergone a total laryngectomy with neck dissection and postoperative radiation therapy and is currently well controlled

THE FUTURE

Recurrent respiratory papilloma is a viral disease and a safe and specific antiviral would probably be a good treatment modality. It is hoped that vaccination over time will bring down the viral presence in individuals and the community as a whole.

Immunomodulation may have a role to play in disease control and genetic predilection in parents is also being studied in a few centers.[13]

REFERENCES

1. San Giorgi M, van den Heuvel ER, Tjon Plan Gi RE, et al. Age of onset of recurrent respiratory papillomatosis: A distribution analysis. Clin Otolaryngol. 2016;41(5):448-53.
2. Omland T, Lie KA, Akre H, et al. Recurrent respiratory papillomatosis: HPV genotypes and risk of high-grade laryngeal neoplasia. PLos One. 2014:9(6):99114.
3. Frederik D. Recurrent respiratory papillomatosis and Narrow Band Imaging. In: Nerurkar NK, Rowchoudhury A, editors. Textbook of laryngology: Official publication of the Association of Phonosurgeons of India. New Delhi: Jaypee Brothers Medical Publishers (P) Ltd.; 2017. pp. 230-6.
4. Farzad I, Rasool H, Hadi G, et al. The role of Human papilloma virus (HPV) genotyping in recurrent respiratory papillomatosis in Rasoul Akram Hospital. Med J Islam Repub Iran. 2012;26(2):90-3.
5. Tjon Pian Gi RE, San Giorgi MR, Slagter-Menkema L, et al. The clinical course of recurrent respiratory papillomatosis: A comparison between aggressiveness of human papilloma virus-6 and human papilloma virus-11. Head Neck. 2015;37(11):1625-32.
6. Kashima HK, Shah F, Lyles A, et al. A comparison of risk factors in juvenile-onset and adult-onset recurrent respiratory papillomatosis. Laryngoscope. 1992;102:9-13.
7. Derkay CS, Malis DJ, Zalzal G, et al. A staging system for assessing severity of disease and response to therapy in recurrent respiratory papillomatosis. Laryngoscope. 1998;108:935-7.
8. Dikkers FG. Treatment of recurrent respiratory papillomatosis with microsurgery in combination with Intralesional cidofovir—A prospective study. Eur Arch Otolaryngol. 2006;263:440-3.
9. Kashima H , Mounts P, Leventhal B, et al. Sites of predilectioninrecurrent respiratory apillomatosis. Ann Otol Rhino Laryngol. 1993;102:580-3.
10. Derkay CS, Task force on recurrent respiratory papillomas. A preliminary report. Arch Otolaryngol Head Neck Surg. 1995;121:1386-91.
11. Strong MS, Vaughan CW, Cooperband SR, et al. Recurrent respiratory papillomatosis:management with the CO2 laser. Ann Otol Rhinol Laryngol. 1976;85:508-16.
12. Weiss MD, Kashima HK. Tracheal involvement in laryngeal papillomatosis. Laryngoscope. 1983;93;45-8.
13. Pawlita M, Gissmann L. Recurrent respiratory papillomatosis—Indication for vaccination?) [Article in German]. Dtsch Med Woche. 2009;134(2): 100-2.

CHAPTER 16

Amyloidosis

DEFINITION

Amyloidosis is an idiopathic disorder where soluble protein is converted into insoluble, fibrillar, and amorphous protein with extracellular deposition within various tissues. It is considered to be a protein misfolding disorder.

Virchow in 1858 described tissue that had a starch-like reaction to iodine and sulfuric acid.[1] Amylon is translated as "starch" and eidos as "similar to" in Greek.

The main components of amyloid are the fibrillary protein, which constitutes the bulk (90%) of the tissue, and is characteristic for each different type of disease. Stacks of doughnut-shaped and rod-shaped proteins, which are common in all types of amyloidosis, form the amyloid P component (10%). Glycosaminoglycan, which forms a fraction of the amyloidosis, is responsible for the positive reaction with iodine.

CLASSIFICATION

Amyloidosis may be classified as localized or systemic, or it may be classified as familial, primary or secondary to underlying chronic infections.

A classification proposed by Symmers[2] is as follows:

- Primary amyloid (localized or general)
- Secondary amyloid (localized or general)
- Amyloid associated with multiple myeloma
- Hereditary or familial amyloid.

The current classification commonly followed is based on the type of protein. Most common amyloid proteins are AL, AA, and A beta.

Classification Based on Amyloid Protein

- AL (amyloid light-chain): Protein is derived from kappa or lambda immunoglobulin light chains of plasma cells. It is postulated that plasma cells located in the periphery of the localized amyloidosis may be the source of the amyloid fibrils. The amyloidosis in this group may be localized, systemic, or seen with multiple myeloma
- AA (amyloid associated): A unique nonimmunoglobulin protein of hepatic origin is found. The amyloidosis is secondary usually associated with inflammatory/infectious diseases
- A beta: Amyloid plaques are deposited in neurons causing Alzheimer's.

LARYNGEAL AMYLOIDOSIS

Though laryngeal amyloidosis constitutes less than 5% of patients with amyloidosis, larynx is the commonest site of isolated amyloid disease in the head and neck. Laryngeal amyloidosis is found to be AL type. Females are more commonly affected with the 50–70 years age group being most commonly involved.

The other head and neck sites are nasopharynx, salivary glands, peripheral nervous system, eye, oral cavity, oropharynx, and tracheobronchial tree. In contrast to other head and neck locations, lingual amyloid is frequently a target organ of systemic amyloidosis

In 1875, Burow and Neumann[3] described the first case of laryngeal amyloidosis. From then until 1990, more than 300 cases of laryngeal amyloidosis have been recorded in the literature.

Hoarseness is the commonest symptom. Occasionally present is dyspnea, globus, hemoptysis, dysphagia, and aspiration

In 1919, New[4] described two types of laryngeal pictures, a discrete tumor nodule or diffuse subepithelial disease.

Multiple areas within the larynx may be involved (75%), with the false vocal folds and ventricle being the commonest. The true vocal folds, arytenoids, and in 30% even the subglottis may be involved. The amyloid tissue is typically firm, nonulcerated submucosal lesion with a yellow-orange or gray hue.

Though systemic involvement and multiple myeloma is very rare with laryngeal amyloidosis, it is still essential to rule it out.

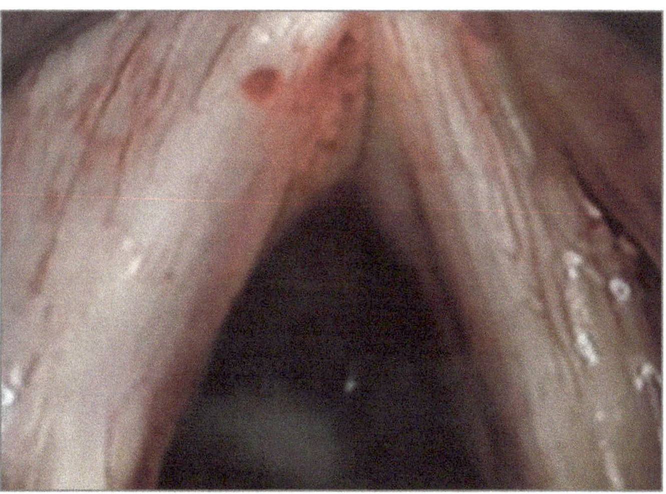

FIG. 16.1: Discrete tumor nodule seen at the left anterior commissure (M-HD)

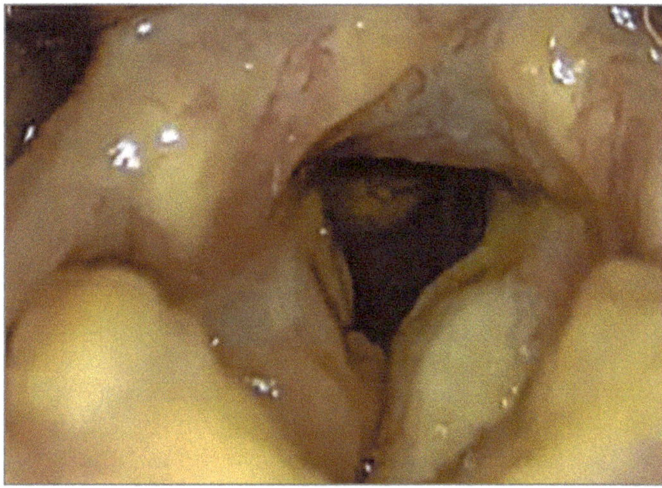

FIG. 16.2: Diffuse subepithelial disease seen on the lateral edges of the laryngeal surface of the epiglottis and both the false vocal folds. The amyloid has a classical yellow hue to it. (70 degree stroboscopy)

Symptoms

Dysphonia without stridor is the commonest presentation of laryngeal amyloidosis. The commonest cause of dysphonia is ventricular phonation pattern due to enlarged ventricular folds that do not permit optimal glottal closure. There is, thus, a hindrance to the formation of a normal mucosal wave. Dyspnea, hemoptysis, and dysphagia may also be seen.

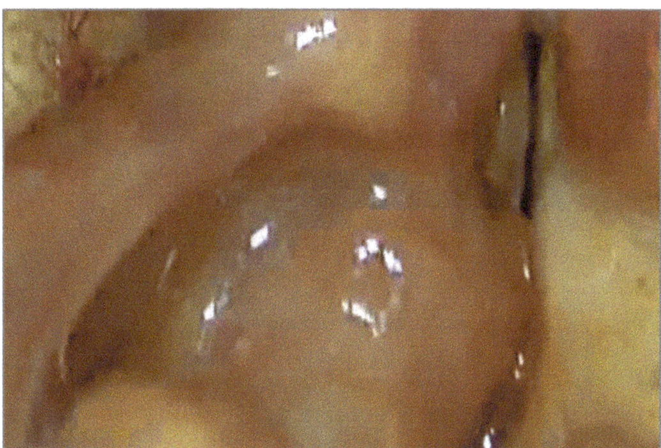

FIG. 16.3: Laryngeal amyloidosis involving the false vocal folds, and resulting in a ventricular phonation pattern. (70° stroboscopy)

Role of CT Scan of the Neck

A CT scan of the neck, in cases of laryngeal amyloidosis, helps to delineate the extent of the lesions. Relatively well-defined mucosal masses, of soft tissue density with variable enhancement, with no associated bone destruction or lymphadenopathy are observed.

The amyloidosis may also present as diffuse intralaryngeal soft tissue infiltration or circumferential glottic or subglottic soft tissue thickening with occasional intralesional calcifications seen.

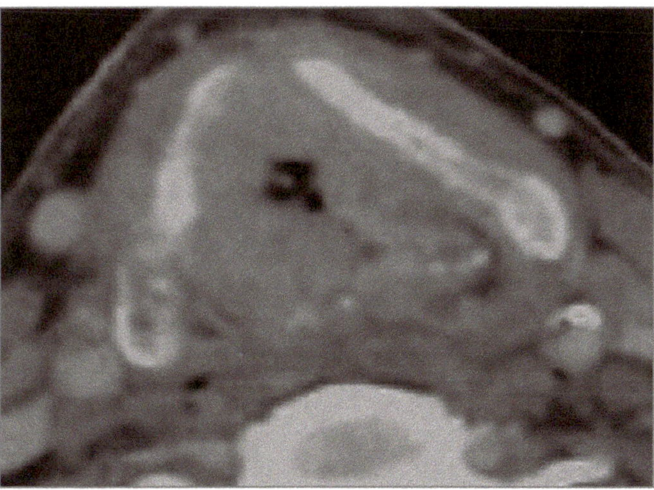

FIG. 16.4: CT scan in a patient of isolated laryngeal amyloidosis revealing circumferential glottic soft tissue thickening with absence of any thyroid cartilage destruction

Philosophy of Surgery

The aim of treatment is to obtain a long disease-free interval, while preserving the voice and swallowing function.

Conservative resection of significantly obstructive lesions using a CO_2 or KTP laser is performed under anesthesia. Staged surgery is performed when indicated to prevent anterior webbing. If a single stage anterior commissure surgery is performed, cleaning up slough tissue 7–10 days postoperatively decreases the web formation.

Today, even a severe, recurrent, transglottic, bilateral, and bulky amyloid can be tackled using multiple resections with the CO_2 laser

HISTOPATHOLOGY

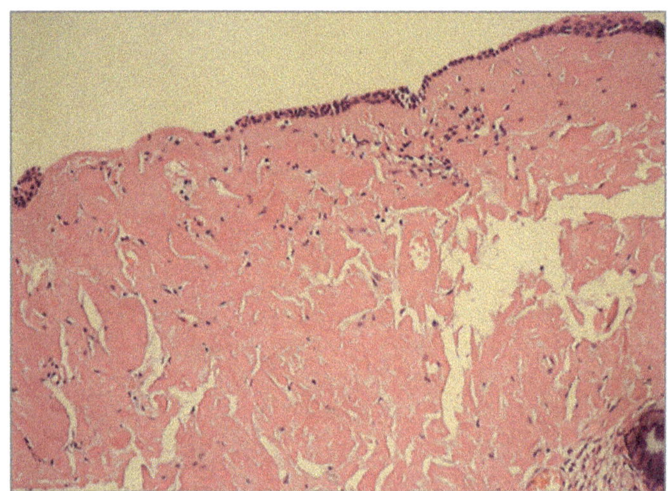

FIG. 16.5: Amyloid deposition on light microscopy with H&E staining reveals subepithelial deposition as sheets or globules of amorphous, homogenous, eosinophilic material

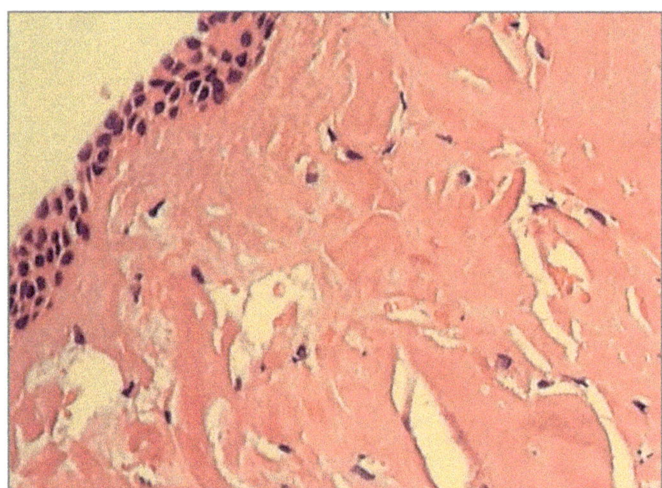

FIG. 16.6: High power image of 16.5

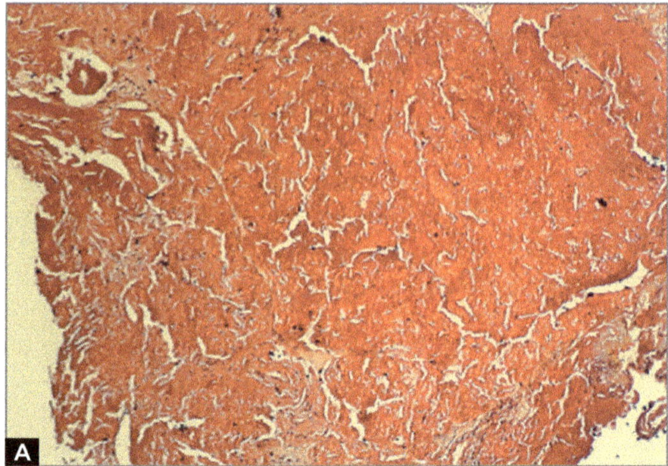

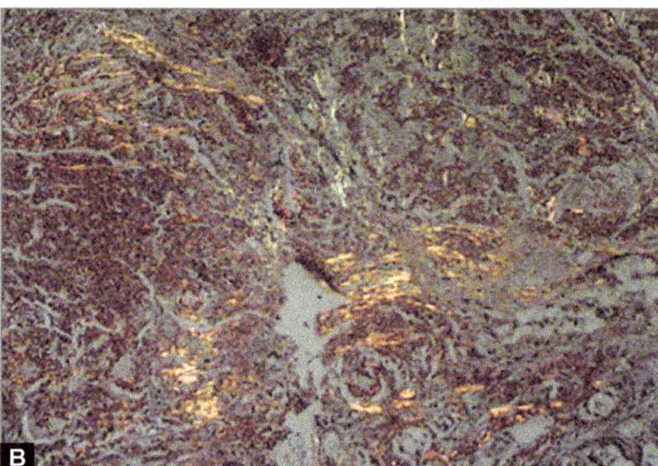

FIG. 16.7: Special stains are to be performed to confirm amyloidosis. The amyloid tissue is stained with Congo red **(A)** and then viewed under polarizing light. A typical apple green birefringence **(B)** is obtained due to the cross-beta-pleated configuration of the amyloid fibrils

ELECTRON MICROSCOPY APPEARANCE OF AMYLOID

Amyloid consists of linear, nonbranching fibrils, 7.5–10 nm in width. The arrangement of the fibrils in a cross beta pleated sheet configuration produces the specific staining properties of amyloid.

DIAGNOSTIC WORKUP

Diagnostic workup to rule out systemic amyloidosis and to rule out multiple myeloma, tuberculosis, rheumatic disease, and medullary thyroid cancer consists of the following:

- Complete blood count, erythrocyte sedimentation rate
- Blood urea nitrogen, creatinine
- Serum glutamic oxaloacetic transaminase, Serum glutamic pyruvic transaminase

- Ultrasound of the abdomen
- Two-dimensional echocardiography
- Chest X-ray
- Computed tomography scan/magnetic resonance imaging
- Tuberculin skin test
- Antinuclear antibody, rheumatoid factor
- Serum and urine immunoelectrophoresis
- Urine analysis for Bence Jones proteins
- Bone marrow biopsy
- Fine-needle aspiration of abdominal fat has been shown to be a simple and effective procedure to rule out systemic amyloidosis.

CASE 1

A 55-year-old lady was diagnosed in another center as amyloidosis and was referred with hoarseness to our center for further management. Three surgeries had been performed on her within a period of 15 months duration. Laryngoscopy revealed amyloid tissue primarily in both the false vocal folds; consequently the false vocal folds were in contact with one another in adduction (16.8A) and abduction (16.8B).

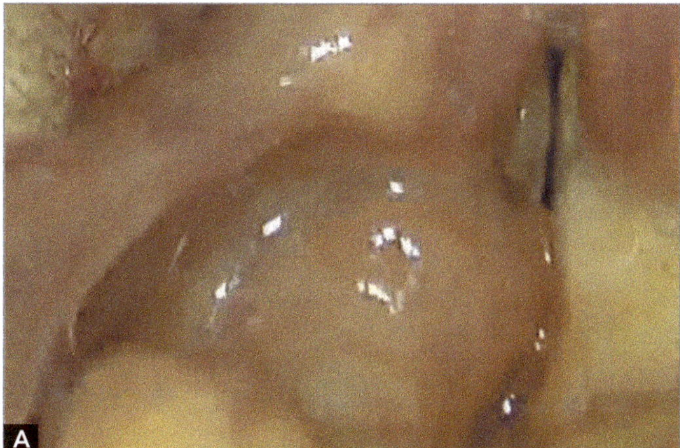

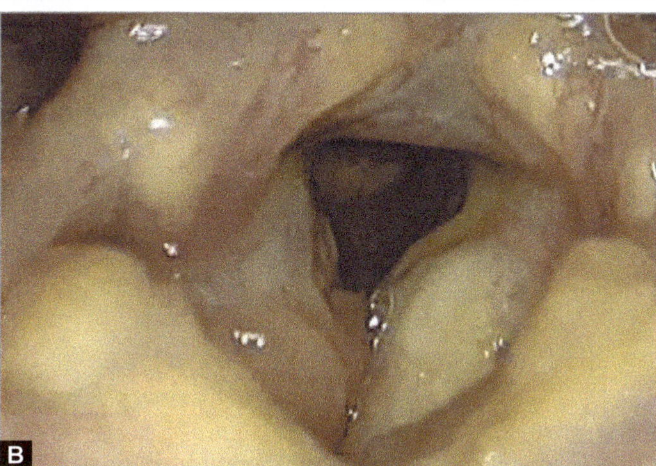

FIG. 16.8: Laryngoscopy in **A,** adduction and **B,** abduction

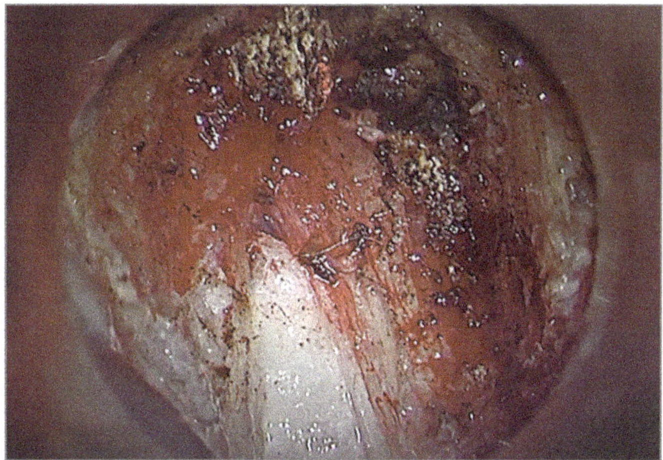

FIG. 16.9: CO_2 laser ablation being performed in a super pulse continuous mode. The disease has been excised even at the anterior commissure necessitating a clean up of the anterior commissure slough in 7–10 days time. (M-CC)

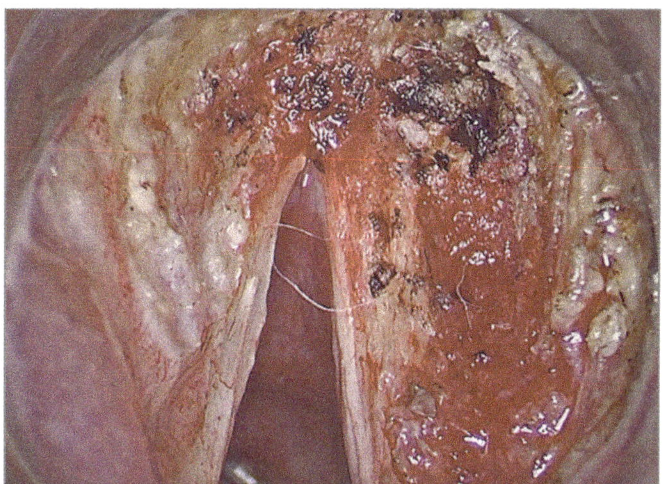

FIG. 16.10: Postoperative image of the debulking performed in both the ventricles and false vocal folds. (E-CC)

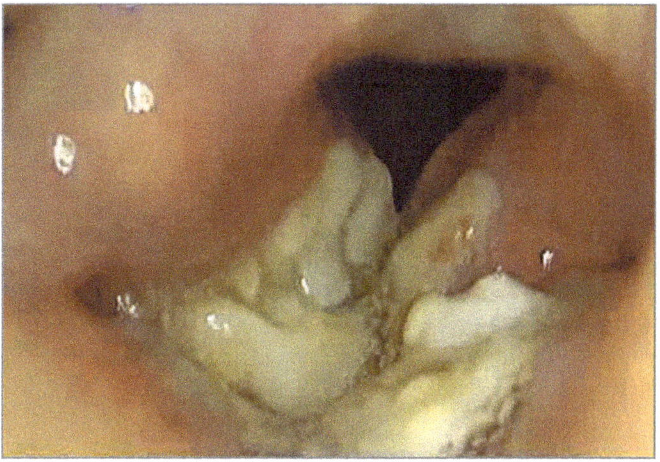

FIG. 16.11: Postoperative slough present 3 weeks later on laryngoscopy. This was cleaned up under general anesthesia. (WL laryngoscopy)

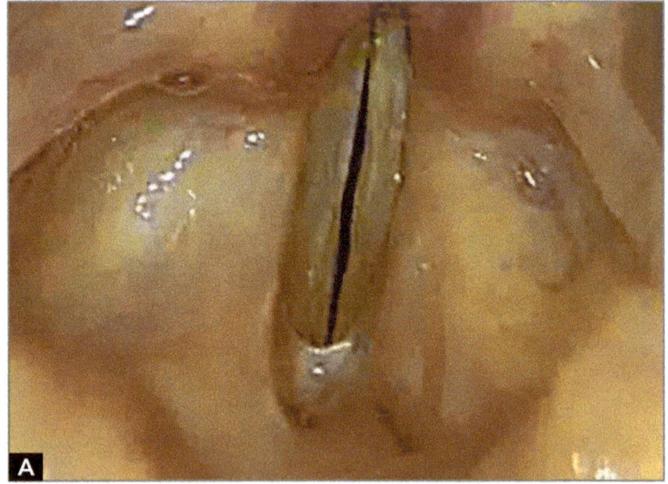

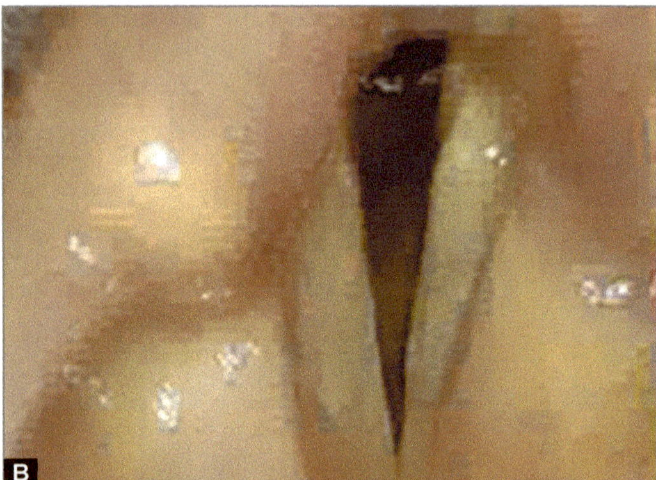

FIG. 16.12: Laryngoscopy in adduction **(A)** and abduction **(B)** 7 months after primary surgery. The false vocal folds do not meet each other even on adduction and the patient has achieved a very serviceable voice quality since then. (70 degree stroboscopy)

CASE 2

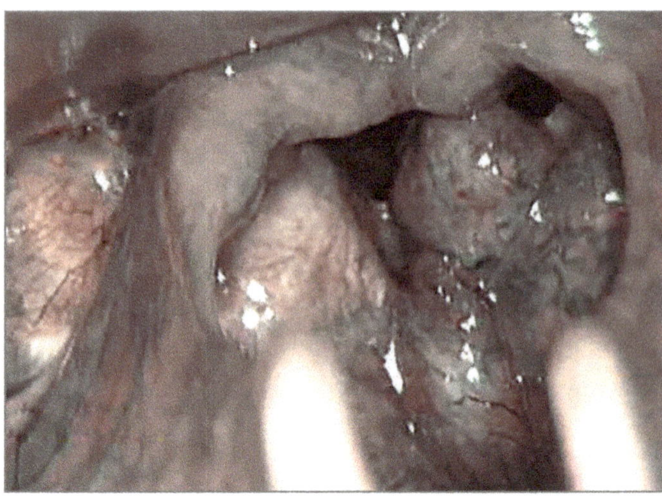

FIG. 16.14: Laryngoscopy with NBI revealed a type 2 Ni pattern of vasculature. (NBI laryngoscopy)

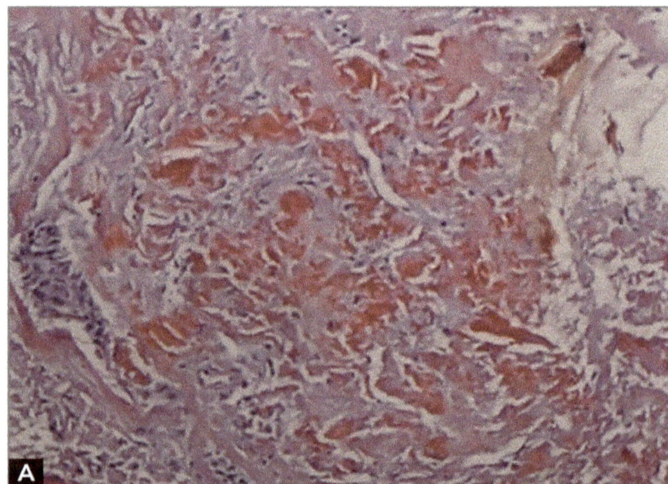

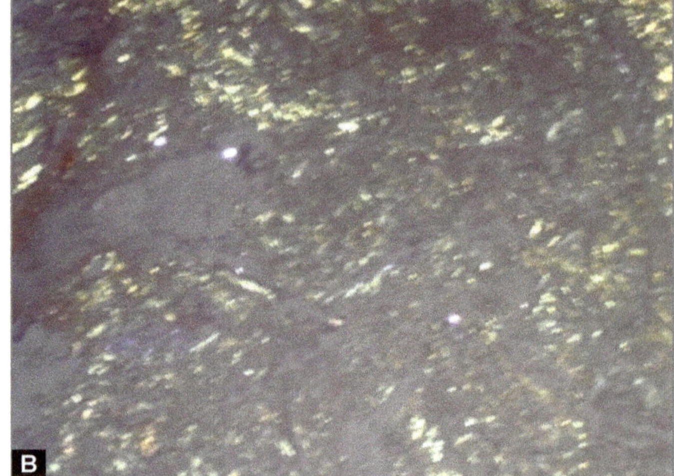

FIG. 16.15: Special stains performed on the tissue excised revealed. **A,** Congo red staining and **B,** apple green birefringence

FIG. 16.13: An adult male patient was referred to our center for hoarseness and dyspnea on exertion. Laryngoscopy revealed pedunculated, firm looking masses of both the vocal folds. (WL laryngoscopy)

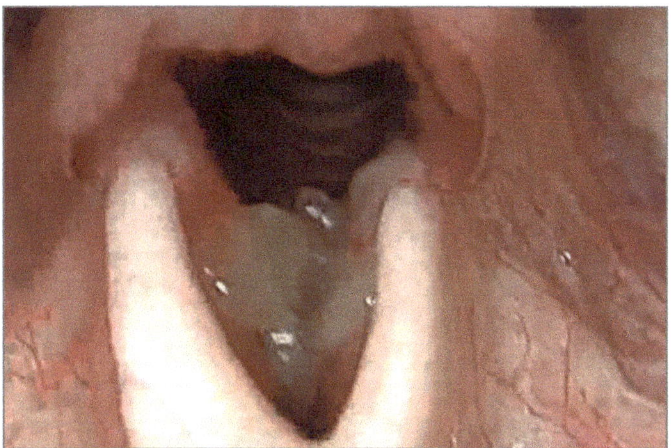

FIG. 16.16: Following CO_2 laser excision, slough is observed on the postoperative laryngoscopy 3 weeks later. This is cleaned under general anesthesia to minimize a web formation. (WL laryngoscopy)

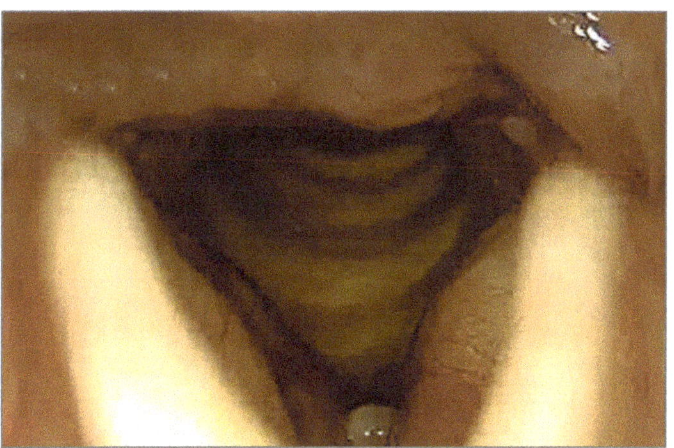

FIG. 16.17: An anterior polypoidal lesion in observed at the 4 month follow up . As the patient has a very serviceable voice, he does not want any further surgical intervention at this time and is under follow up. (WL-laryngoscopy)

CASE 3

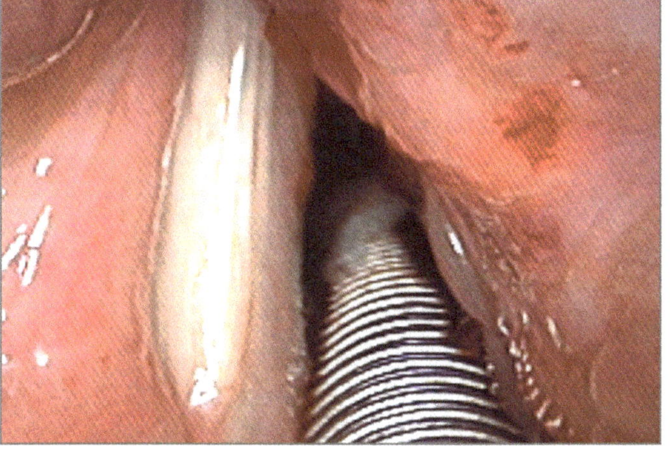

FIG. 16.18: An adult female patient was referred to us for persistent hoarseness. A right false vocal fold bulge suggesting a subepithelial lesion was observed. (E-CC)

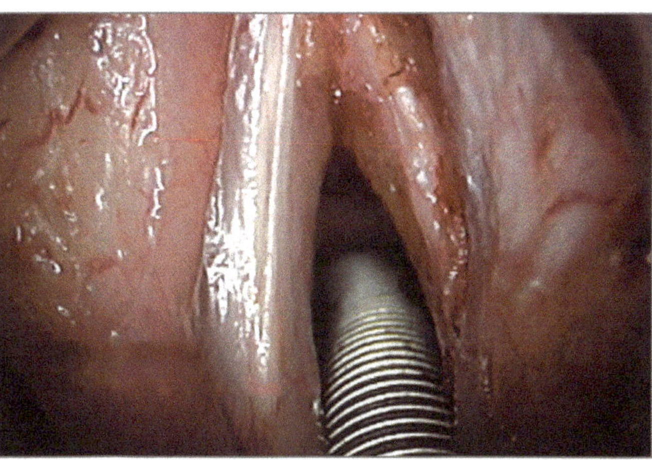

FIG. 16.19: CO_2 laser excision was performed and the histopathology and special stains revealed amyloidosis. This is the postoperative image. (E-WL)

CASE 4

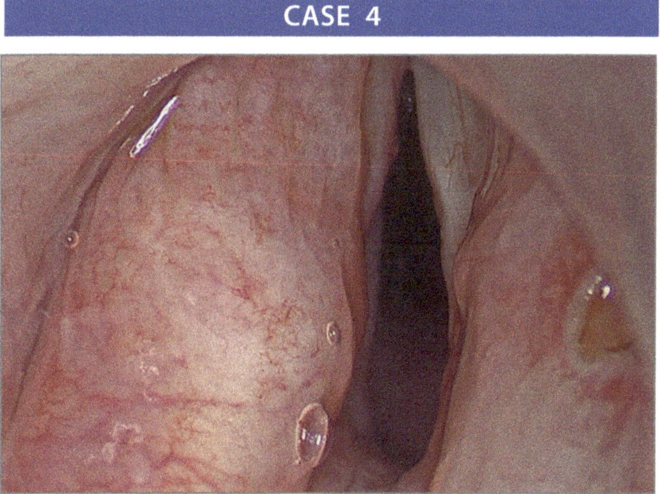

FIG. 16.20: An adult male patient presents with hoarseness and a left false vocal fold bulge is seen. (M-CC)

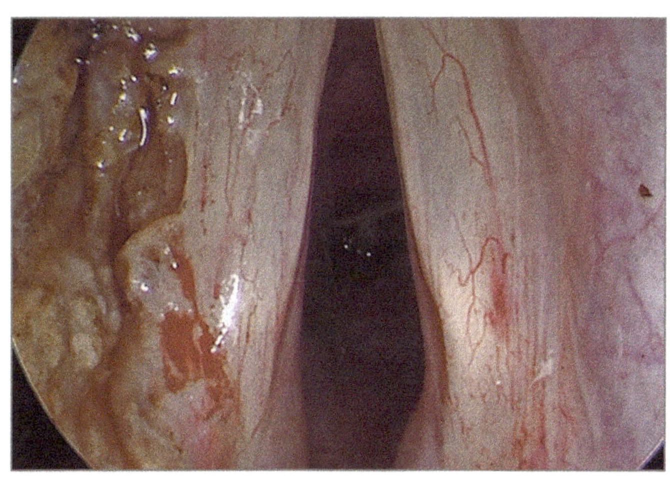

FIG. 16.21: Laser excision was performed revealing amyloidosis on histopathology. (M-CC)

CASE 5

An adult male patient presents with hoarseness and dyspnea on exertion of 4-5 months duration.

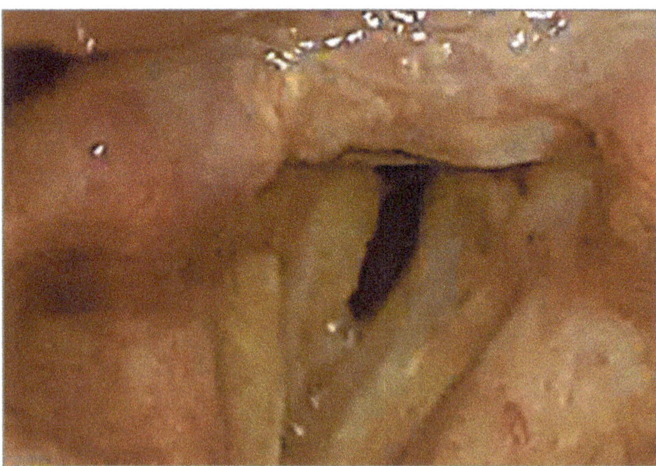

FIG. 16.22: Laryngoscopy reveals a circumferential infraglottic swelling

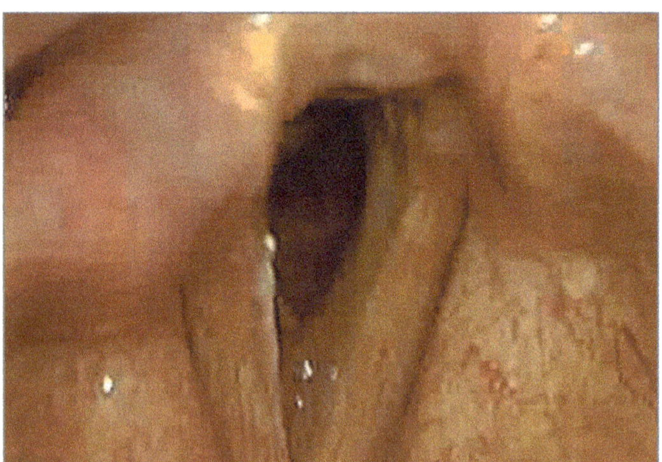

FIG. 16.23: Histopathology following laser excision reveals amyloidosis. This is the postoperative laryngoscopic image. The patient is on regular follow up for an early pick up of any recurrence. (WL-laryngoscopy)

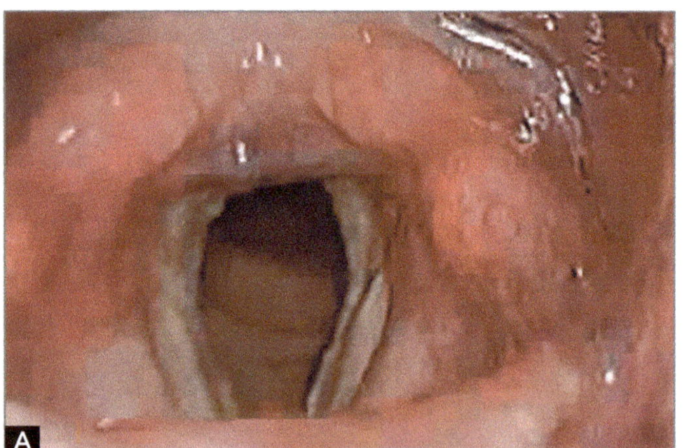

Continued

Continued

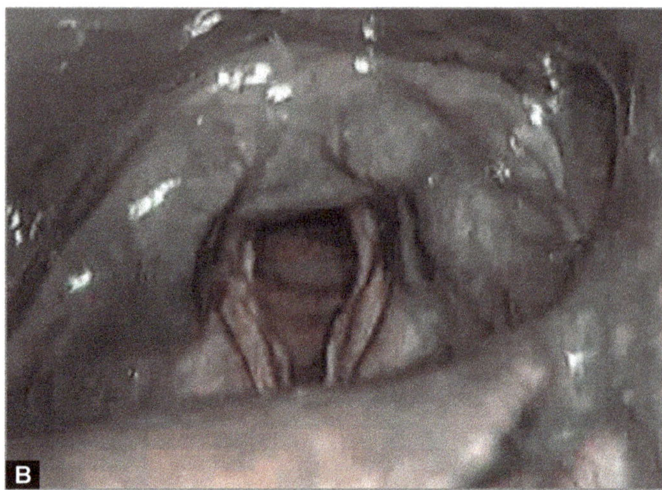

FIG. 16.24: A, WL laryngoscopy; **B,** NBI laryngoscopy

A pseudosulcus is due to an infraglottic swelling which may be due to laryngopharyngeal reflux, malignancy, tuberculosis, amyloidosis, and sarcoidosis. It should not be mistaken to be a sulcus. The laryngoscopy of a female patient with infraglottic amyloidosis is shown in figure 16.24. This may be mistakenly diagnosed as a sulcus.

FOLLOW-UP

The patients are advised a follow-up at 1-3 weeks, 3 and 6 months in the first year and then yearly. Most patients require a total of 1-2 revision surgeries.

Typically, disease progression stops after 7 years, possibly due to slowing-down of the disease, which may be caused by exhaustion of the underlying clonal plasma cells.

REFERENCES

1. Aterman K. A historical note on the iodine-sulphuric acid reaction of amyloid. Histochemistry. 1976;49(2):131-43.
2. W. St. C. Symmers, Primary Amyloidosis: A Review, J Clin Pathol. 1956;9(3):187-211.
3. Burow A, Neumann L. Amyloide degeneration von larynx tumoren, canule sieben jahre lang gretagen. Arch Clin Chir. 1875;18:242-6.
4. New GB. Amyloid tumors of the upper air passages. Laryngoscope. 1919;29:327-41.

CHAPTER 17

Fungal Laryngitis

INTRODUCTION

Fungi are organisms of low pathogenicity, manifesting as opportunistic infections, typically in an immunocompromised host.[1] Fungal laryngitis historically has been labeled as uncommon in immunocompetent patients. The commonest type of fungus to infect the larynx is *Candida albicans* seen most commonly in immunocompromised patients and those using inhaled corticosteroids.[2] Patients developing laryngeal candidiasis may also give a history of having received oral steroids for asthma or cough. Other fungi like *Aspergillus, Histoplasma, Coccidioimycosis, Blastomycosis,* and *Cryptococcus* have also been implicated.

The clinical hallmark of fungal laryngitis (especially *Candida* infection) is bilateral white plaques on a bed of severe erythema. Diagnosis should be considered in any immunocompetent patient with refractory laryngitis and with risk factors predisposing to local mucosal barrier impairment, e.g., gastropharyngeal reflux, smoking, or inhaled steroid use.[3]

Clinically, suspicion is based on white cheesy plaques seen on the vocal fold, surrounded by congestion. Most patients have an elevated ESR. Patients respond to 200 mg once a day oral fluconazole, and any previously recommended antibiotics or steroids are discontinued if feasible. In patients who show no improvement at 2 weeks, complete excision of the lesion is performed. The tissue is sent for fungal hyphae and culture, histopathology, and *Mycobacterium tuberculi* testing. Previous reports have outlined the importance of biopsy in making the diagnosis of laryngeal candidiasis.[4] However, current opinion does not feel this is necessary in most cases because clinical findings and treatment response can confirm the diagnosis.[5] Furthermore, a premature biopsy might cause vocal fold scarring, which can be extremely difficult to treat.[6]

In a study by Wong et al.,[2] 54 patients of laryngeal candidiasis were reviewed, 89% of the patients were on steroid inhalers and 7% were on oral steroids. The success rate with the first course of oral antifungals was as high as 96%.[2]

An NBI reveals an absence of type 4 and type 5 (Ni classification) vascular pattern at the periphery of the white plaques.

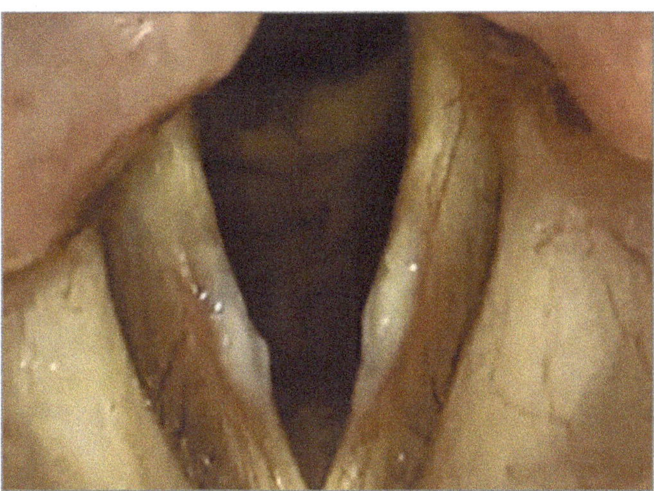

FIG. 17.1: Laryngeal candidiasis is typically seen as flaky white plaques on the vocal folds surrounded by erythema. (70 degree stroboscopy)

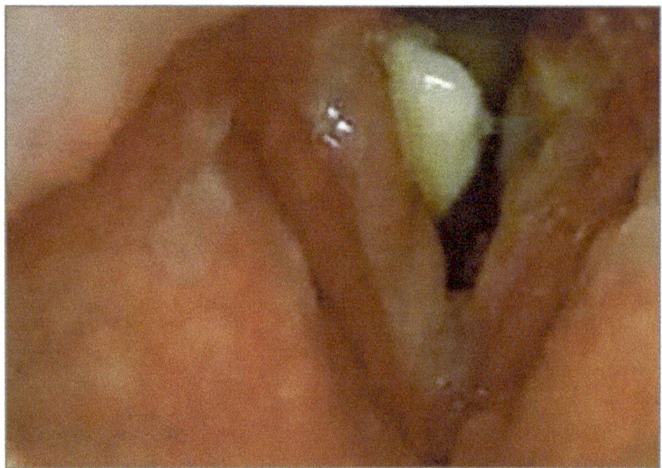

FIG. 17.2: Laryngeal aspergillosis may mimic candidial infection and even occasionally appear as a malignancy. This is the image of a patient who had concurrent tuberculosis with aspergillus infection of the larynx

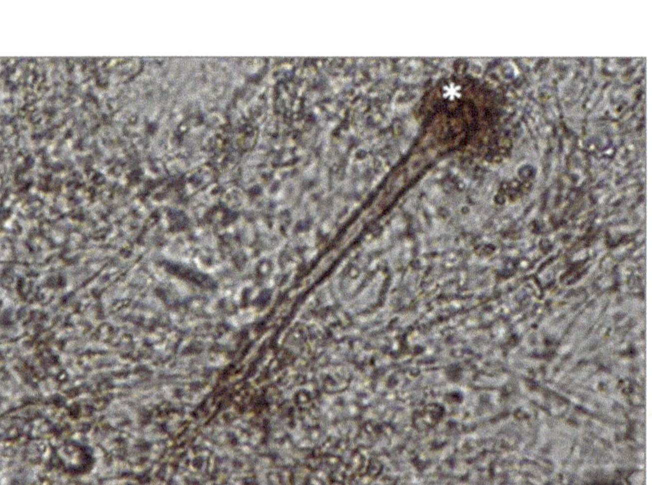

FIG. 17.3: The KOH mount revealing an unbranched conidiophore of *Aspergillus* terminating in a globose vesicle (white asterisk "*"). This patient had concurrent tuberculosis

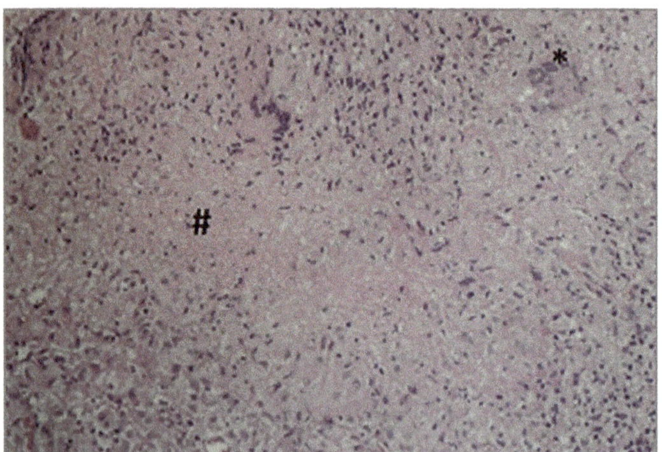

FIG. 17.4: Histopathology of the patient showing subepithelial infiltration with multinucleated giant cells (*) and necrotizing granulomas (#)

CASE 1

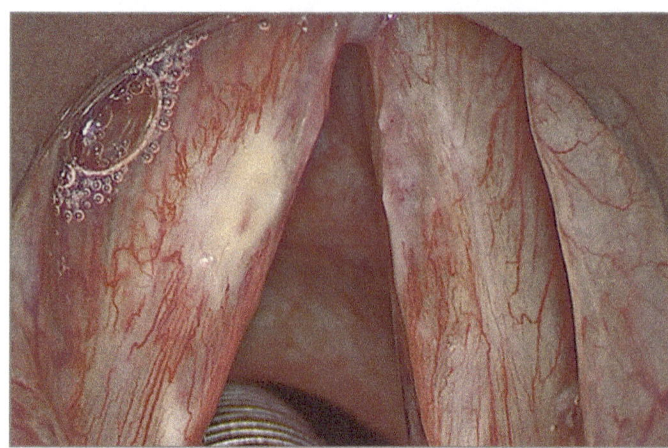

FIG. 17.5: Left vocal fold midmembranous white plaque surrounded by inflammation in a patient who complaints of persistent hoarseness. He has received 2 weeks of daily 200 mg fluconazole with no improvement. (E-CC)

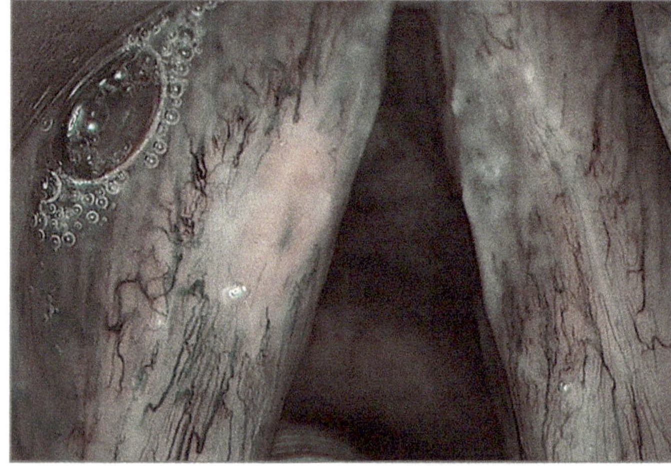

FIG. 17.6: SA image reveal an absence of type 4 or 5 Ni vascular pattern at the periphery of the white plaques. A type 1 Ni pattern is observed. (E-SA)

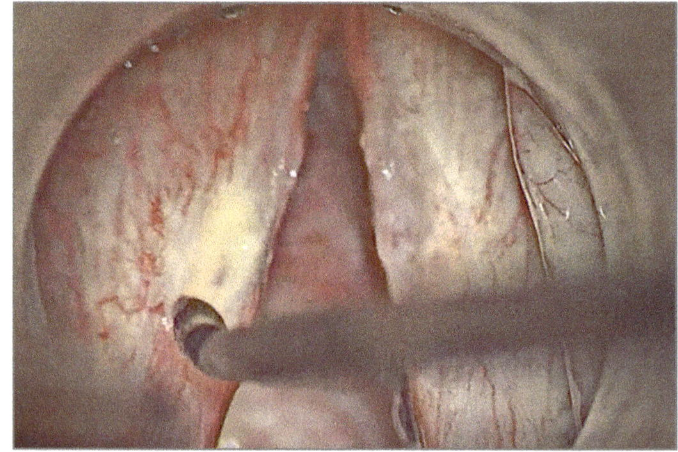

FIG. 17.7: Palpation of the lesion with a blunt microflap elevator. (M-CC)

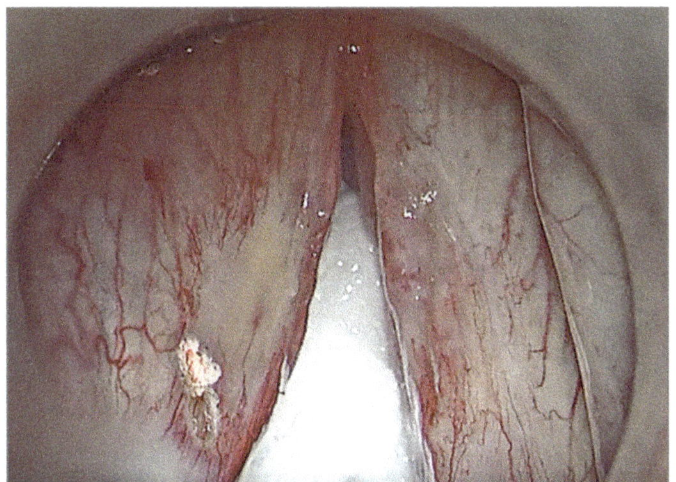

FIG. 17.8: CO_2 laser acublade being used to perform an epithelial cordotomy just lateral to the lesion. (M-CC)

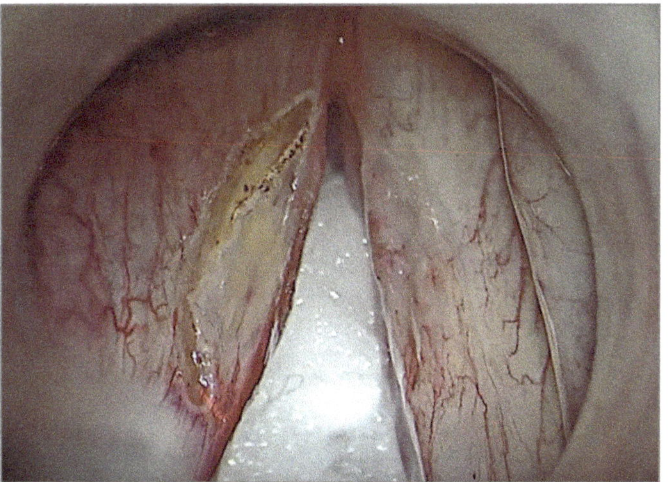

FIG. 17.9: Completion of the epithelial cordotomy from posterior to anterior. (M-CC)

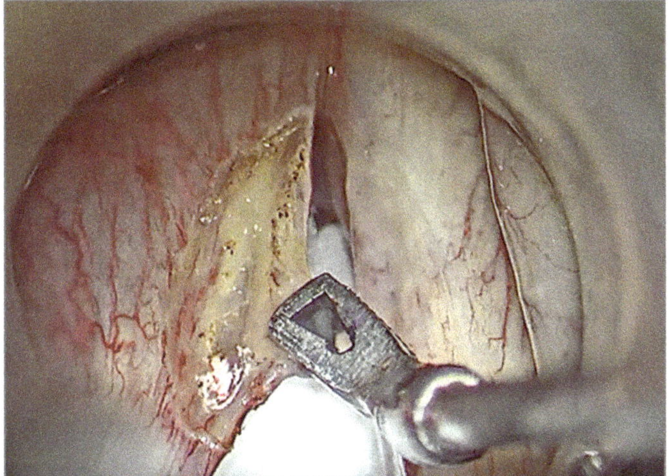

FIG. 17.10: A Bouchayer forceps is holding the epithelial lesion and gently retracting it medially while the laser excision of the microflap is being completed. A healthy SLP can be appreciated. (M-CC)

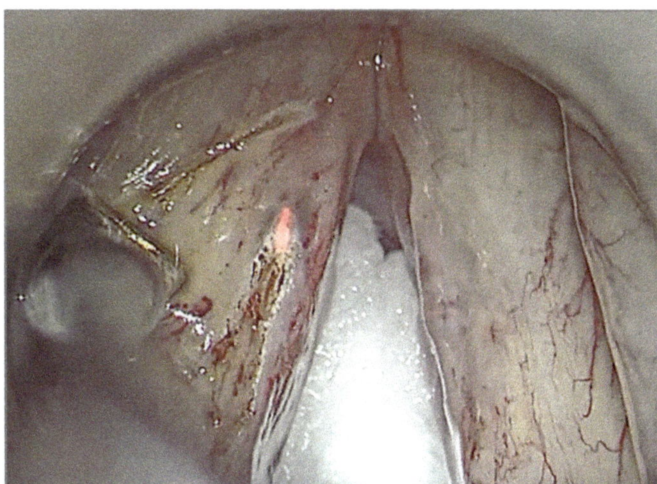

FIG. 17.11: The Bouchayer forceps is now retracting the epithelial flap laterally, such that the infraglottic laser cut may be accurately made. (M-CC)

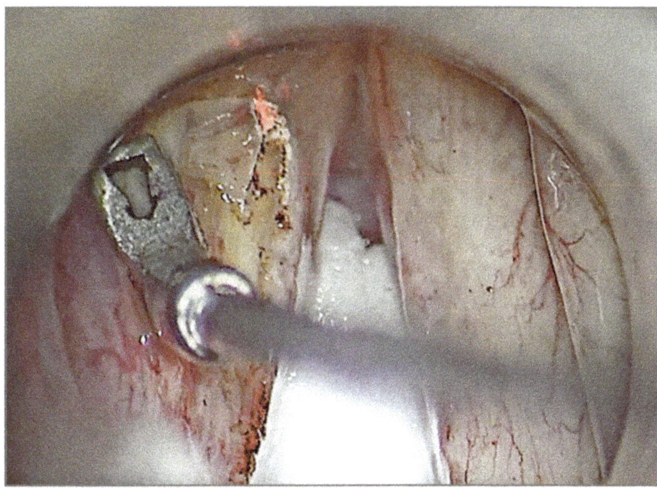

FIG. 17.12: Final anterior excision of the lesion. The anterior commissure has not been made raw. (M-CC)

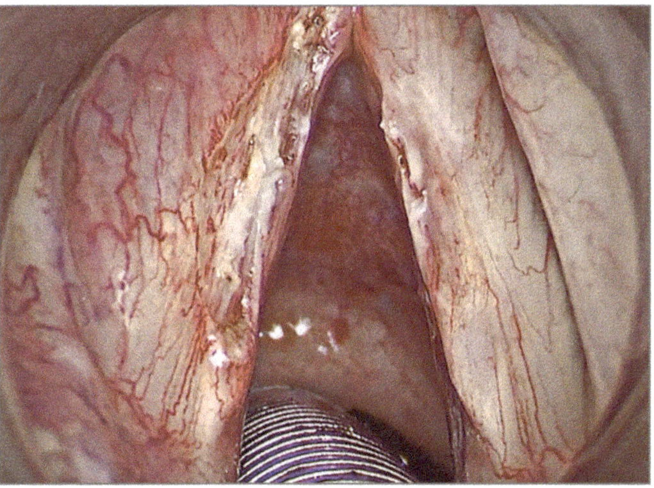

FIG. 17.13: Final postoperative image following complete excision of the left plaque and a small right contact lesion. This was a case of Candidiasis

CASE 2

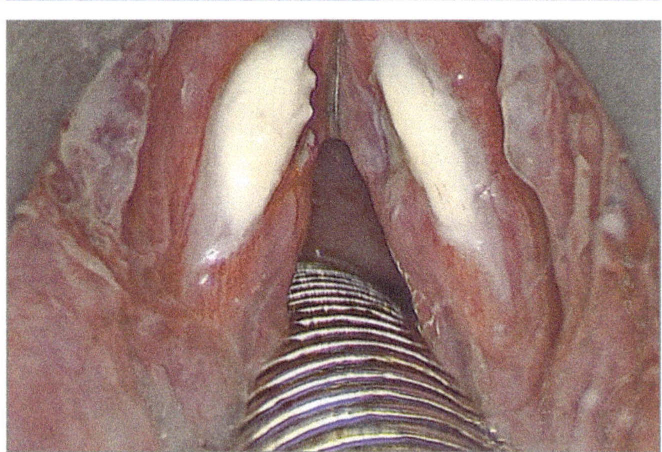

FIG. 17.14: White flaky plaques seen on both the vocal folds with surrounding erythema. This patient has history of taking oral steroids and was empirically treated with 2 weeks of fluconazole at our center, with no improvement. (E-CC)

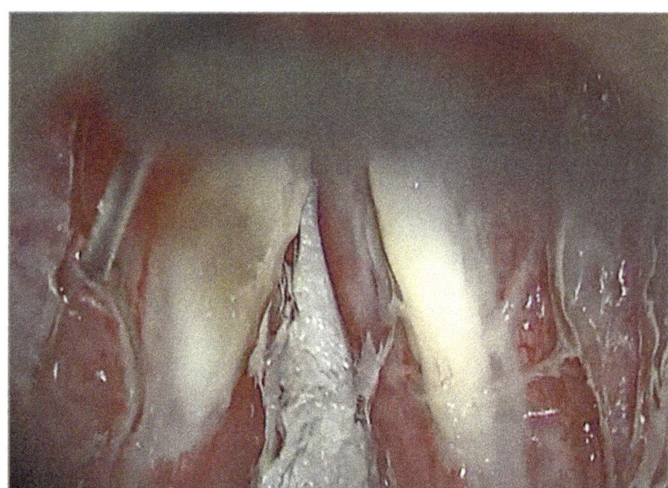

FIG. 17.17: SEIT being used with a 27-gauge needle

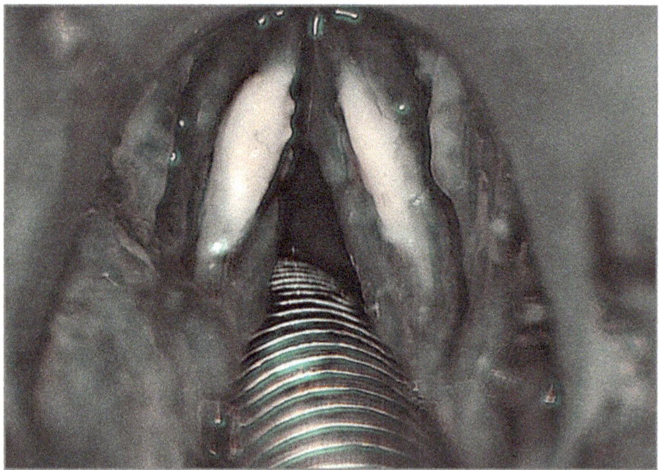

FIG. 17.15: SA image of 17.15. The plaques appear as a brilliant white against a bluish-gray background

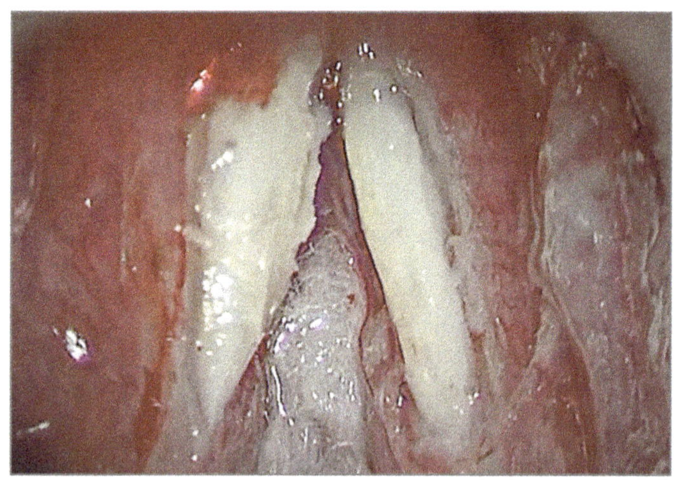

FIG. 17.18: CO_2 laser acublade incision being made just lateral to the lesion on the left vocal fold

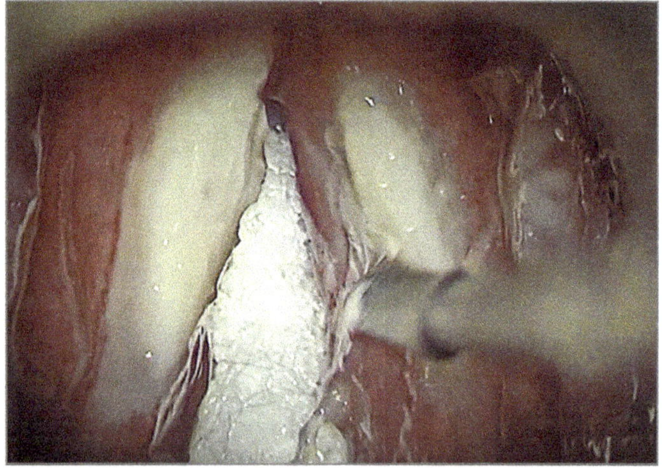

FIG. 17.16: Palpation of the vocal folds with a blunt microflap elevator. (M-CC)

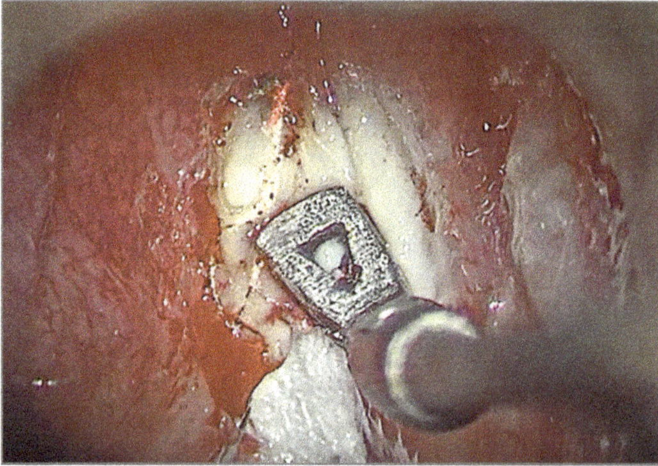

FIG. 17.19: Upward bouchayer forceps holding the left epithelial lesion with gentle medial retraction

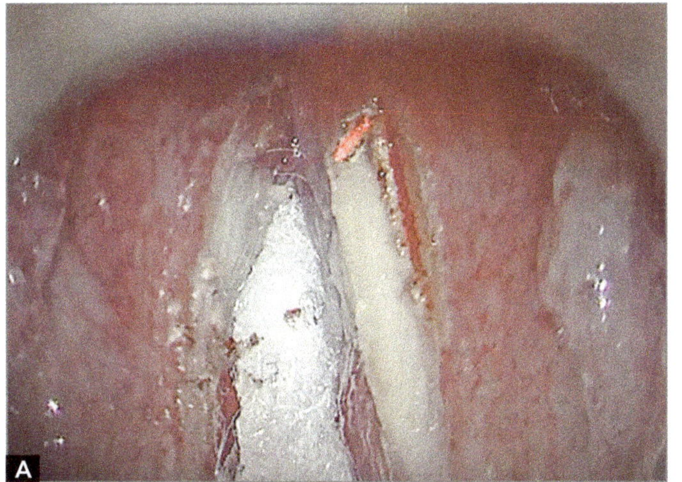

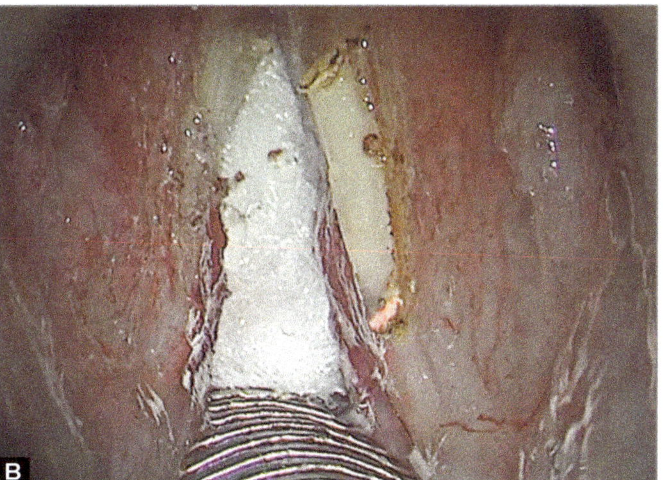

FIG. 17.20: Right laser excision of the lesion. The laser cuts are made without taking any extra margin of healthy tissue in order to preserve maximum epithelium

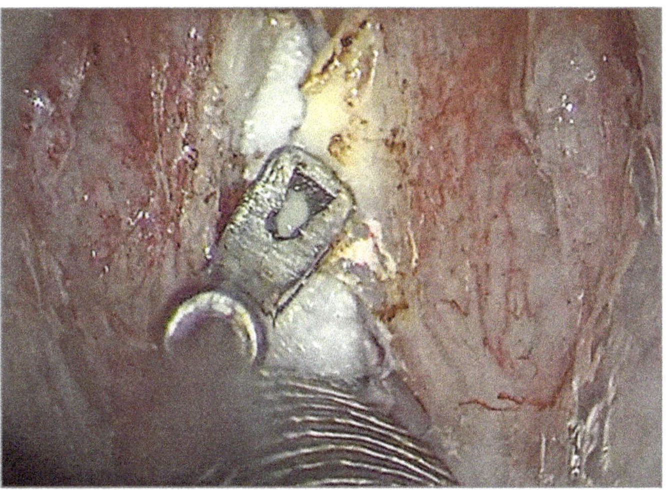

FIG. 17.21: An upward Bouchayer forceps, holding and gently retracting the right epithelial lesion. The tension on the tissue aids in optimal laser excision

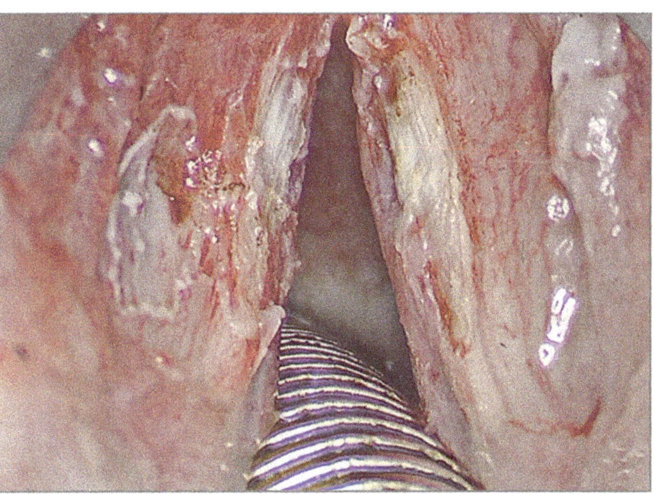

FIG. 17.22: Final postoperative image. The tissue from both vocal folds is sent for histopathology, fungal KOH mount, fungal culture and mycobacteria studies. This patient had laryngeal candidiasis

CASE 3

A young male patient complained of longstanding hoarseness with an occasional dry cough. A right-sided congested vocal fold was observed on laryngoscopy and a workup of pulmonary tuberculosis (sputum acid-fast bacilli, complete blood count, and chest X-ray) was unremarkable. The erythrocyte sedimentation rate (ESR), however, was grossly elevated.

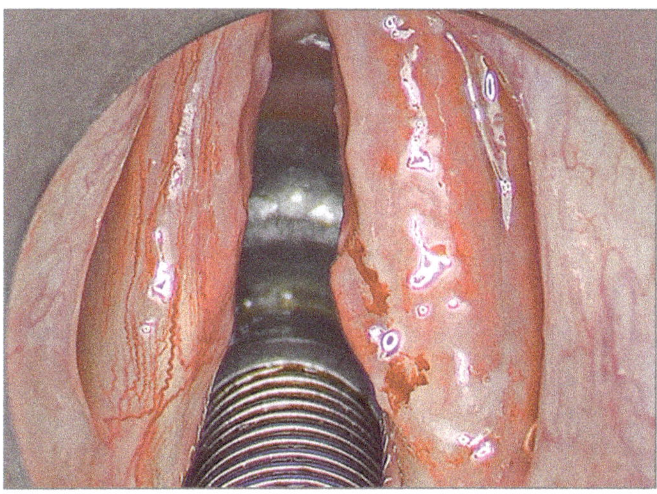

FIG. 17.23: Under the microscope the right congested vocal fold seems to be an erythroplasia with some white areas over it. Also seen is a left vocal fold congestion. (E-CC)

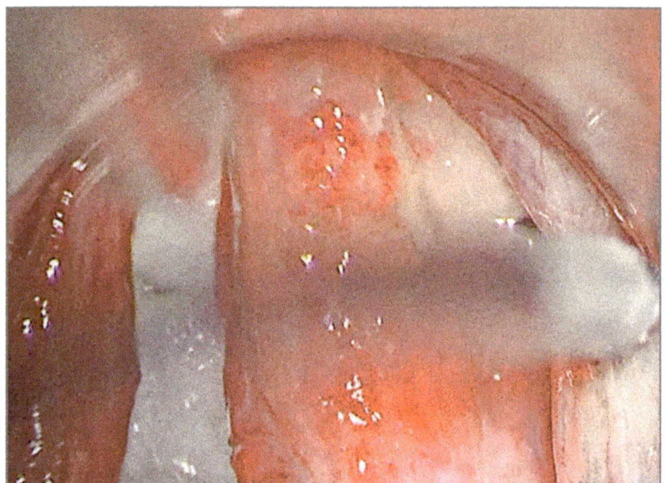

FIG. 17.24: SEIT being used prior to left microflap excision of the erythroplastic epithelium. (M-CC)

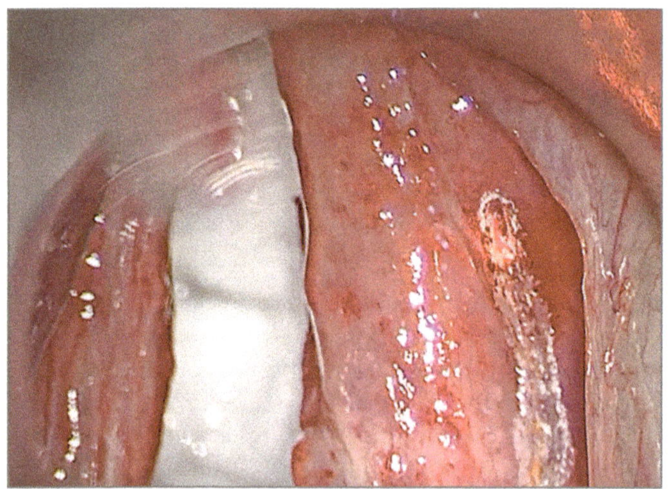

FIG. 17.25: A right laser epithelial cordotomy is being made from a posterior to anterior direction. (M-CC)

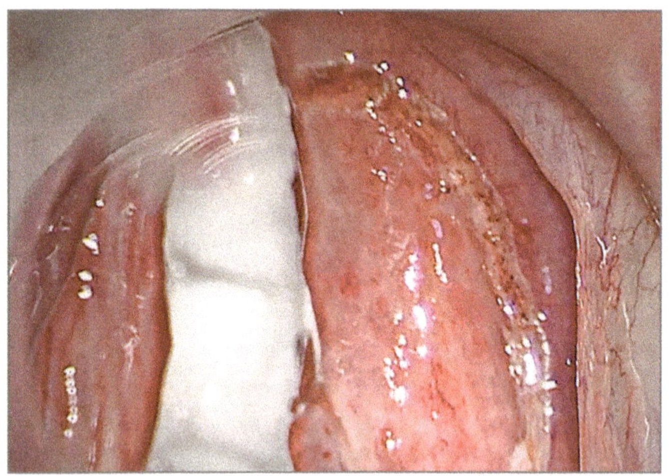

FIG. 17.26: Completion of the right epithelial cordotomy. (M-CC)

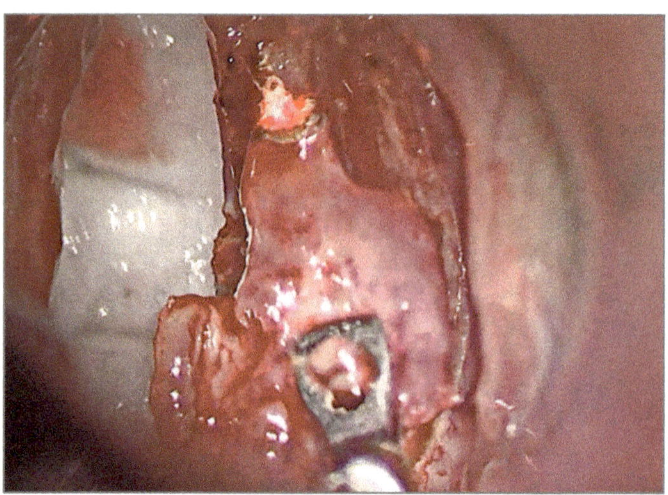

FIG. 17.27: Anterior excision of the epithelial microflap which has been elevated with the CO_2 acuBlade. (M-CC)

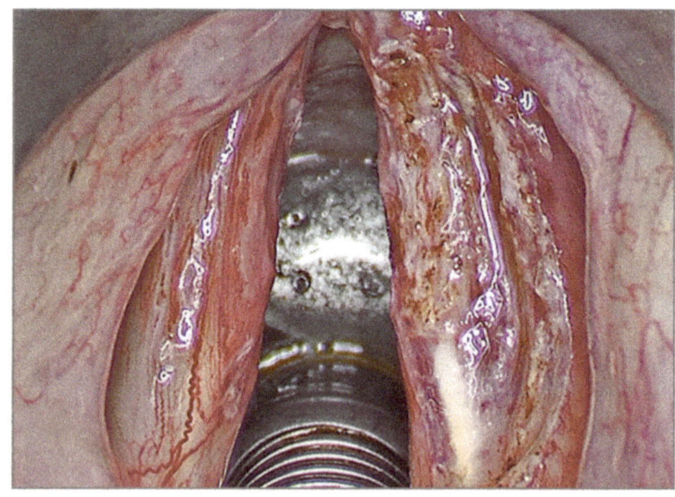

FIG. 17.28: Final postoperative image. This patient had laryngeal Candidiasis with concurrent laryngeal tuberculosis. (E-CC)

CASE 4

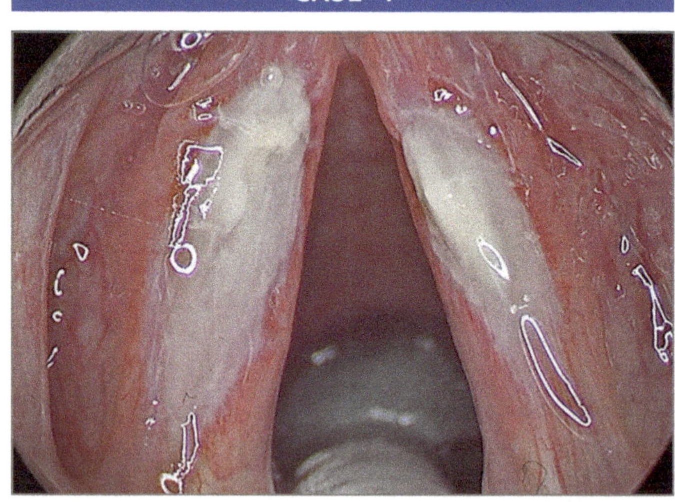

FIG. 17.29: A patient with hoarseness since 3–4 months has a bilateral chalky plaque with surrounding erythema. (E-CC)

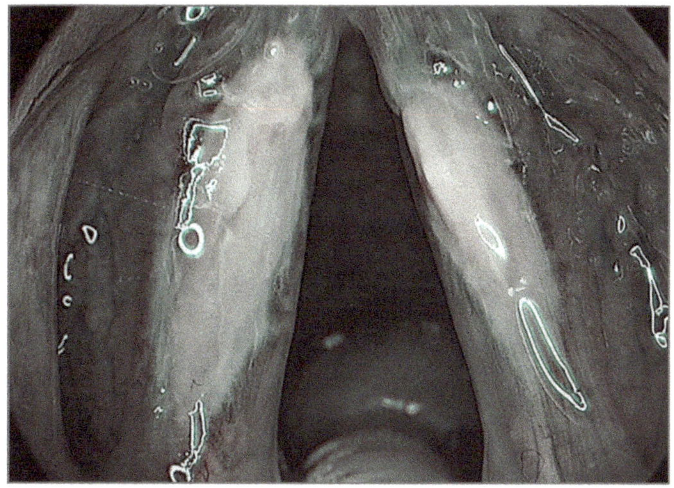

FIG. 17.30: Image 17.29 in SA mode. (E-SA)

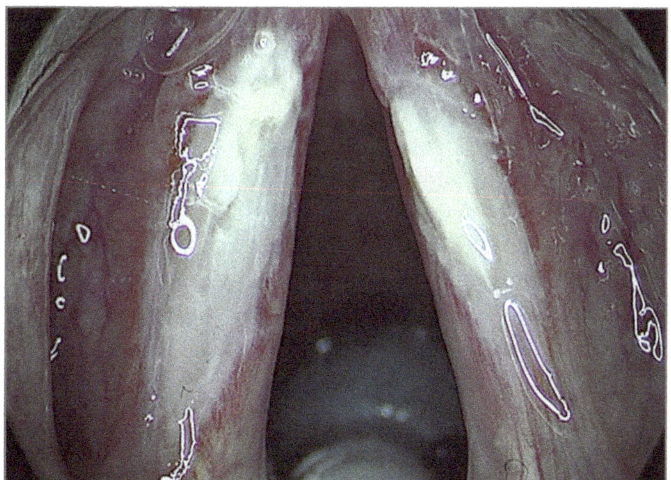

FIG. 17.31: Image 17.29 in SB mode. (E-SB)

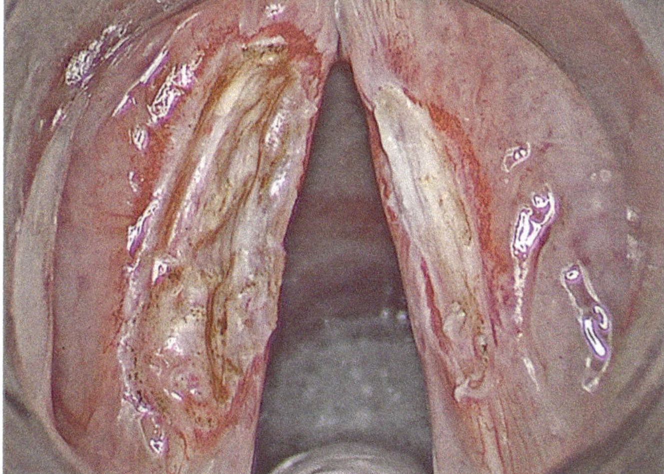

FIG. 17.32: Final postoperative image. Anterior commissure has not been touched. This was a case of laryngeal Candidiasis

CONCLUSION

The diagnosis of fungal laryngitis should be considered in cases where laryngoscopy reveals white, smooth plaques surrounded by erythema. An elevated ESR and history of steroid use are helpful diagnostic pointers. A trial of oral antifungals such as fluconazole is recommended. Some patients require surgical excision, especially in the case of thick avascular fungal plaques. In case of extensive lesions or no response to treatment, a possibility of concomitant tuberculosis should be considered.

REFERENCES

1. Vrabec DP. Fungal infections of the larynx. Otolaryngol Clin North Am. 1993;26(6):1091-114.
2. Wong KK, Pace-Asciak P, Wu B, et al. Laryngeal candidiasis in the outpatient setting. J Otolaryngol Head Neck Surg. 2009;38:624-7.
3. Mehanna HM, Kuo T, Chaplin J, et al. Fungal laryngitis in immuno-competent patients. J Laryngol Otol. 2004;118(5):379-81.
4. Forrest LA, Weed H. Candida laryngitis appearing as leukoplakia and GERD. J Voice. 1998;12:91-5.
5. Neuenschwander MC, Cooney A, Spiegel JR, et al. Laryngeal candidiasis. Ear Nose Throat J. 2001;80(3):138-9.
6. Sataloff RT. Vocal fold scar. In: Sataloff RT, editor. Professional voice: The science and art of clinical care. San Diego: Singular Publishing Group; 1997. pp. 555-7.

CHAPTER 18

Laryngeal Tuberculosis

INTRODUTION

Tuberculosis (TB) is an infectious disease caused by the bacillus *Mycobacterium tuberculosis*. It most commonly affects the lungs, with pulmonary TB accounting to 80% of the cases,[1] however, it can also affect any other organ of the body.

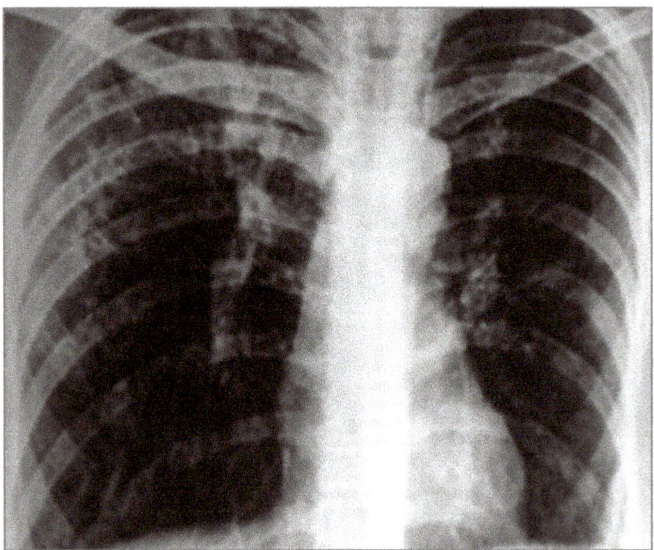

FIG. 18.1: Chest X-ray of a pulmonary tuberculosis patient, who had also developed secondary laryngeal tuberculosis. A right upper lobe cavitatory lesion can be identified

Laryngeal tuberculosis is a rare form of extra-pulmonary TB and constitutes less than 1% of all tuberculosis cases.[2,3] Laryngeal TB is the most common granulomatous disease of the larynx.[4] With the increasing number of immunocompromised hosts and development of multidrug-resistant cases of TB, today otolaryngologists are seeing increasing number of laryngeal TB cases.

Most commonly the larynx is involved secondarily. The larynx may be affected by TB in three ways:

1. The patient has advanced pulmonary disease, usually fibrocavitary with larynx being inoculated by the infected sputum
2. Hematogenous spread
3. Lymphatic drainage seeds the larynx.[5]

Primary TB of larynx is rare and is caused by direct invasion of inhaled bacilli.[6]

In the past, laryngeal TB most commonly affected the younger age group with advanced pulmonary TB. Symptoms like cough, hemoptysis, fever, weight loss, and night sweats were common.[7] The classic presentation was that of multiple ulcers involving the posterior part of the larynx due to pooling of secretions in recumbent patients.[8] However, today variable clinical patterns are emerging. The most common symptom is hoarseness.[8] Other symptoms includes odynophagia, dysphagia, referred otalgia, cough, and stridor.[3] Any site of the laryngeal framework may be involved including the true vocal folds, false vocal folds, epiglottis, aryepiglottic folds, arytenoids, and the subglottis.[9] Grossly the lesions may appear as ulcerative, ulcerofungative, nonspecific inflammatory, or polypoid.[8] Unilateral vocal fold congestion should also alert the clinician for the possibility of TB.

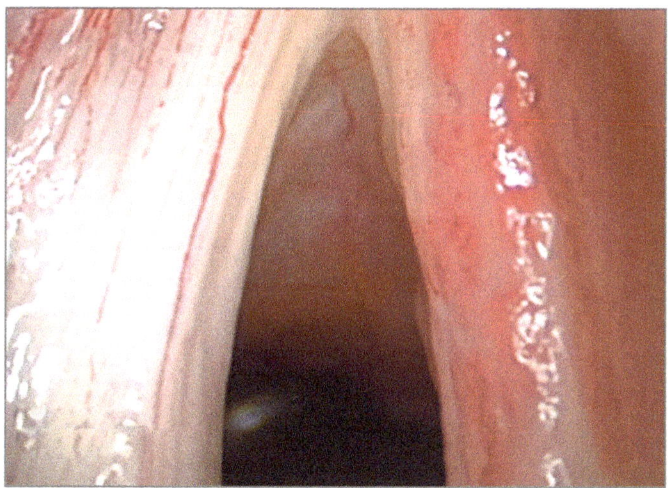

FIG. 18.2: Right vocal fold congestion is seen in a patient of primary TB laryngitis. This is not an infrequent appearance of laryngeal TB today. (E-CC)

Starting empirical steroids in such cases can lead to a flare up of underlying TB. The diagnosis of TB is mainly based on a positive mycobacterial smear of acid fast bacilli and culture or the histopathological demonstration of multinucleate giant cells and granulomatosis with chronic caseating granulomas.

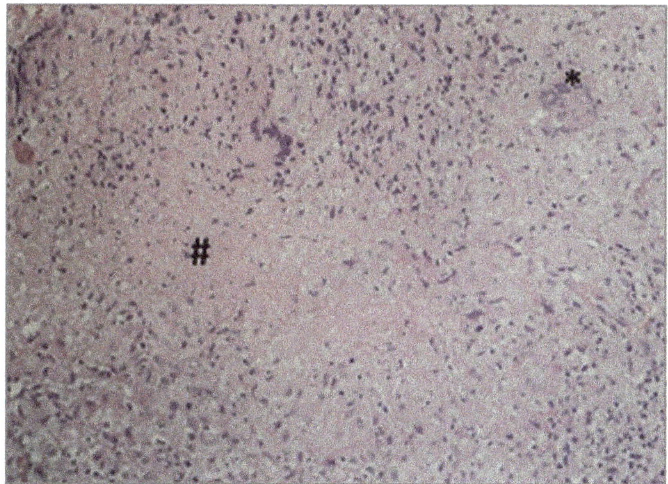

FIG. 18.3: Histopathology of a patient of laryngeal TB. Subepithelial infiltration with multinucleated giant cells (*) and granulomas (#) are seen on the H&E stain

Sputum microscopy is positive in 20% of the cases of laryngeal TB and most of the patients have chest radiograph findings consistent with pulmonary TB.[10] The computed tomography (CT) scan findings of laryngeal TB described are bilateral involvement, lobulated thickening of the free epiglottic margin, and an absence of extra- or paralaryngeal fat space infiltration.[11] However, CT findings can sometimes be nonspecific and even misleading.[12]

An important differential of laryngeal TB is laryngeal carcinoma. Both the conditions have similar clinical, laryngoscopic, and radiological features, but majority of cases of laryngeal TB cases will be associated with pulmonary TB.[12]

Therefore, an abnormal chest X-ray, if not compatible with pulmonary metastasis, should alert the clinician to the possibility of TB, especially when former chest X-rays were normal.[7] However, it is possible for laryngeal TB to coexist with laryngeal cancer, though uncommon.

Laryngeal TB should also be differentiated from other chronic infections such as syphilis, fungal infections, and granulomatous conditions like Wegener's granulomatosis and sarcoidosis.

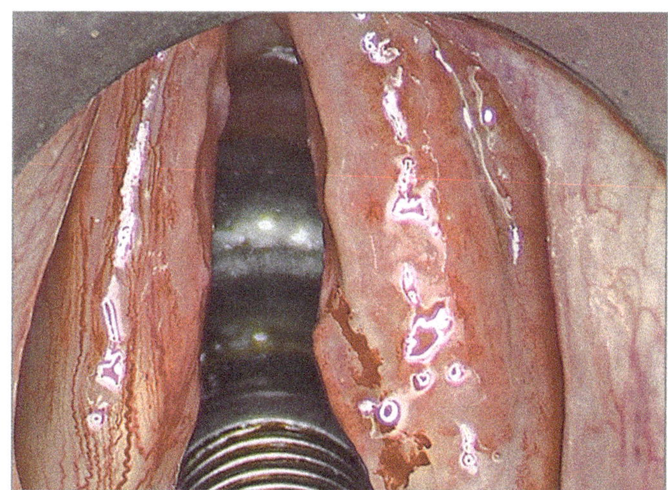

FIG. 18.4: Congestion with a granulomatous appearance of both the vocal folds in a patient of concurrent laryngeal TB with fungal infection. (E-CC)

The classic presentation of the past no longer holds true today and a changing trend in its pattern of presentation is observed. Unless a high index of suspicion is maintained, these cases often get misdiagnosed as nonspecific laryngitis.[13]

Patients with laryngeal TB respond well to antitubercular treatment. A 6 month course is sufficient and gives remarkable results.[14] If not treated early, laryngeal TB can result in glottic stenosis, subglottic stenosis, muscular involvement, and vocal cord paralysis due to invasion of cricoarytenoid joint or recurrent laryngeal nerve.[14,15] It can also lead to fibrosis in the layers of the lamina propria of the vocal folds causing irreversible changes in the quality of the voice.[16]

CASE 1

A young female presented with hoarseness since 4–5 months. Conservative management did not benefit her and a TB work up was unremarkable.

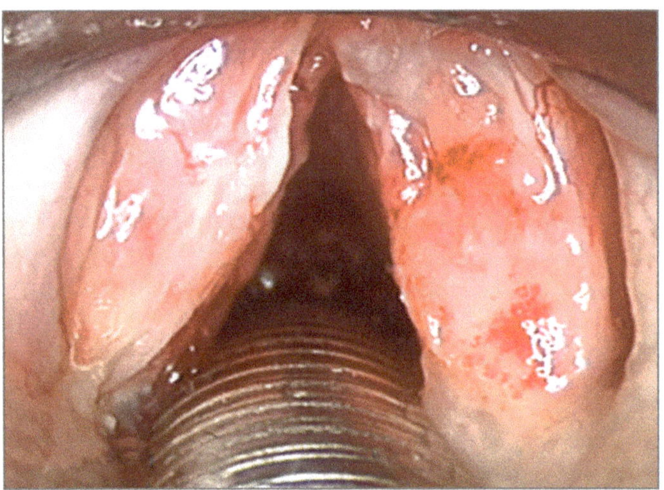

FIG. 18.5: Bilateral vocal folds appearing congested and edematous with a granulomatous appearance of the right vocal fold. This is a patient of primary laryngeal TB. (E-CC)

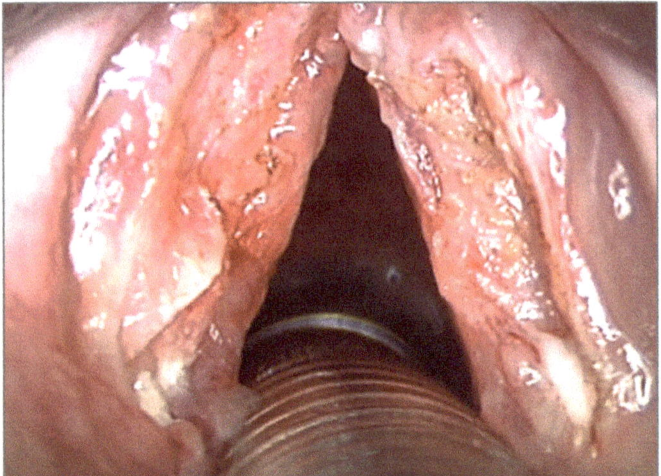

FIG. 18.6: CO_2 Laser excision from the superior surface of the right vocal fold. Histopathology revealed TB and the patients lesions and voice improved within 2–3 months of commencement of antitubercular treatment. (E-CC)

CASE 2

A 19-year-old female patient was referred with history of chronic hoarseness over 4–5 months and she was almost aphonic on presentation.

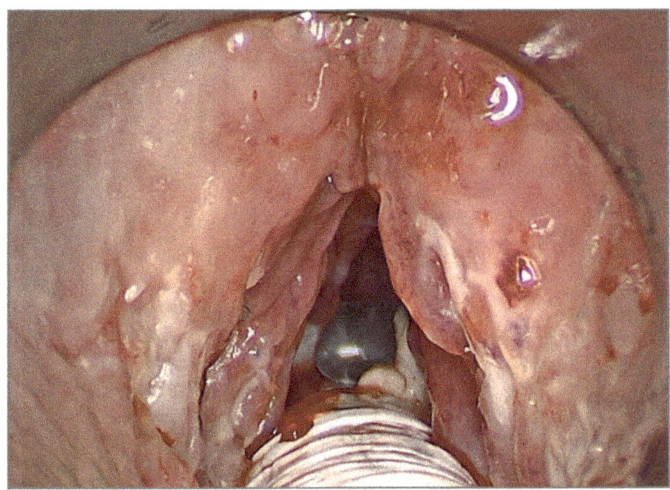

FIG. 18.7: Laryngoscopy revealed a very congested, edematous larynx with a granulomatous appearance. There appeared to be areas of sloughing tissue in the infraglottic area. She was investigated for laryngeal TB however, barring a highly elevated ESR and anemia all other reports were unremarkable. (E-CC)

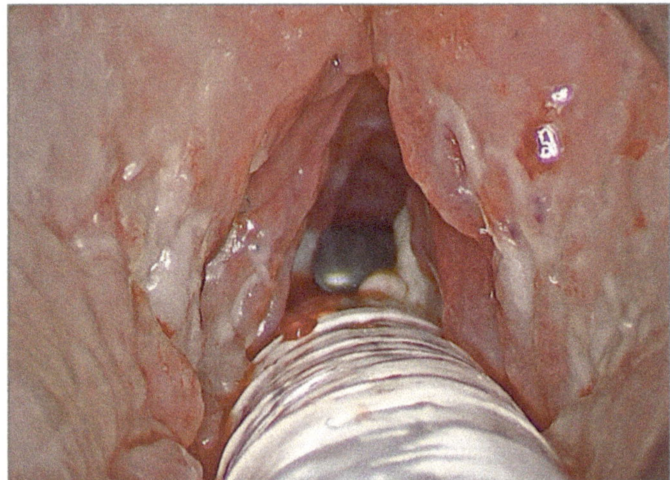

FIG. 18.8: High power image of 18.6. The granulomatous appearance of the larynx can be appreciated. (E-CC)

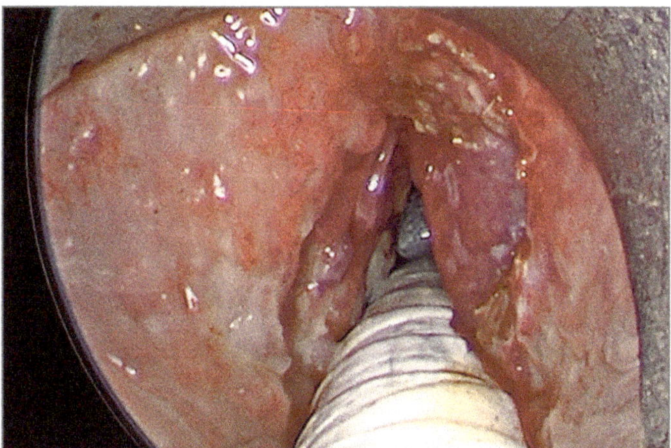

FIG. 18.9: A large piece of granulomatous tissue was excised from the right false vocal fold and ventricle and sent for histopathology, fungal tests, and *Mycobacterium tuberculi*. The true vocal folds should preferably not be operated upon when a diagnosis is being established, as many granulomatous conditions can be treated medically

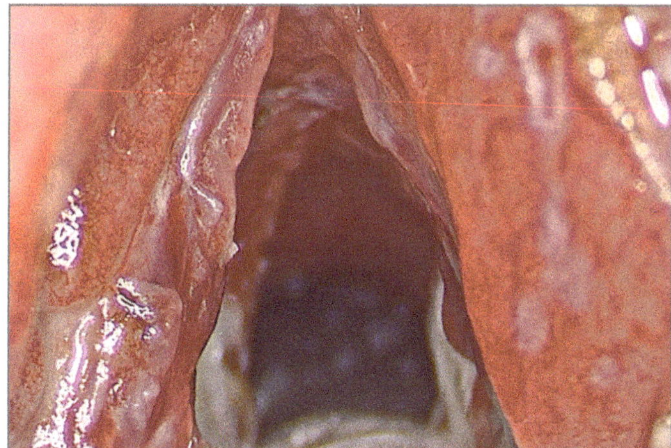

FIG. 18.10: A zoomed image of the true vocal folds, which appear very friable, congested and granulomatous. The histopathology revealed laryngeal TB and the patient achieved a serviceable though rough voice within 3–4 months of initiating the anti-tubercular treatment regimen

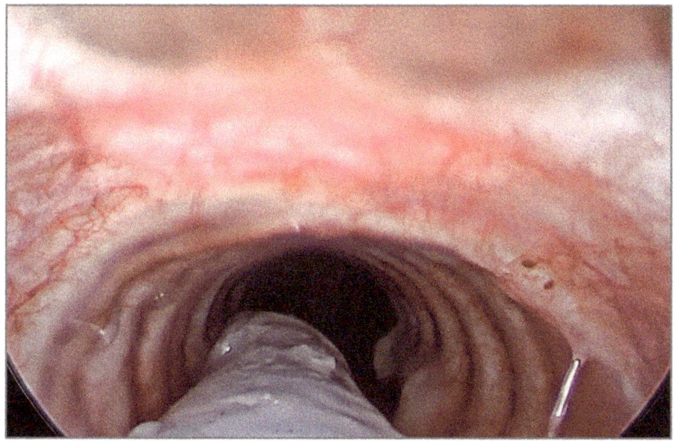

FIG. 18.11: A telescopic bronchoscopy being performed on the patient, to evaluate the lower airway, after deflating the cuff of the laser endotracheal tube. (E-CC)

CASE 3

A 45-year-old female patient presented with hoarseness of more than a years duration and no other complaints.

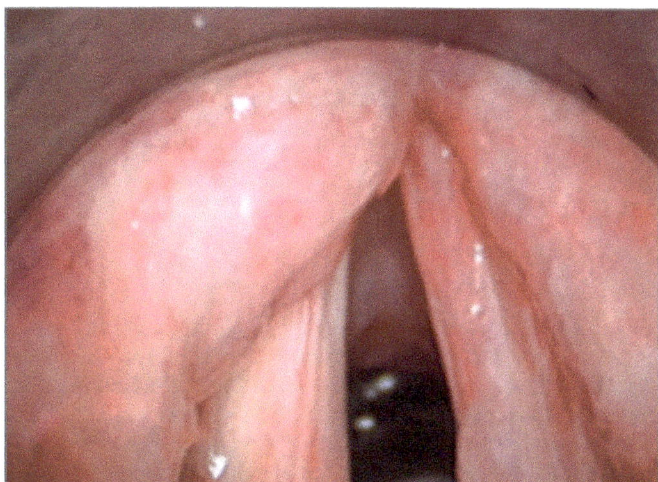

FIG. 18.12: Microlaryngeal examination reveals a left anterior ventricular bulge and a right true vocal fold congestion. (M-3 chip)

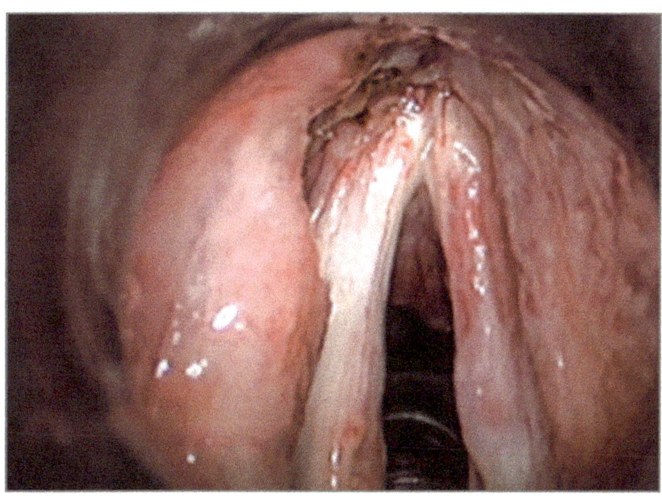

FIG. 18.13: Laser excision of the left ventricular bulge provides sufficient representative tissue for histopathology, fungal culture and AFB testing. The congested right vocal fold is not biopsied, in an order to maximally preserve voice. Histopathology confirms TB and the patient improves within 2 months of starting treatment. (M-3 chip)

CASE 4

A young female patient presented with history of cough and hoarseness since 3–4 months. She had been given a course of oral steroids by an earlier treating physician, following which her symptoms worsened.

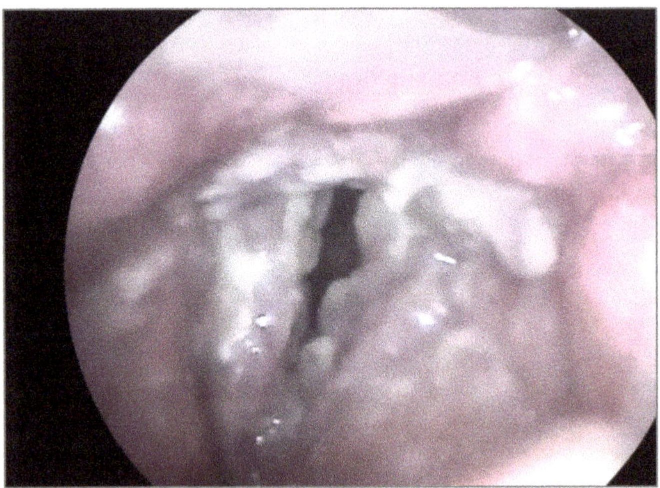

FIG. 18.14: Stroboscopy revealed granulomatous lesions over the entire larynx, covered with slough. Her sputum was positive for AFB and she slowly improved with antitubercular treatment. She was thus diagnosed as secondary laryngeal TB. Steroids should be given with caution when the diagnosis has not been reached, as they may flare up conditions such as laryngeal TB. (70 degree stroboscopy)

REFERENCES

1. World Health Organization, Global tuberculosis control, Geneva, Switzerland, WHO Report 2010.
2. Uslu C, Oysu C, Uklumen B. Tuberculosis of the epiglottis: A case report. Eur Arch Otorhinolaryngol. 2008;265:599-601.
3. Williams RG, Tony DJ. Mycobacterium marches back. J Laryngol Otol. 1995;109:5-13.
4. Caldarelli DD, Freidberg SA, Haris AA. Medical and surgical aspects of the granulomatous diseases of the larynx.Otolaryngol Clin North Am. 1979;12:767-81.
5. Ramadan HH, Wax MK. Laryngeal tuberculosis: A cause of stridor in children. Arch Otolaryngol Head Neck Surg. 1995;121:109-12.
6. Mehndiratta A., Bhat P, D'Costa L, et al. Primary tuberculosis of larynx. Indian J Tuberc. 1997;44:211-2.
7. Smulders YE, De Bondt BJ, Lacko M, et al. Laryngeal tuberculosis presenting as a supraglottic carcinoma: A case report and review of the literature. J Med Case Rep. 2009;3:9288.
8. Shin JE, Nam SY, Yoo SJ, et al. Changing trends in clinical manifestations of laryngeal tuberculosis. Laryngoscope. 2000;110:1950-3.
9. Munck K, Mandpe AH. Mycobacterial infections of the head and neck. Otolaryngol Clin North Am. 2003;36(4):569-76.
10. Nishiike S, Irigune M, Kubo T. Laryngeal tuberculosis: A report of 15 cases. Ann Otol Rhinol Laryngol. 2002;111:916-8.
11. Kim MD, Kim DI, Yune HY, et al. CT findings of laryngeal tuberculosis: Comparison to laryngeal carcinoma. J Comput Assist Tomogr. 1997;21:29-34.
12. Harney M, Hone S, Timon C, et al. Laryngeal tuberculosis: An important diagnosis. J Laryngol Otol. 2000;114:878-80.
13. Nerurkar NK, Singh S, Nerurkar R. Tubercular laryngitis-A rebirth? Int J Phonosurg Laryngol. 2016;6(1);17-9.
14. Lim JY, Kim KM, Choi EC, et al. Current clinical propensity of laryngeal tuberculosis: review of 60 cases. Eur Arch Otorhinolaryngol. 2006;263:838-42.
15. Yencha MW, Linfesty R, Blackmon A. Laryngeal tuberculosis. Am J Otolaryngol. 2000;21:122-6.
16. Özüdogru E, Çakli H, Altuntas EE, et al. Effects of laryngeal tuberculosis on vocal fold functions: Case report. Acta Otorhinolaryngol Ital. 2005;25(6):374-77.

CHAPTER 19

Plexiform Neurofibromatosis

INTRODUCTION

Neurofibromatosis is classified as type 1 and 2. Neurofibromatosis type 1 (NF1) is also known as Von Recklinghaussen's disease in which plexiform neurofibromas (PN) may occur.[1]

Suchanek reported the first case of an endolaryngeal neurofibroma in 1925.[2] The neurofibromas in NF1 could be plexiform or nonplexiform. Plexiform neurofibromas are generally congenital and hence present early on in life. They are diffuse and ill localized and thought to involve terminal fibers of multiple nerve branches.

Potential for malignant transformation has been reported at around 5%.[3] Since they are locally infiltrating, complete resection is often thought to be difficult. The usual site of occurrence of a laryngeal neurofibroma is in the supraglottis, probably since this area is rich in terminal nerve plexuses of the superior laryngeal nerve. These tumors are usually seen as large smooth submucosal masses located in the supraglottis resulting in difficulty in breathing and swallowing as has been the case in most reported pediatric laryngeal neurofibromas.

The management of PN is challenging due to the diffuse involvement of surrounding tissues. A long-term follow up in these patients is essential for an early pick up of recurrence and potential malignant transformation.

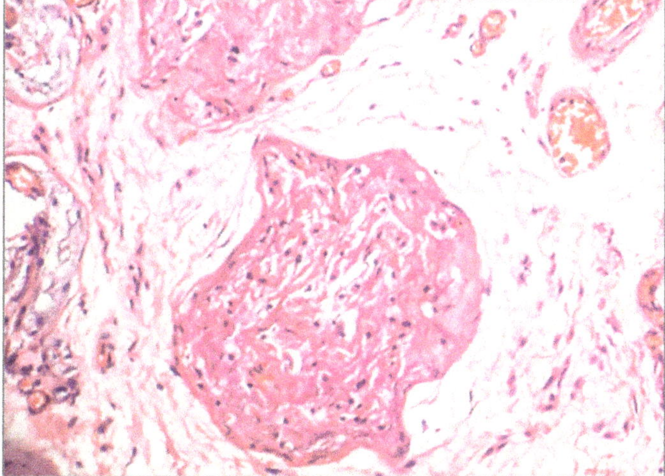

FIG. 19.1: Histopathology of a PN showing intertwined spindle shaped cells with dense surrounding connective tissue on H&E staining

CASE 1

A 3-year-old boy was referred from another center for definitive management of his right supraglottic swelling.

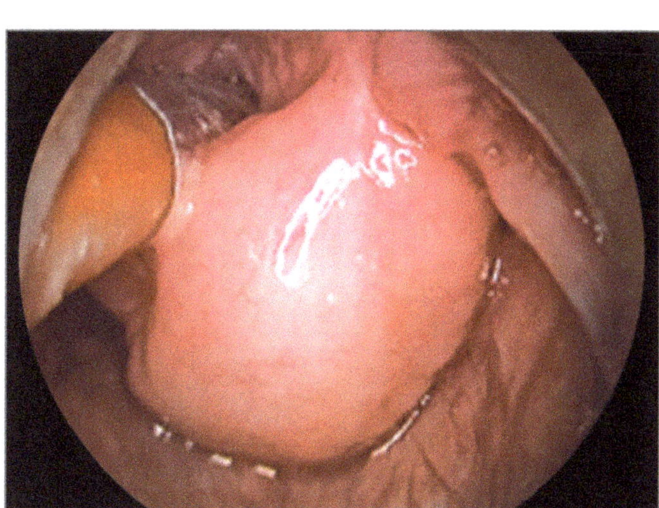

FIG. 19.2: Laryngoscopy reveals a right large, smooth, submucosal arytenoid mass, extending to the medial pyriform sinus and aryepiglottic fold. The vocal folds are normal. (M-3 chip)

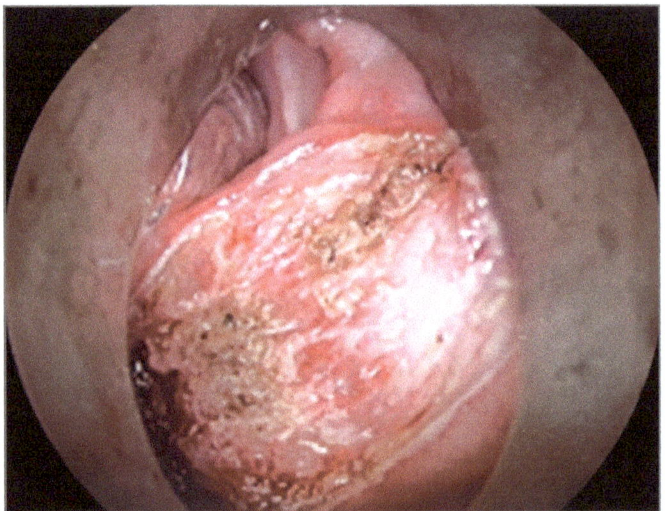

FIG. 19.3: Endolaryngeal CO_2 laser excision is appropriate for medium sized tumors. Histopathology confirmed PN. This is the postlaser excision image. (M-3 chip)

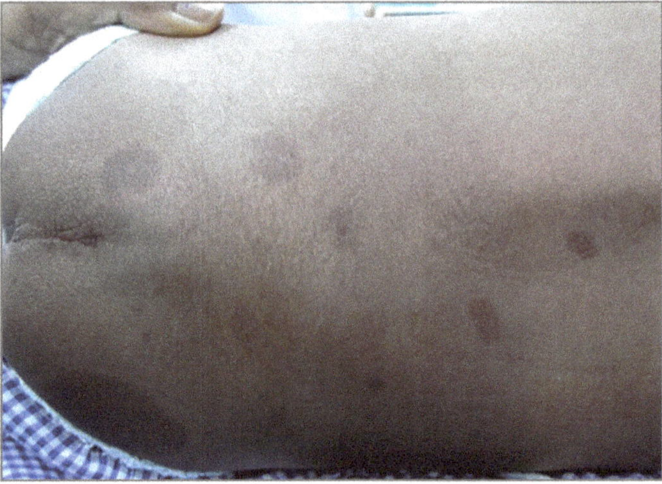

FIG. 19.4: A thorough clinical examination for signs of NF1 was done in collaboration with a pediatric ophthalmologist, orthopedic surgeon, and pediatric surgeon. The child had obvious café-au-lait spots on his lower back (total 7 in number), with the largest one being around 4 cm in diameter

CASE 2

A 4-year-old boy was sent to our center with a tracheostomy *in situ*. The child had been referred for definitive management of an extremely large right supraglottic mass.

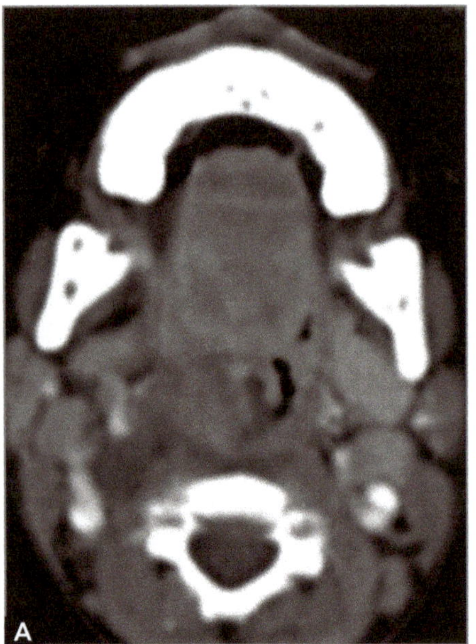

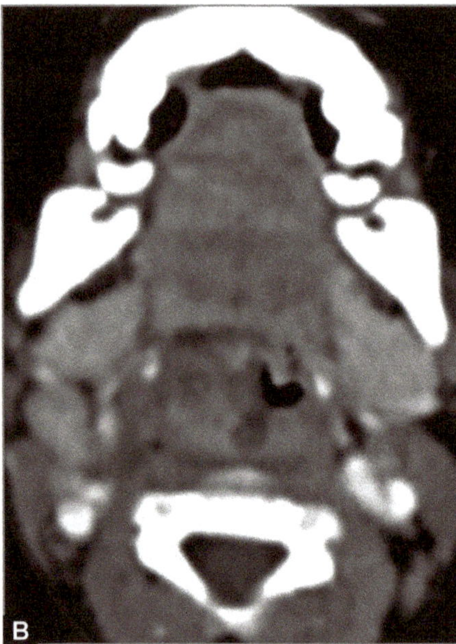

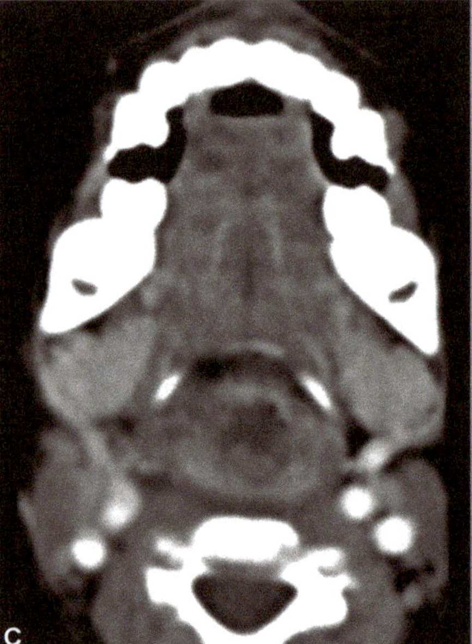

Continued

Continued

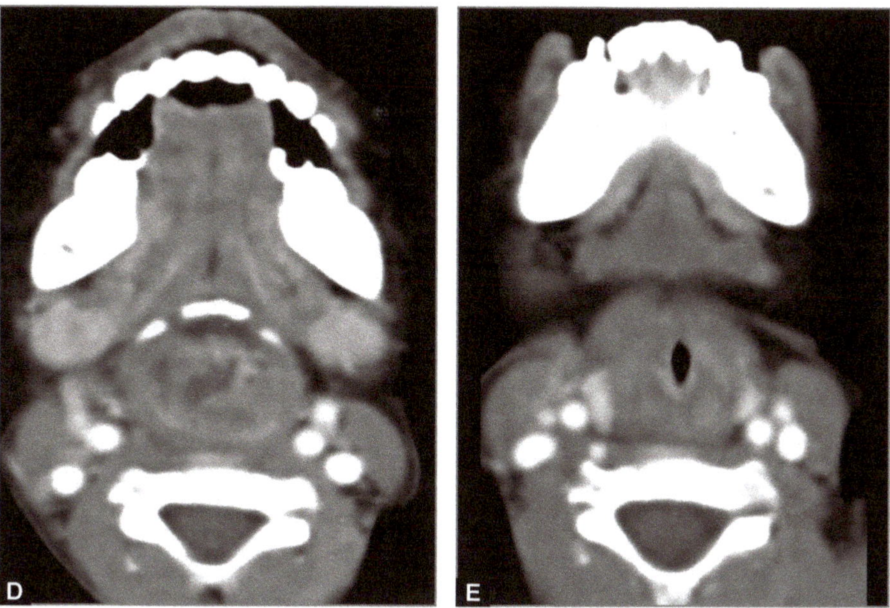

FIG. 19.5: The consecutive axial computed tomography scans of the neck with contrast reveal a large, centrally necrosed, moderately vascular lesion, originating from the right supraglottis and almost totally occupying the supraglottic lumen. The vocal folds appear uninvolved

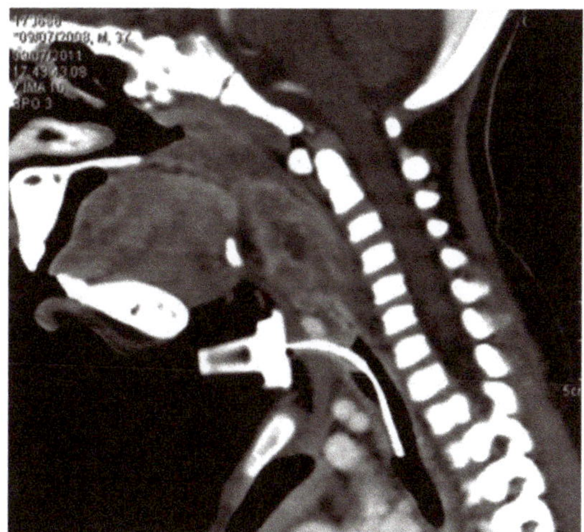

FIG. 19.6: The sagittal computed tomography scan reveals an almost completely blocked airway due to the mass lesion above the tracheostomy

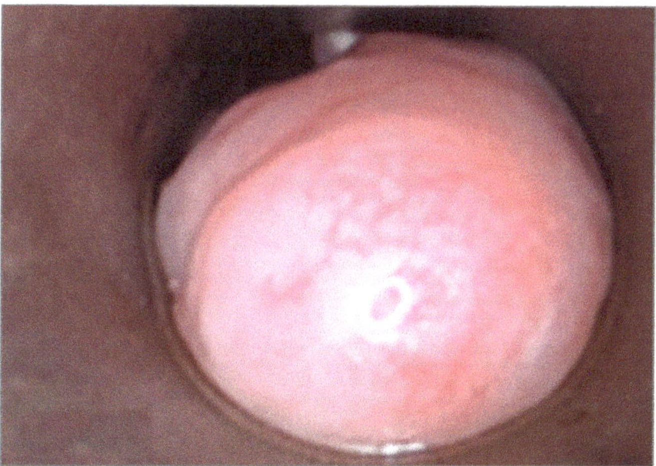

FIG. 19.7: As expected, a large right supraglottic lesion is seen on microlaryngeal surgery. The posterior part of the right normal vocal fold can be observed in this image (M-3 chip)

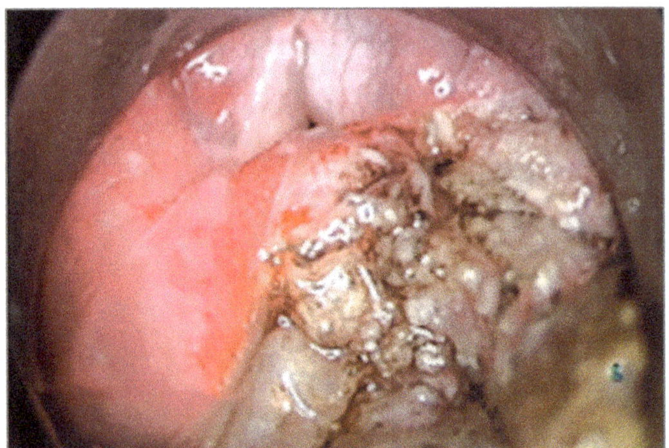

FIG. 19.8: Carbon dioxide laser excision was performed for the lesion in combination with laryngeal microdebrider debulking. Both the true vocal folds can be appreciated postoperatively (M-3 chip)

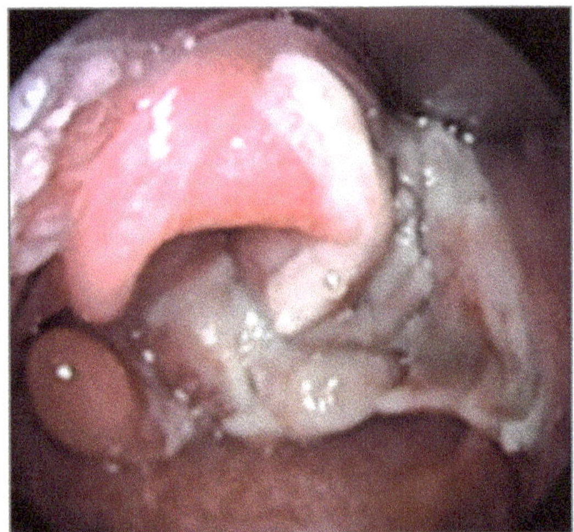

FIG. 19.9: Microlaryngeal surgery performed 2 weeks post-surgery reveals extensive slough which is cleaned with moist cotton pledgets for better healing

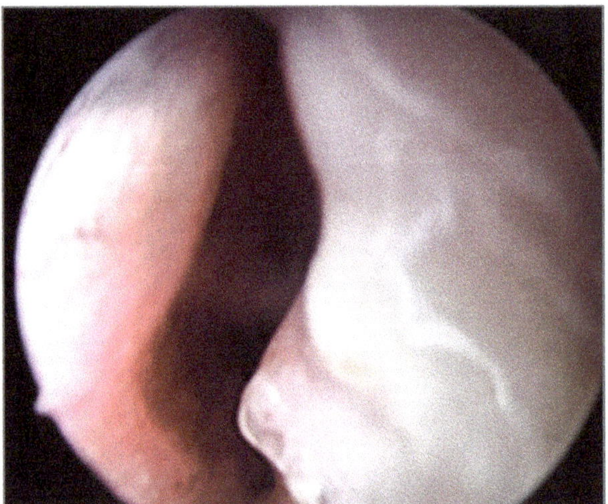

FIG. 19.10: Slough over the right vocal fold at 2 weeks, though no direct laser surgery was performed on the vocal fold. This healed well over the next 6–8 weeks (M-3 chip)

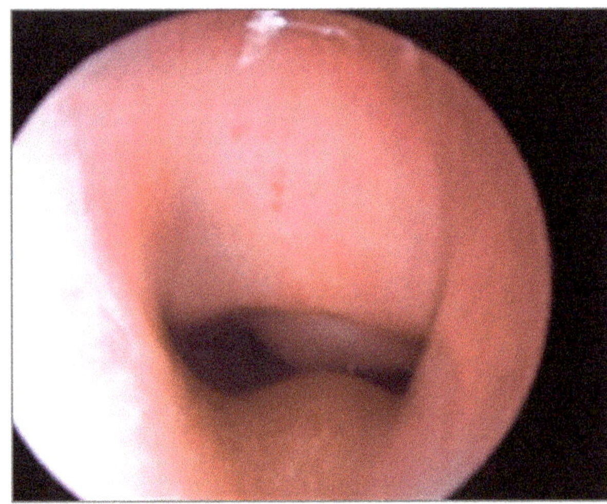

FIG. 19.11: A clear subglottis with the tracheostomy tube is visible. The patient was decannulated after 2 years and needed a total of three surgical procedures (M-3 chip)

REFERENCES

1. Wise JB, Cryer JE, Belasco JB, et al. Management of head and neck plexiform neurofibromas in pediatric patients with neurofibromatosis type 1. Arch Otolaryngol Head Neck Surg. 2005;131:712-8.
2. Dave SP, Farooq U, Civantos FJ. Management of advanced laryngeal and hypopharyngeal plexiform neurofibroma in adults. Am J Otolaryngol. 2008;29:279-83.
3. Ducatman BS, Scheithauer BW, Piepgras DG, et al. Malignant nerve sheath tumors. Cancer. 1986;57:2006-21.

CHAPTER 20

Granulomatosis with Polyangiitis (Wegener's Granulomatosis)

INTRODUCTION

Wegener described the entity known as Wegener's Granulomatosis in 1936 and then again in 1939.[1] Wegener's granulomatosis has now been renamed granulomatosis with polyangiitis (GPA). It is a rare disease defined by the triad of:

1. Necrotizing granulomatosis of the upper and/or lower airways
2. Generalized vasculitis primarily of the small arteries and veins
3. Focal necrotizing glomerulitis.

Involvement of the upper respiratory tract occurs in 95% of the patients.

Subglottic stenosis occurs in approximately 16% of patients in GPA and may result in severe airway obstruction, which does not typically respond to medical line of treatment.[2]

Diagnosis is made by demonstration of necrotizing granulomatous vasculitis on tissue biopsy. The characteristic laboratory findings include a positive anti-proteinase 3 anti-neutrophil cytoplasmic antibody, anemia, elevated erythrocyte sedimentation rate and mildly elevated rheumatoid factor. Granulomatosis with polyangiitis is treated with daily steroids with or without cyclophosphamide.

Subglottic stenosis in GPA is due to necrotizing vasculitis, so any mucosal trauma resulting from major surgery, laser, and stents leads to worse stenosis and should be avoided.[3,4] Microlaryngoscopy and dilatation with local steroid, mitomycin C gives a good result in subglottic stenosis due to GPA.[5]

CASE 1

A 12-year-old girl, diagnosed 6 months back as GPA, presented with severe stridor with a history of respiratory distress since 6 months. Flexible laryngoscopy revealed a pinhole opening in the subglottis. An emergency tracheostomy was performed and she was subsequently taken under general anesthesia for microlaryngoscopy with dilatation.

Case 1 has required serial dilations but her stenosis has progressed to involve the entire larynx. She remains on a tracheostomy tube.

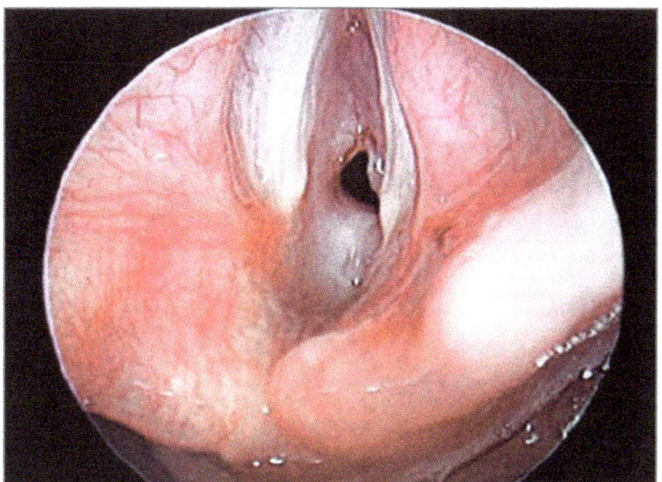

FIG. 20.1: Pinhole opening is seen during microlaryngoscopy. (E-3 chip)

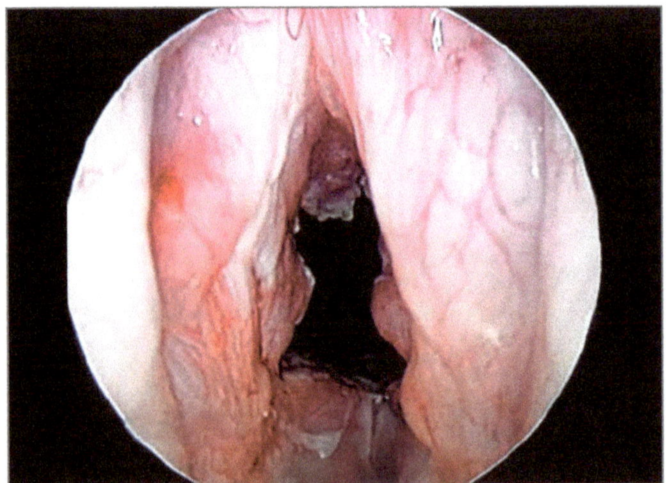

FIG. 20.2: Four radial cuts were made at the site of stenosis followed by dilation, injection of steroids locally, and mitomycin C local application. (E-3 chip)

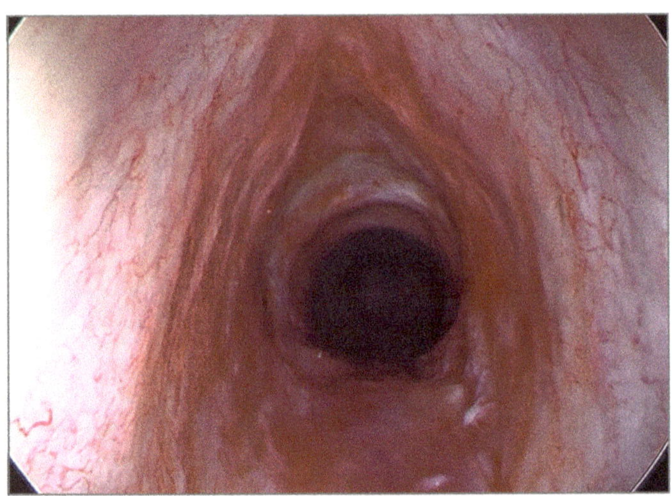

FIG. 20.4: Dilation with gum-elastic-bougies coated with jelly, is performed with apnea technique. The final subglottic airway can be seen. (E-CC)

CASE 2

An 18-year-old girl with GPA was referred by the treating physician for respiratory distress.

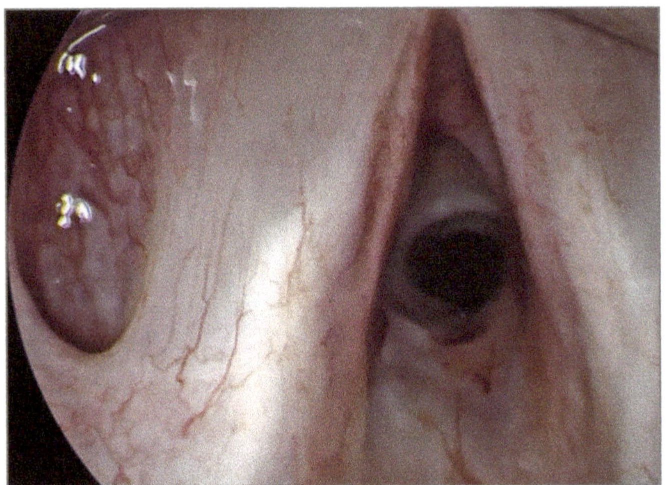

FIG. 20.3: A subglottic stenosis of 2 cm length is seen during microlaryngoscopy. (E-CC)

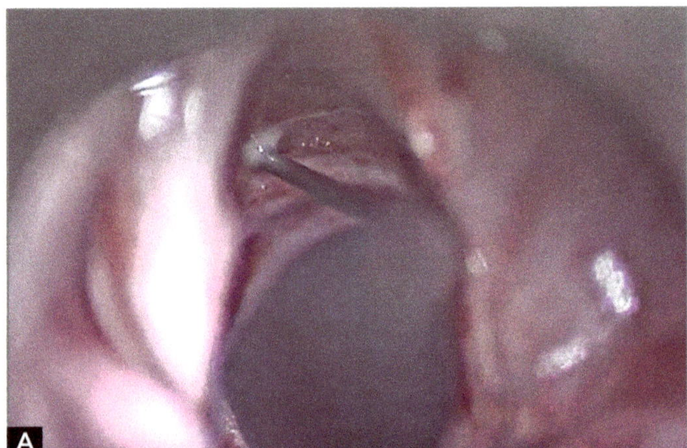

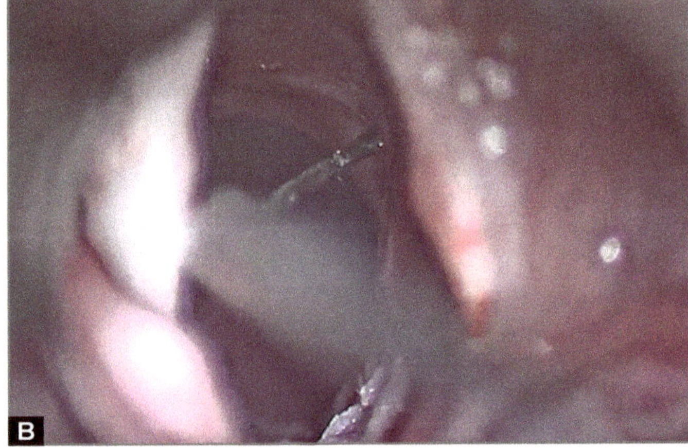

FIG. 20.5: Subepithelial methylprednisolone (60–80 mg) is injected circumferentially at the site of stenosis

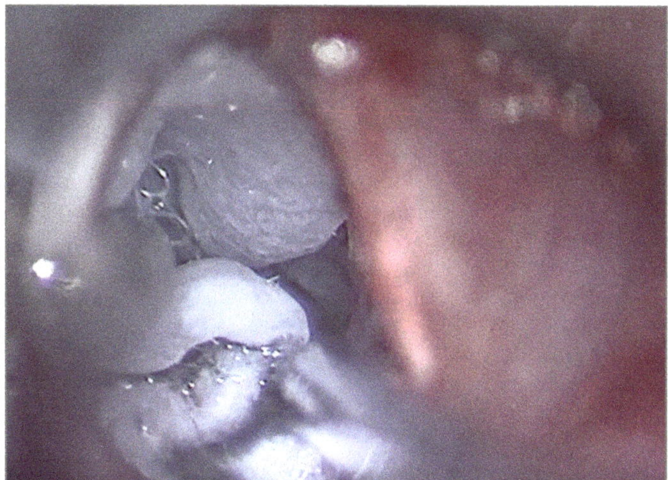

FIG. 20.6: Local application of 4 mg of mitomycin C in 1 mL dilution is applied for 5 minutes. A large saline soaked cotton pledget(with a thread attached) is placed below this mitomycin pledget, to make sure that the mitomycin does not trickle into the distal airway, since the procedure is taking place in apnea

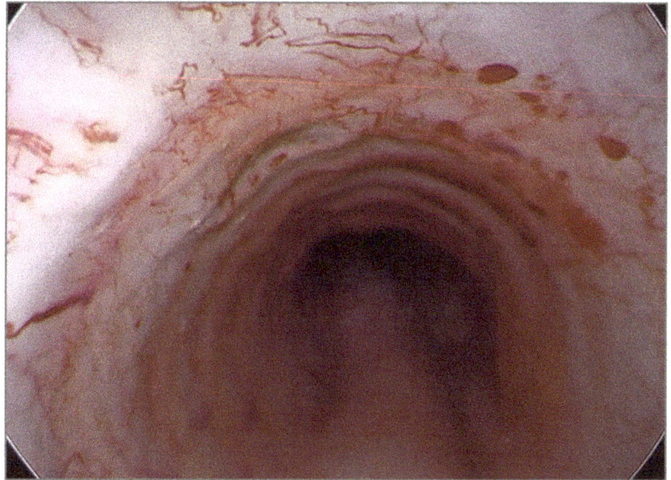

FIG. 20.7: The trachea is inspected and appears essentially normal. (E-CC)

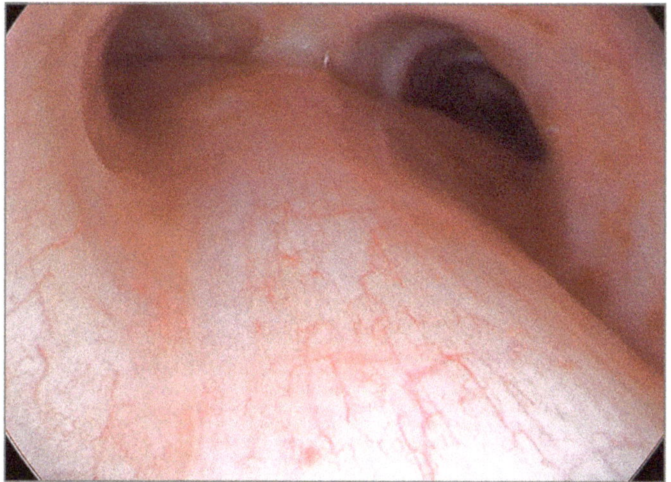

FIG. 20.8: The carina and bronchii also appear unremarkable. (E-CC)

CASE 3

A 19-year-old girl of GPA is referred to our center for management of her respiratory distress.

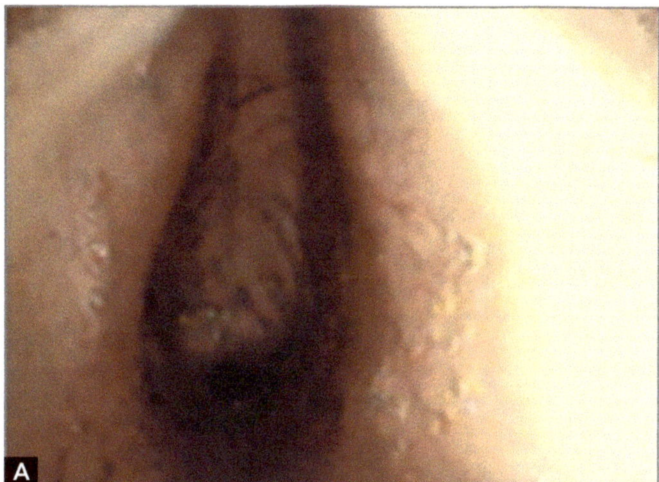

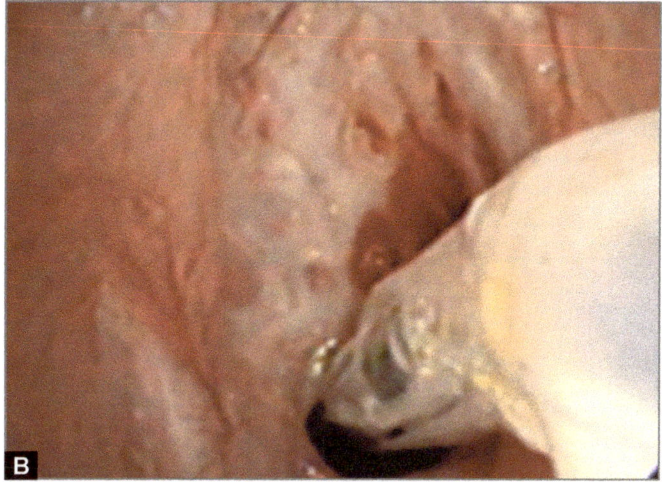

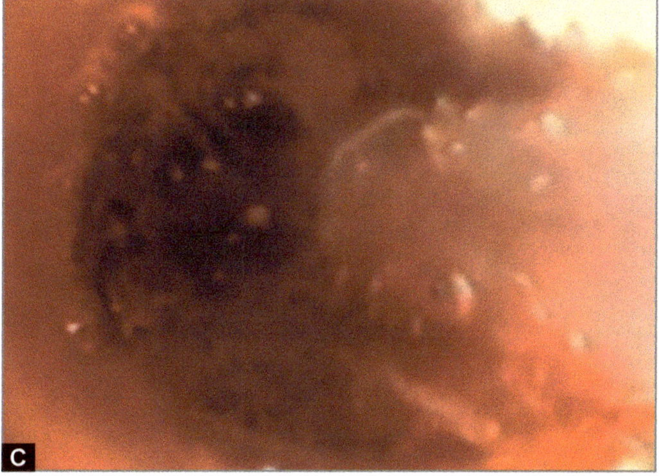

Continued

Continued

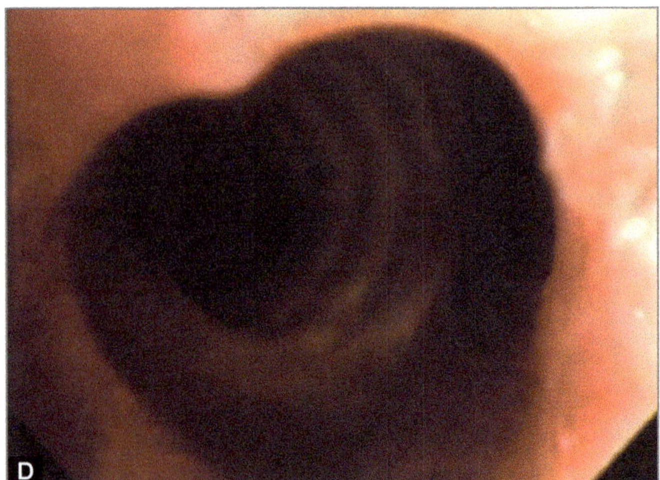

FIG. 20.9: An airway balloon catheter, 40 mm x 10 mm is guided under vision to the site of stenosis and dilated up to 12 atmospheric pressure for 1 minute. Following this, 60 mg methylprednisolone is injected at the stenotic site. Finally, mitomycin C is applied locally for 5 minutes

REFERENCES

1. Djalilian M, McDonald TJ, Devine KD, et al. Nontraumatic, nonneoplastic subglottic stenosis. Ann Otol. 1975;84:757-63.
2. Michael C Sneller, et al. Vasculitis syndrome. Harrison's principle of internal medicine 2005; 2:2004-07.
3. Shvero J, Shitrit D, Koren R, et al. Endoscopic laser surgery for subglottic stenosis in Wegener's Granulomatosis. Yonsei Med J. 2003;48(5):748-53.
4. Watters K, Russell J. Subglottic stenosis in Wegener's Granulomatosis and the nitinol stent. Laryngoscope. 2003;113(12):2222-24.
5. Hoffman GS, Thomas-Golbanov CK, Chan J, et al. Treatment of subglottic stenosis due to Wegener's granulomatosis, with intralesional corticosteroids and dilation. J Rheumatol. 2003;30(5):1017-21.

CHAPTER 21

Bilateral Vocal Fold Paralysis

INTRODUCTION

When both the vocal folds do not have any adduction or abduction (no movement), the condition is referred to as bilateral immobile vocal folds. One of the commonest causes of this is a bilateral vocal fold paralysis, although arytenoid dislocation, posterior glottic stenosis, and cricoarytenoid joint fixation may also be responsible. The final confirmation can be performed under general anesthesia by inspecting and palpating the crico-arytenoid joint and posterior glottic area. A laryngeal electromyography is another way to test for vocal fold paralysis.

The commonest mode of presentation of patients with bilateral vocal fold paralysis (BLVFP) is stridor in the emergency unit, often necessitating immediate tracheostomy. Unlike unilateral vocal fold paralysis, where patients might not require surgery, patients with BLVFP almost always warrant some intervention. Occasionally, patients present with dyspnea of long-standing duration.

The causes of BLVFP include a long list, the commonest being open surgery of the neck or chest, especially for malignancies of the thyroid, esophagus, or lungs. Many a times, even after diligent clinical work-up, the cause may remain undiagnosed and such cases are labeled as idiopathic.

Management of bilateral vocal fold paralysis is a balancing act between comfortable breathing and a serviceable voice. Over the past decades, several options for surgery in bilateral vocal fold paralysis have emerged, from suture lateralization to renervation and even laryngeal pacing. Jackson introduced ventriculocordectomy in 1922,[1] where he removed the entire vocal fold and the ventricle. In 1939, King suggested extralaryngeal arytenoidectomy.[2] Endoscopic arytenoidectomy developed in 1948.[3] Ossoff et al. in 1983 mentioned the use of CO_2 laser in endoscopic arytenoidectomy.[4] However, the most commonly employed treatment worldwide is the Dennis and Kashima's posterior laser cordotomy.[5] Most surgeons prefer to do a unilateral procedure with the view point that it is minimally destructive with a better postoperative voice than that with a bilateral procedure. Burian and Hofler (1979) first suggested operating both the vocal folds in the primary stage.[6]

The author prefers the Kashima procedure, performed unilaterally, with the patient informed about a 20–30% chance of second side surgery at 4–6 weeks.

All our patients of BLVFP are offered a unilateral laser assisted Kashima's posterior cordotomy. The CO_2 AcuBlade laser is used at 10 W power setting and superpulse mode, depth 2 and length 2 mm. The side of surgery is determined by the presence of a flickering movement perceived in any of the vocal folds. The vocal fold with no flickering motion is selected for surgery in such cases.

The vocal fold is palpated on both sides at the level of the vocal process to confirm that there is no fixation of the cricoarytenoid joint and posterior glottic stenosis is also ruled out. The Kashima cordotomy is then commenced just anterior to the vocal process. This horizontal cordotomy is extended up to the inner thyroid perichondrium of the thyroid cartilage, so that the entire width of the vocal fold can be cut for maximum airway benefit. The false vocal fold may be retracted or cut, to facilitate this. Once this end-point is reached, some brisk bleeding is frequently encountered, which can be controlled with an insulated suction cautery.

As the formation of a granuloma is a known complication once cartilage is exposed, it is preferred to leave the perichondrium intact.

CASE 1

An adult female patient was referred to us for management of progressively increasing respiratory distress over 4–5 months, following a near total thyroidectomy. On laryngoscopy, she had bilateral immobile vocal folds with a slight flicker of her left vocal fold. She was planned for a right Kashima cordotomy.

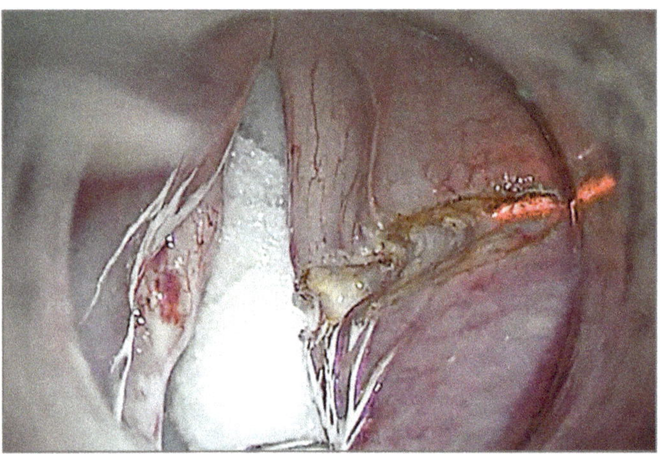

FIG. 21.1: The CO_2 laser AcuBlade is being used in superpulse, repeat mode with a 10 W power, 2 mm blade size and depth 2 (500 microns). The AcuBlade is seen making a horizontal cut anterior to the vocal process and cutting the true and false vocal fold on the right side. A Mallinckrodt laser tube with a moist cotton pledget is seen in the subglottis. (M-CC)

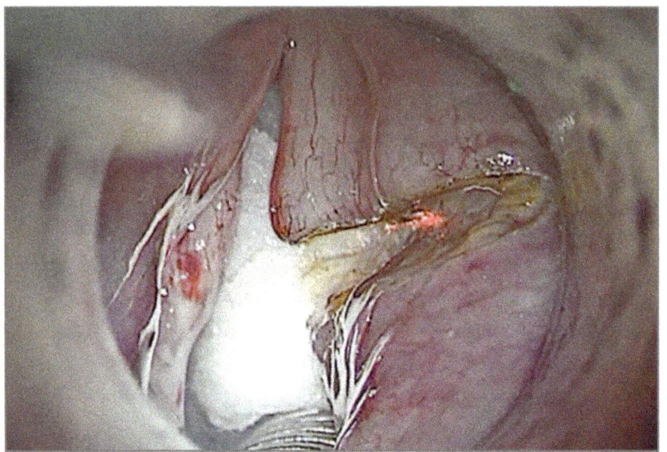

FIG. 21.2: The laser has now cut the entire depth of the true vocal fold medially and the underlying cotton pledget can be seen in that area. The left corner of the image has the laser suction plume in place. (M-CC)

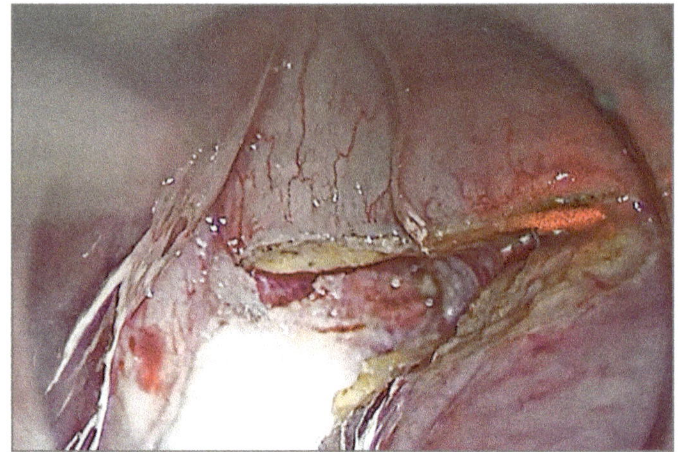

FIG. 21.3: The true vocal fold lying deep to the false vocal fold can be cut under direct vision, once the false vocal fold cut is complete. (M-CC)

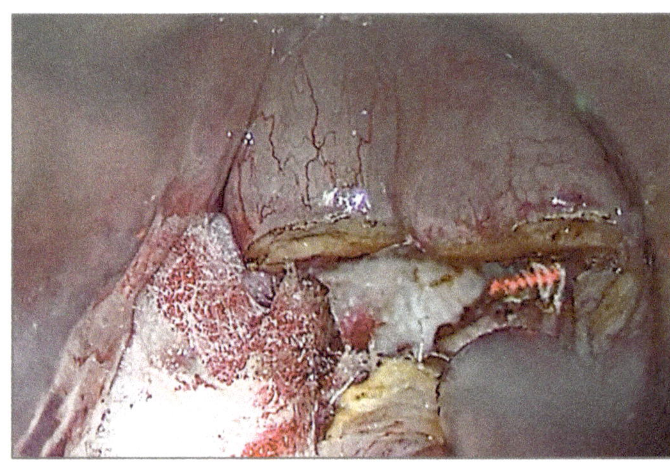

FIG. 21.4: The final cut nearing the inner perichondrium of the thyroid cartilage. (M-CC)

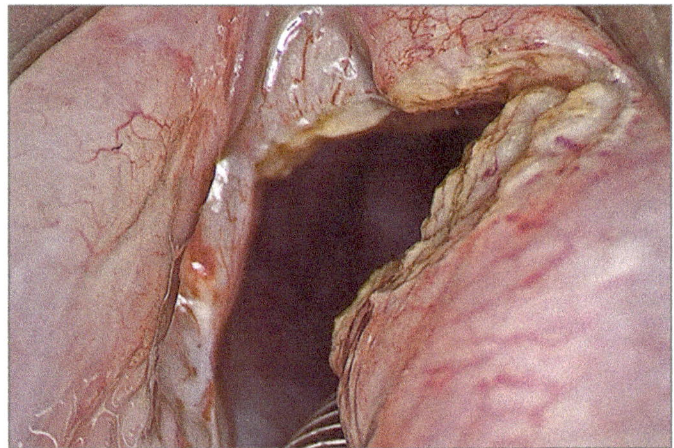

FIG. 21.5: Final postoperative image showing the airway created and the thicker right vocal fold (due to its anterior retraction). (E-CC)

CASE 2

An adult male patient presented with history of respiratory distress since over a year, with an episode of hospitalization for what was felt to be severe asthma.

Flexible laryngostroboscopy revealed bilateral immobile vocal folds and the workup of the patient including computed tomography scan (base skull to mediastinum) was unremarkable. The patient was posted for a left Kashima cordotomy.

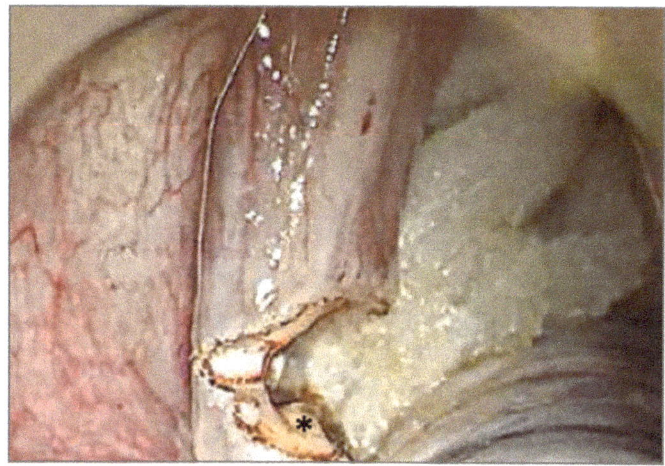

FIG. 21.8: Extension of the horizontal cordotomy. A hint of the exposed vocal process tip can be seen (*). (M-CC)

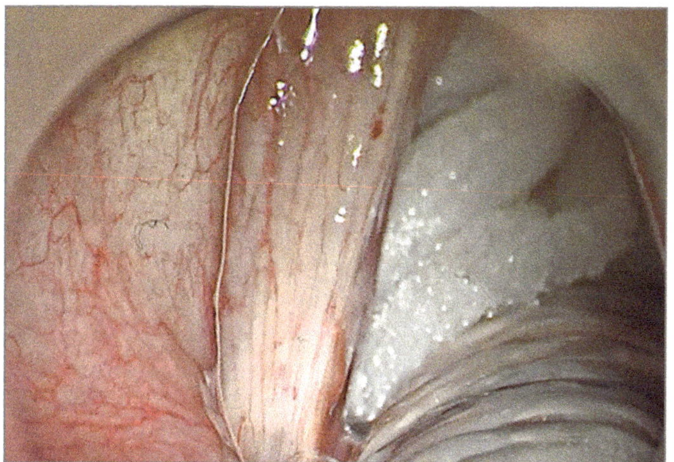

FIG. 21.6: The microlaryngoscope is positioned such that the left true and false vocal fold are in clear vision. (M-CC)

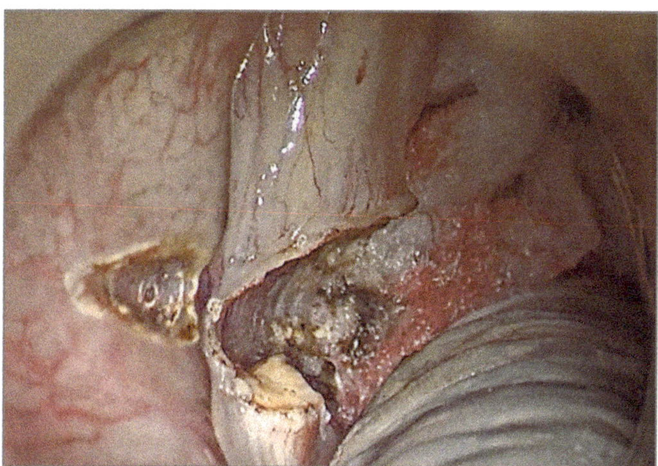

FIG. 21.9: In order to cut the true vocal fold lying below the false vocal fold, a cut is first made on the false vocal fold in the line of surgery. (M-CC)

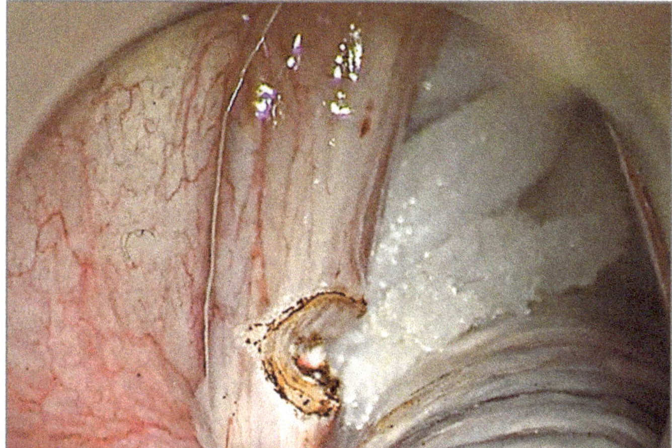

FIG. 21.7: The horizontal laser cut is made to separate the left vocal process from the vocal fold. The natural tensile strength of the vocal fold results in an anterior retraction of the vocal fold, consequently producing a triangular gap rather than a slit. (M-CC)

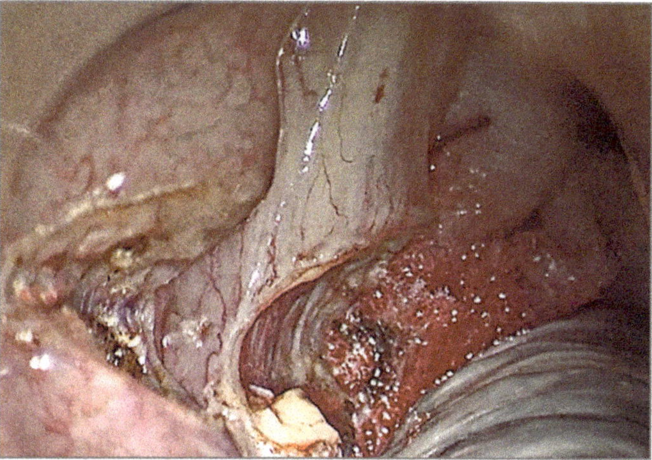

FIG. 21.10: It can clearly be appreciated that one-third of the true vocal fold lies hidden by the false vocal fold. Once the false vocal fold is cut, completion cordotomy of the true vocal fold can be performed easily. (M-CC)

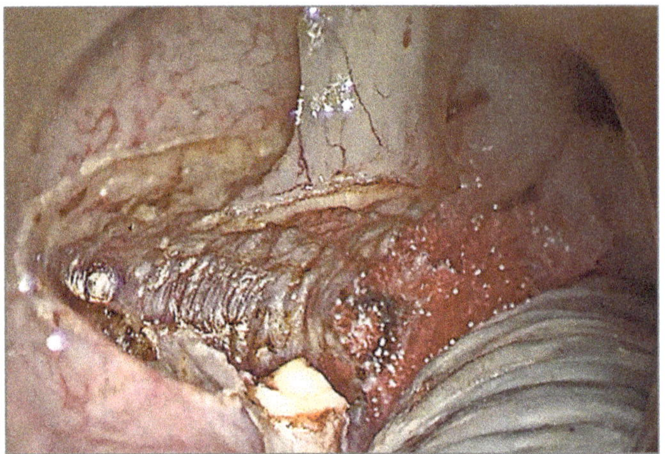

FIG. 21.11: Both the true and false vocal fold have been cut to their lateral extent. It is possible to retract the false vocal fold with an elevator and cut the entire width of the true vocal fold if preferred by the surgeon. (M-CC)

CASE 3

A 9-year-old boy is referred with history of dyspnea on exertion during the day and severe intercostal and suprasternal in drawing with a loud sterterous sound at night. Bilateral immobile vocal folds, with a right flicker of motion, is observed on flexible laryngoscopy. The diagnostic workup is unremarkable and the child is maintained conservatively for 5 months but worsens especially with every upper respiratory tract infection. A decision to perform left Kashima's cordotomy is taken. The parents are counseled regarding permanent slight breathiness to the voice.

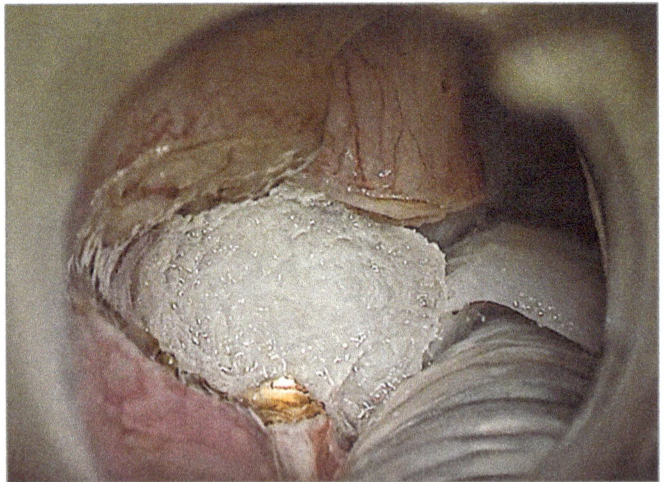

FIG. 21.12: Since the vocal process has been exposed in this case, we prefer to laser ablate it. Exposed cartilage can provide a nidus for infection and granuloma formation. (M-CC)

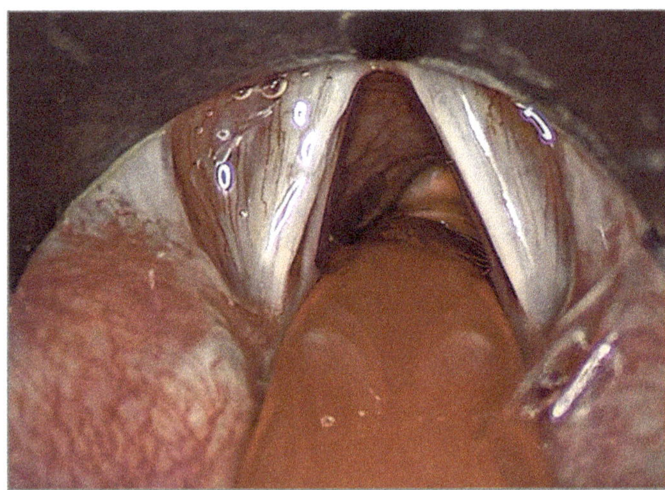

FIG. 21.14: A 3 number red-rubber tube with a cuff is used in this patient. (E-CC)

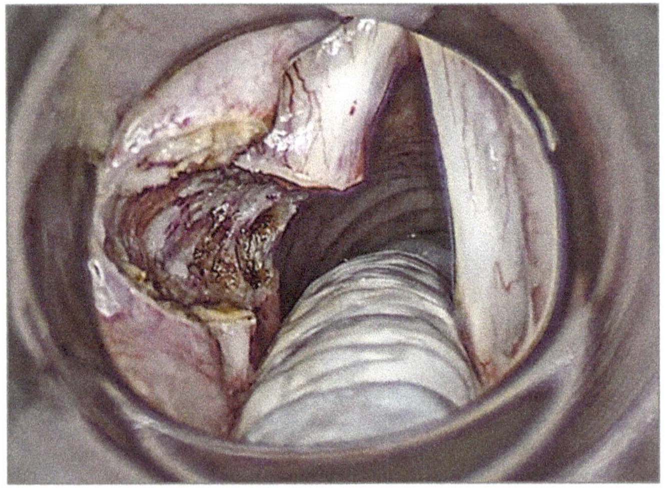

FIG. 21.13: The final postoperative image. (E-CC)

A

Continued

Continued

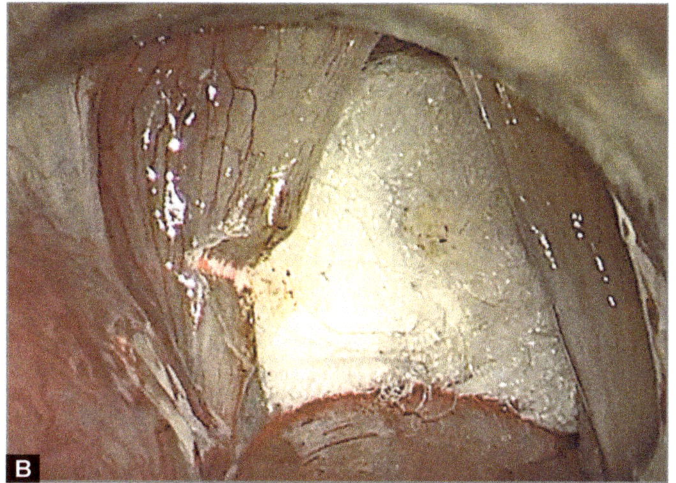

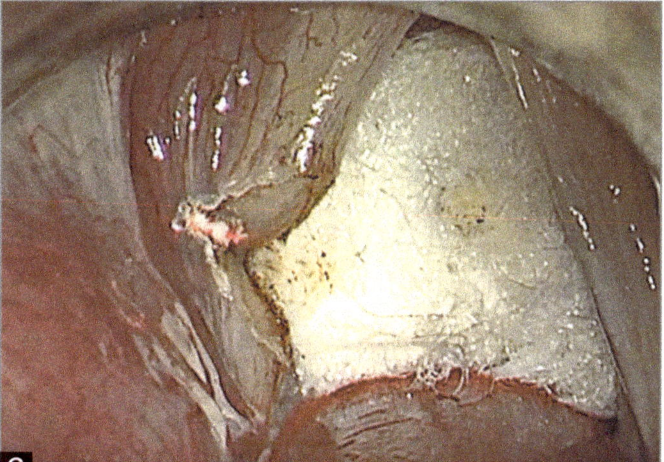

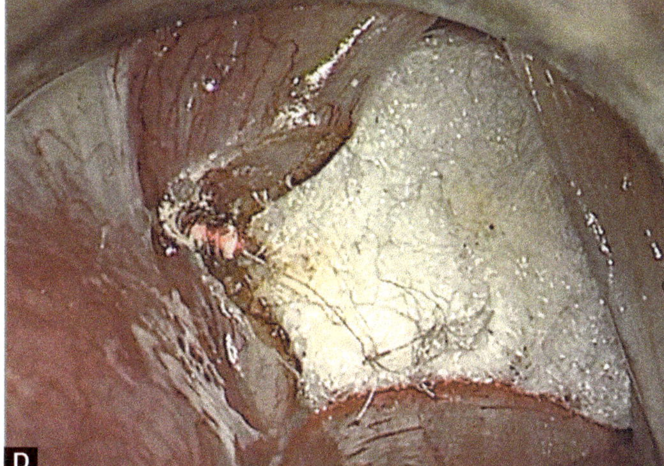

FIG. 21.15: A left Kashima cordotomy is commenced using 1 mm length AcuBlade, 1 depth, 10 w in superpulse, repeat mode. A moist cotton pledget is protecting the cuff. (M-CC)

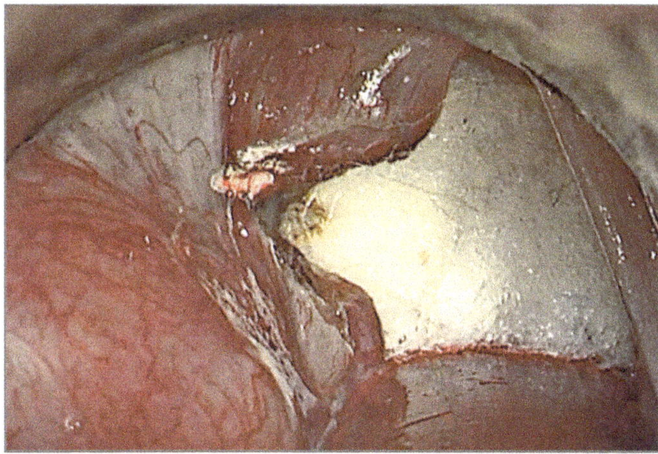

FIG. 21.16: The procedure is complete once the thyroid cartilage can be palpated. (M-CC)

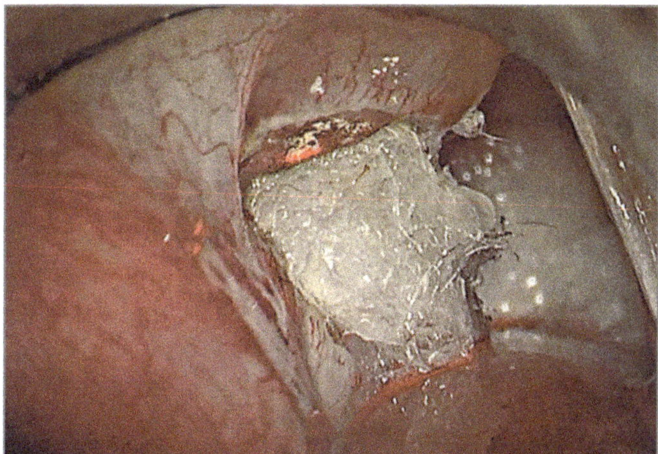

FIG. 21.17: The false vocal fold has not been cut in this case, only retracted during surgery. (M-CC)

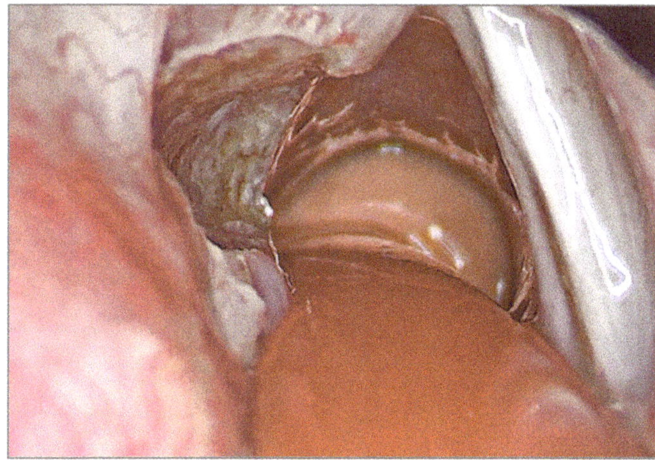

FIG. 21.18: Final postoperative airway. (E-CC)

POSTOPERATIVE CARE

After surgery, patients receive antibiotics for 1 week and proton pump inhibitors for 6 weeks. Patients who do not have a tracheostomy, receive a short course of steroids in tapering doses. In patients with a tracheostomy, the glottic chink is examined on the 7th day and if found to be adequate, the tracheostomy is blocked for progressively increasing lengths of time. This is done over a period of 1 week and eventually the tube is kept completely blocked. Once the patient can tolerate a fully blocked tube for 1–2 months, they are decannulated. In case the patient still has respiratory distress, 4–6 weeks postoperatively, despite good healing at the operated side, the opposite vocal fold is operated upon.

In case of a granuloma developing at the operative site, steroid inhalation is added onto the proton-pump inhibitor and oral steroids.

REFERENCES

1. Jackson C. Ventriculocordectomy. A new operation for the cure of goitrous glottic stenosis. Arch Surg. 1922;4:257-74.
2. King BT. A new and function restoring operation for bilateral abductor cord paralysis. JAMA. 1939;112:814-23.
3. Thornell WC. Intralaryngeal approach for arytenoidectomy in bilateral abductor vocal cord paralysis. Arch Otolaryngol. 1948;47:505-08.
4. Ossoff RH, Karlan MS, Sisson GA. Endoscopic laser arytenoidectomy. Lasers Surg Med. 1983;2:293-9.
5. Dennis DP, Kashima H. Carbon dioxide laser posterior cordectomy for treatment of bilateral vocal cord paralysis. Ann Otol Rhinol Laryngol. 1989;98:930-4.
6. Burian K, Höfler H. Zur mikrochirurgischen Therapie von Stimmband-Karzinomen mit dem CO_2-laser. Laryngol Rhinol Otol (Stuttg). 1979;58:551-6.

CHAPTER 22

Early Glottic Malignancy

INTRODUCTION

The treatment options for early glottic malignancy are transoral laser microsurgery (TLM) or radiation therapy. Very infrequent situations today warrant partial laryngectomy for early glottic malignancy.

Laser surgery has gained sufficient acceptance as an oncologically safe, less morbid, and functionally equivalent modality to conventional radiotherapy. It is also cost-effective and repeatable with the option of open surgery and radiotherapy in the event of recurrence or a new primary.[1]

The TNM staging of glottic malignancy as defined in the 6th edition of the American Joint Committee on Cancer (AJCC) staging system is given in table 1.[2]

TABLE 22.1: The TNM staging of glottic malignancy as defined in the 6th edition of the American Joint Committee on Cancer (AJCC) staging system

Tis	Carcinoma *in situ* of the vocal fold(s)
T1	Tumor limited to the vocal fold(s), may involve anterior or posterior commissure with normal mobility
T1a	Tumor involves one vocal fold
T1b	Tumor involves both vocal folds
T2	Tumor extends to supraglottis and/or subglottis, or with impaired vocal fold mobility
T3	Tumor limited to larynx with vocal fold fixation
T4a	Tumor invades cricoid or thyroid cartilage and/or invades tissues beyond the larynx (e.g., trachea, soft tissues of neck including deep extrinsic muscles of the tongue, strap muscles, thyroid, or esophagus)
T4b	Tumor invades prevertebral space, encases carotid artery, or invades mediastinal structures

The prognostic significance of involvement of the paraglottic space by glottic tumors is acknowledged in the sixth edition of the AJCC staging, and these tumors are now staged T3. Tumors that have caused minor cartilage erosion (e.g., inner cortex of the thyroid lamina) are now staged T3, while the T4a category is reserved for tumors that actually penetrate through the cartilage.[3]

Early glottic malignancies are considered to be carcinoma *in situ*, T1a, T1b, and T2 malignancy.

According to the European Laryngological Society (2000, 2007) there are nine types of cordectomy.[4,5]

- Type 1 cordectomy: Subepithelial for dysplasia and carcinoma *in situ*
- Type 2 cordectomy: Subligamental for microinvasive carcinoma and invasive carcinoma not involving the ligament
- Type 3 cordectomy: Transmuscular for cancers infiltrating the ligament and reaching the vocalis muscle but not affecting the mobility of the vocal fold.
- Type 4 cordectomy: Total cordectomy for cancers involving the thyroarytenoid muscle

Extended cordectomies involve excision of the vocal fold and extension of the excision beyond the ipsilateral side. There are four subtypes:

- Type Va: Extended cordectomy with anterior commissure
- Type Vb: Extended cordectomy with arytenoidectomy
- Type Vc: Extended cordectomy with ventricular fold resection
- Type Vd: Extended cordectomy with subglottic resection
- Type VI: Anterior commissure and unilateral/bilateral anterior vocal folds.

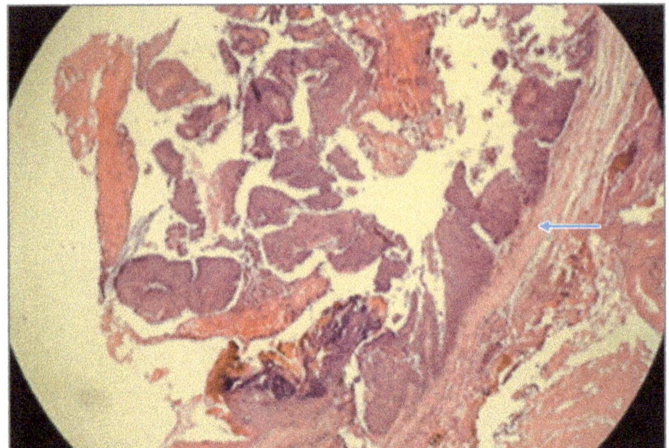

FIG. 22.1: Carcinoma *in situ* of the true vocal fold (H&E staining). An intact basement membrane is noted (blue arrow)

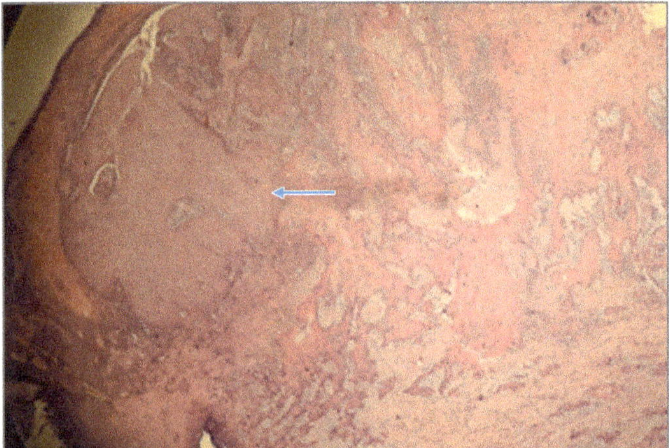

FIG. 22.2: Invasive squamous cell carcinoma where the basement membrane and superficial lamina propria is involved in the malignancy (blue arrow)

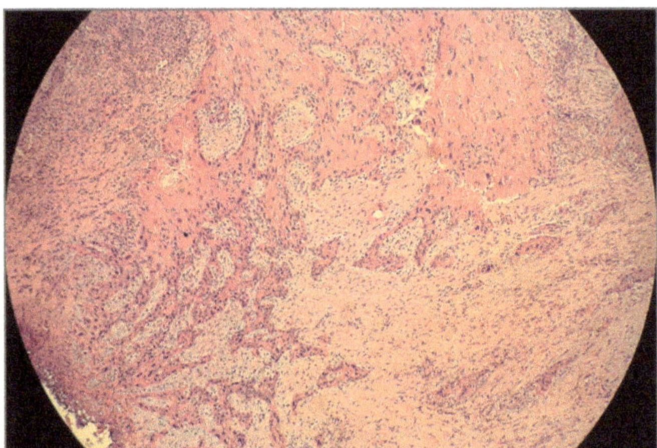

FIG. 22.3: High power of 22.2

Appearance of transglottic carcinoma *in situ* in a 40-year-old lady (Figs 22.4 to 22.7). She had history of a renal transplant 2 years back with hoarseness since 3–4 months. Presence of koilocytes in the histopathology was suggestive of human papillomavirus (HPV) infection.

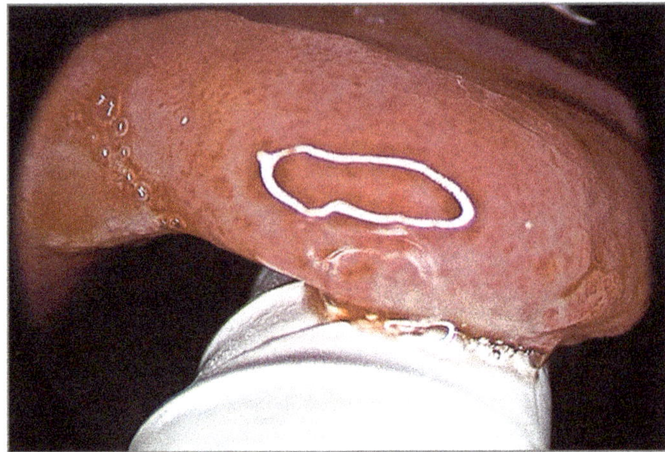

FIG. 22.4: Mottled appearance of the lingual surface of the epiglottis. (E-CC)

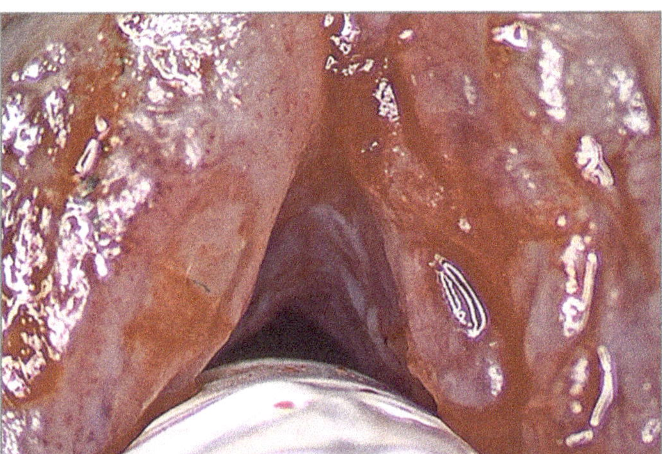

FIG. 22.5: Mottled and irregular appearance of the false and true vocal folds. (E-CC)

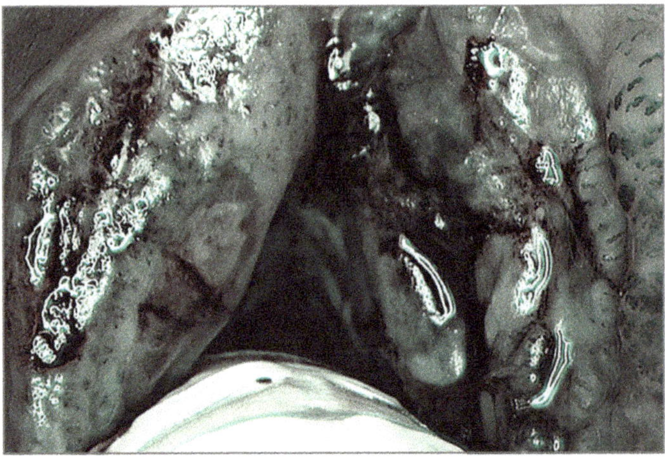

FIG. 22.6: Type 5a Ni pattern on the left true vocal fold and type 5b Ni pattern on the right false vocal fold. (E-SA)

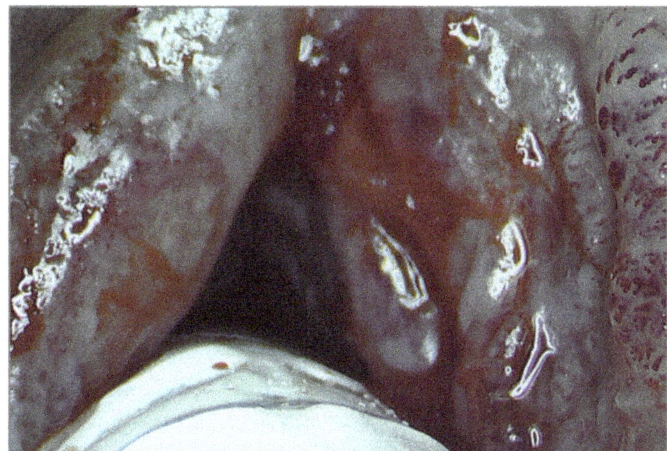

FIG. 22.7: Spectra B image of 22.6. The clarity and contrast of the aberrant blood vessels on the right false vocal fold are well appreciated. (E-SB)

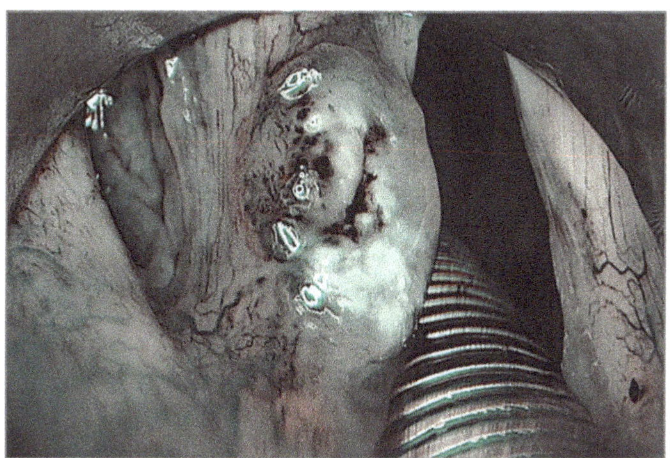

FIG. 22.8: The type 5c Ni pattern observed over the left posterior vocal fold growth in a male patient helped rule out a benign contact granuloma. The lesion was an invasive squamous cell carcinoma. (E-SA)

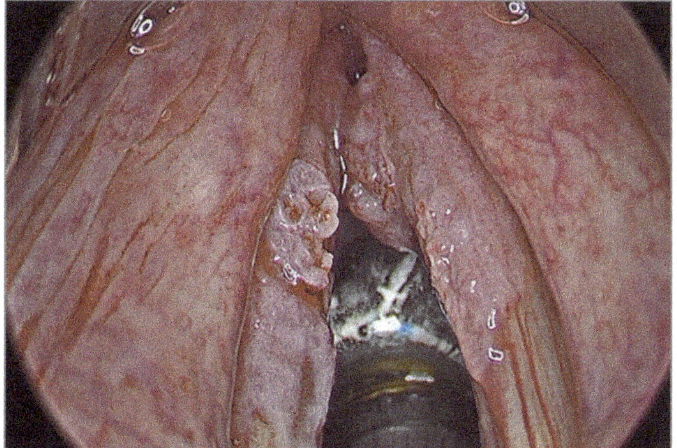

FIG. 22.9: A carpet-like growth is seen on both the vocal folds in an elderly male patient with the disease getting bulkier anteriorly. (E-CC)

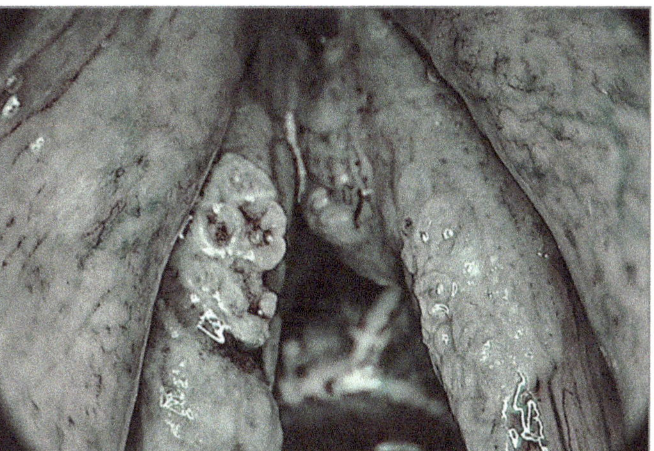

FIG. 22.10: The spectra A image of this lesion cannot clearly identify the type of vascular pattern by Ni staging. This is due to an apparent layer of keratosis over the lesion. The vascular pattern around the lesion on the right vocal fold posteriorly is unremarkable. (E-SA)

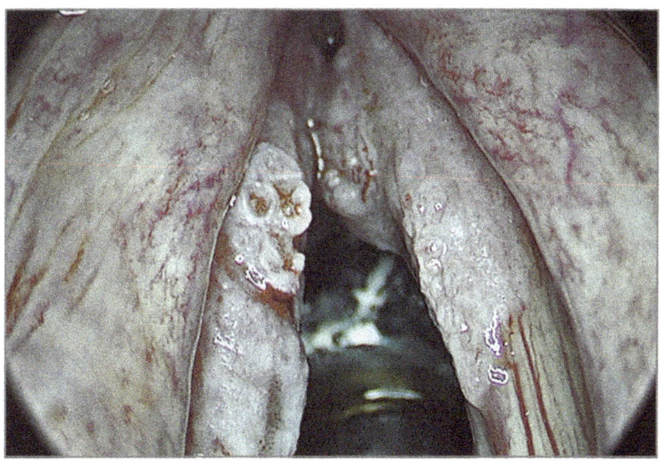

FIG. 22.11: The SB image of the lesion reveals a distinct margin of the growth but the vascular pattern cannot be clearly commented upon. The histopathological report revealed an Invasive squamous cell carcinoma. Keratosis is known to be a condition that may result in a false negative for cancer on both narrow band imaging light or SA/SB imaging. (E-SB)

PHILOSOPHY OF SURGERY

A stroboscopy with narrow band imaging (NBI) testing is performed for all glottic lesions at our Voice Clinic. With anterior commissure lesions, bulky disease, decreased or absent vocal fold mobility, a preoperative computed tomography scan of the neck to rule out cartilage destruction and lymphadenopathy is performed.

During micro laryngeal surgery, inspection under magnification and palpation of the lesion and surrounding structures is the first step followed by the subepithelial infiltration technique. A 27 gauge needle is used to infiltrate 1-2 cc of 1 in 10,000 saline adrenaline in the subepithelial space. A good elevation of the superficial lamina propria rules out ligament involvement. A doughnut sign with infiltration collecting all around the lesion suggests ligament or even muscle involvement.

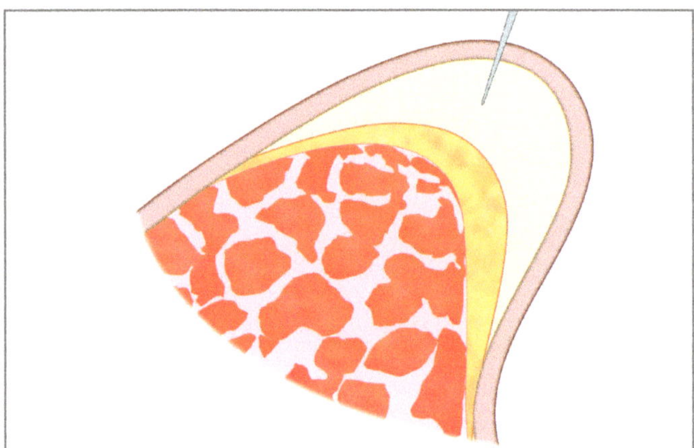

FIG. 22.12: Diagrammatic representation of 27 gauge infiltration needle in the subepithelial space causing a temporary increase in superficial lamina propria volume in a normal vocal fold

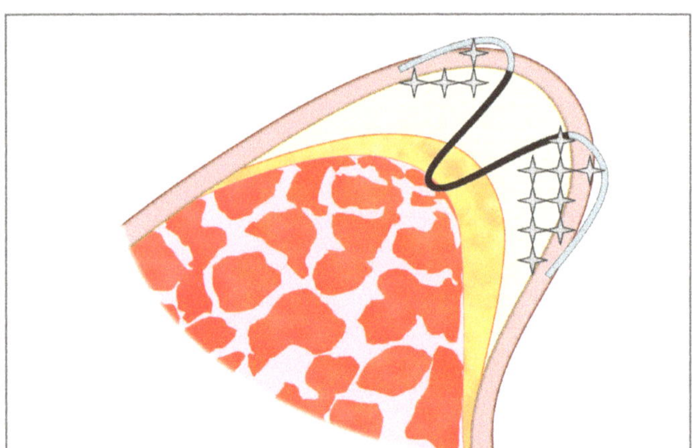

FIG. 22.13: Diagrammatic representation of a vocal fold lesion infiltrating the vocal ligament with subepithelial infiltration ballooning up superficial lamina propria around the lesion (doughnut effect)

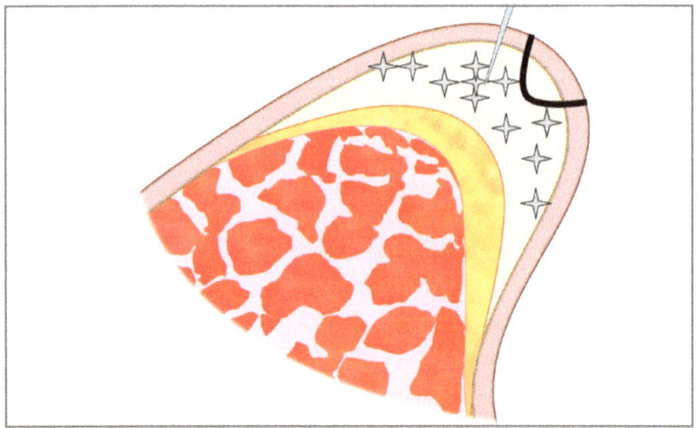

FIG. 22.14: Diagrammatic representation of vocal fold lesion involving the epithelium and superficial lamina propria (SLP) with subepithelial infiltration ballooning up the entire SLP and lifting up the lesion

The lesion is then excised, usually in toto, with the help of the AcuBlade CO_2 laser in superpulse, repeat mode at 10 W with the AcuBlade length varying from 1-2 mm and a depth of 2-3 (500-750 microns). In case of large lesions, they are removed in 2 or more parts.

The author sends margins from the patient's side for frozen histopathology. The reasoning behind this is the natural shrinkage of tissue once excised, especially with a laser. This leads to the false appearance of close margins. Thus, the lesion is first sent for frozen (not if a positive biopsy is already present). Following this, the peripheral margins for 1-2 mm and the entire depth of the next uninvolved layer of the vocal fold is excised and sent for frozen confirmation of the free margins. No malignant cells should be seen in this carpet of tissue, which is marked anteriorly with methylene blue, and placed on a filter paper placed in a Petri dish. A diagram of the vocal folds is made on the filter paper and the tumor placed/pinned on this diagram to best represent the way it was placed anatomically in the larynx.

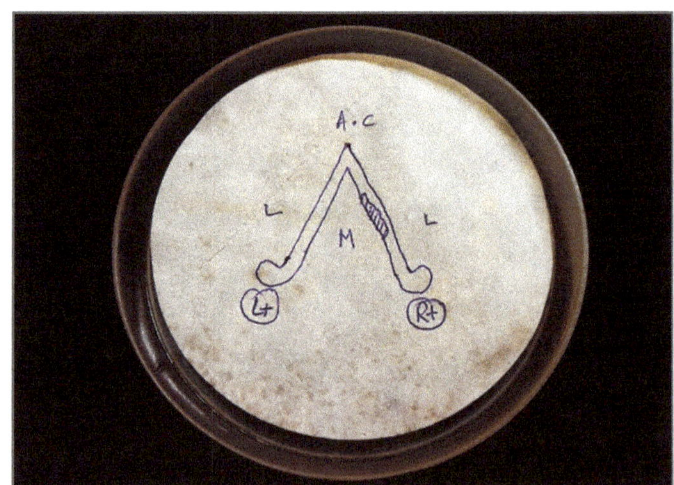

FIG. 22.15: A diagram of the vocal folds made on the filter paper and the tumor placed/pinned to best represent the way it was placed anatomically in the larynx

During a cordectomy, if it becomes apparent that a type 4 or 5 cordectomy is warranted, we prefer to abandon the procedure in favor of radiation therapy, in order to optimize the patient's vocal outcomes. This decision is taken after a detailed preoperative discussion with the patient and relatives' regarding this scenario has been already discussed.

However, in the situation of history of radiation failure, we do not follow this dictum and proceed with type 4 or 5 cordectomy. Though technically, a medialization laryngoplasty can be performed following type 4 or 5 cordectomy, it is not typically successful as there is no bulk of tissue to medialize. Various flap surgeries may be also attempted in this scenario.

In our experience, the final voice after a type 6 cordectomy is serviceable. If the anterior commissure is adequately accessible, type 6 cordectomy is a good option to offer the patient for anterior commissure malignancies.

CASE 1

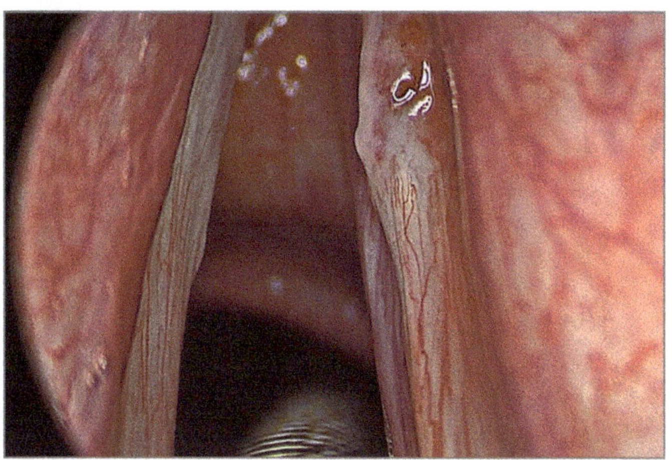

FIG. 22.16: Type 1 cordectomy being performed for a right vocal fold carcinoma *in situ*, where the anterior commissure is free of disease. (E-CC)

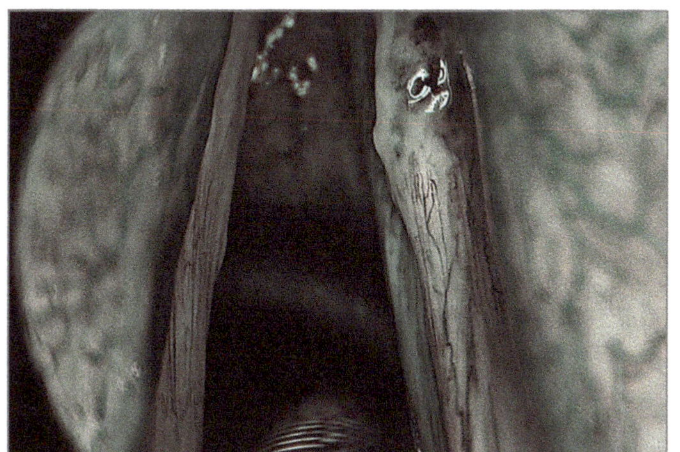

FIG. 22.17: Image of 22.16 in spectra A mode. A type 4 Ni pattern is seen anteriorly on the lesion. (E-SA)

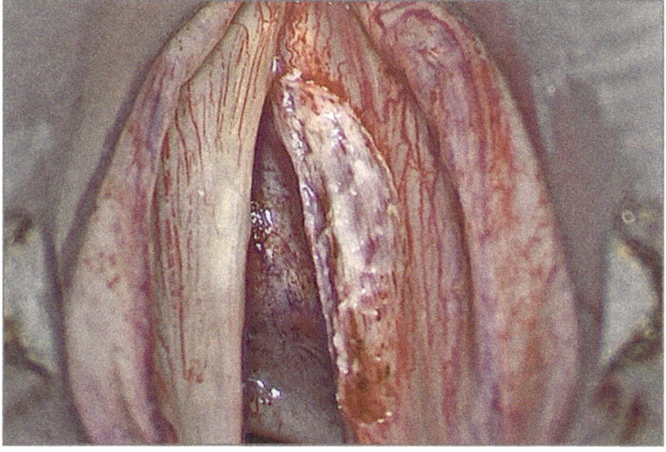

FIG. 22.18: Image following the right subepithelial cordectomy with the exposed right vocal ligament seen. A 1 mm margin has been taken at the tumor periphery. The anterior commissure (anterior-most 3 mm of the vocal fold) are free of disease. (E-CC)

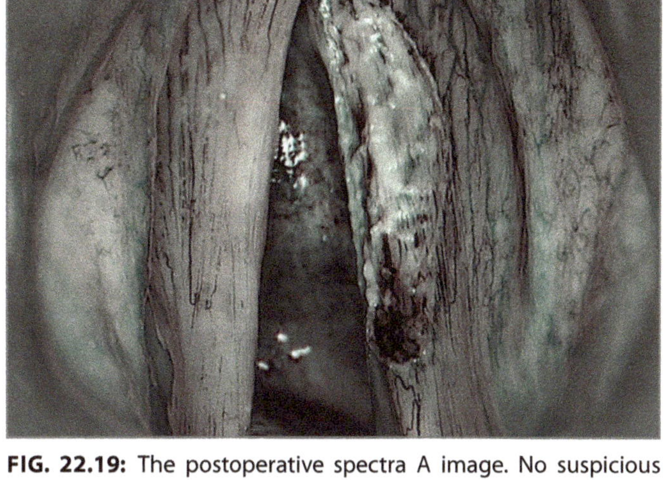

FIG. 22.19: The postoperative spectra A image. No suspicious vascular patterns are visible. (E-SA)

CASE 2

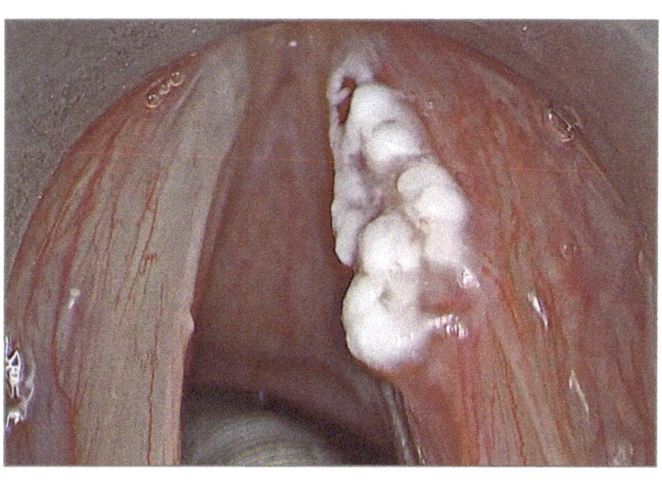

FIG. 22.20: Right type 2 cordectomy being performed for a T1aN0M0 microinvasive squamous cell carcinoma in an adult male patient. The growth appears keratotic in nature. (E-CC)

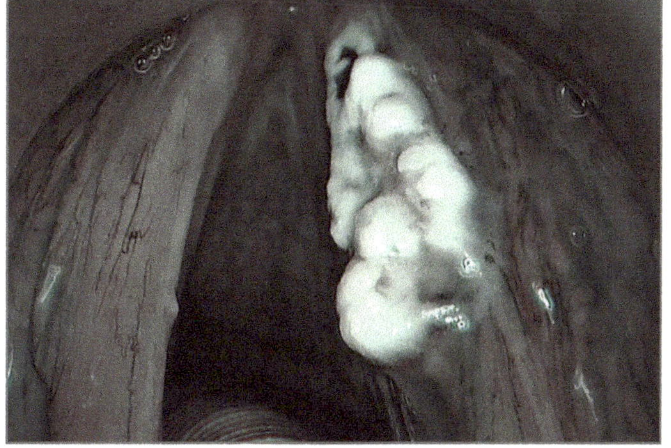

FIG. 22.21: Spectra A image of 22.20 does not reveal any aberrant vascular pattern on the surface of the cancer or the margins. A false negative impression on spectra A or narrow band imaging is known with keratotic lesions and is to be kept under consideration at all times. (E-SA)

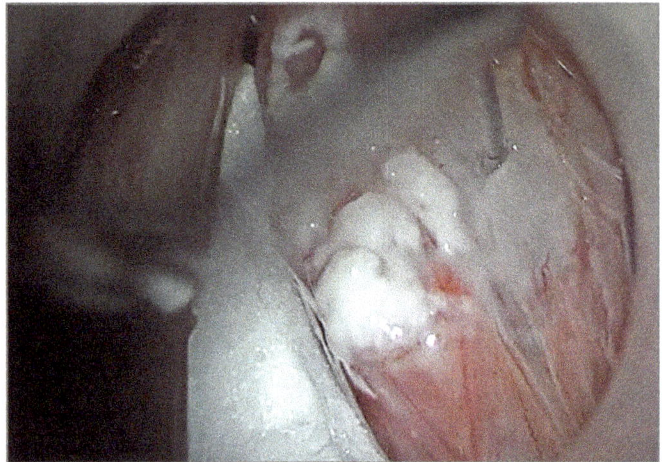

FIG. 22.22: Subepithelial infiltration technique being performed with a 27 gauge needle. The blanching of the infiltrate is seen. (M-CC)

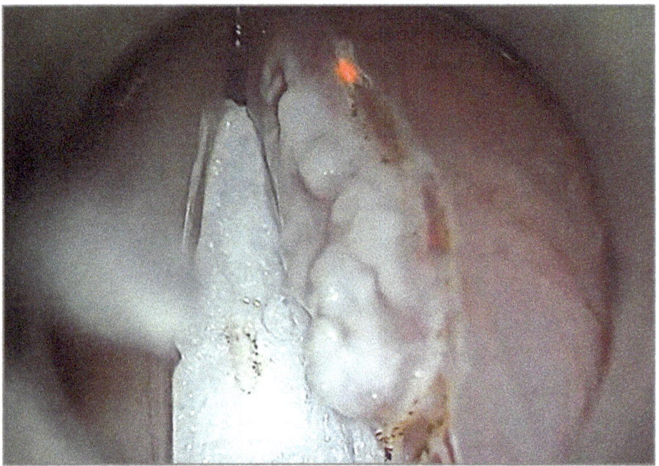

FIG. 22.23: Laser epithelial cordotomy lateral to the tumor. (M-CC)

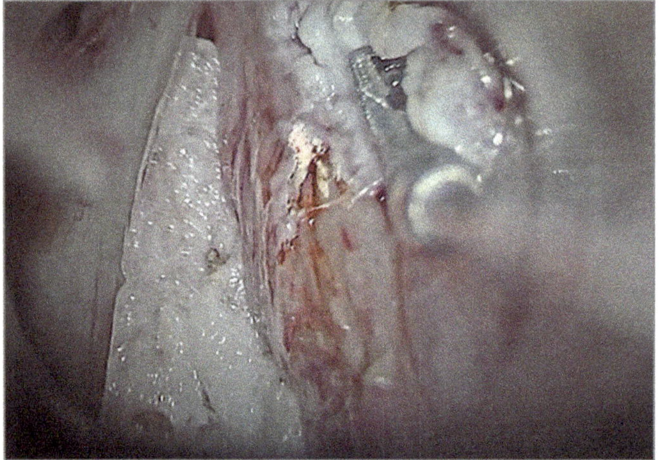

FIG. 22.24: Laser epithelial cordotomy being performed medial to the tumor, at its infragltiic edge. To facilitate this the tumor is laterally retracted with a bouchayer. (M-CC)

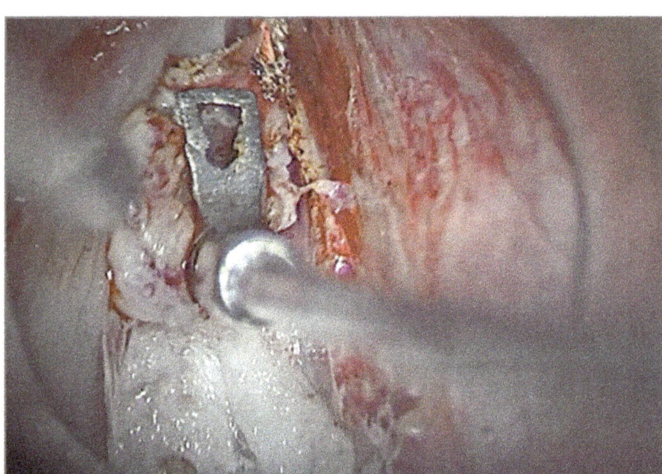

FIG. 22.25: Anterior attachment of the tumor being excised by the acublade. (M-CC)

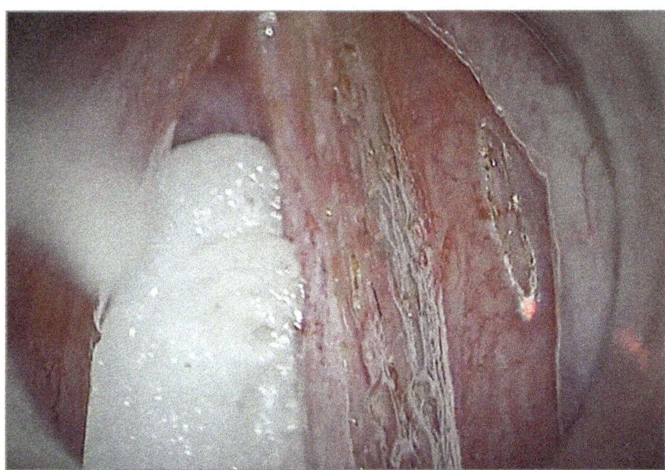

FIG. 22.26: Following tumor excision, the margins are now excised from the patient side, 1–2 mm all around the periphery and one uninvolved layer in depth. The AcuBlade is seen making a lateral cut 1.5 mm from the edge of the excised tumor. (M-CC)

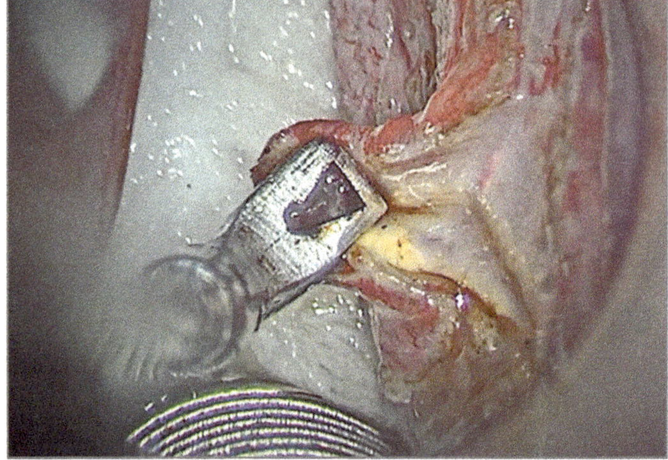

FIG. 22.27: The depth margin (ligament) is now being excised from a posterior to anterior direction. After making a cut with the laser to separate the vocal process from the vocal ligament, the ligament is held medially with a Bouchayer and excised in an anterior direction, in this case. (M-CC)

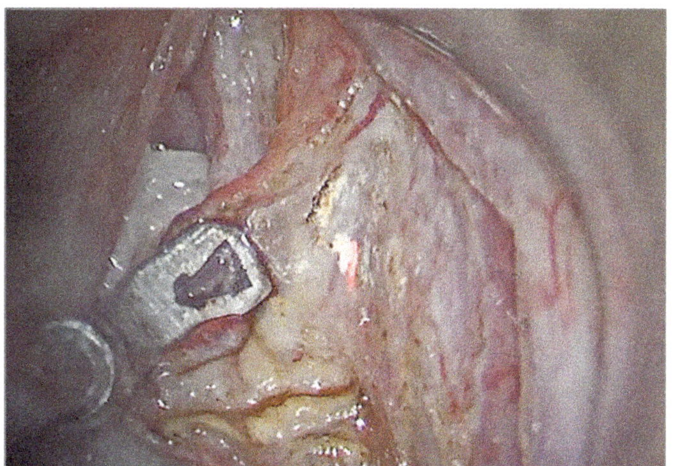

FIG. 22.28: The AcuBlade is seen in the plane of dissection, between the ligament and the vocalis muscle. (E-CC)

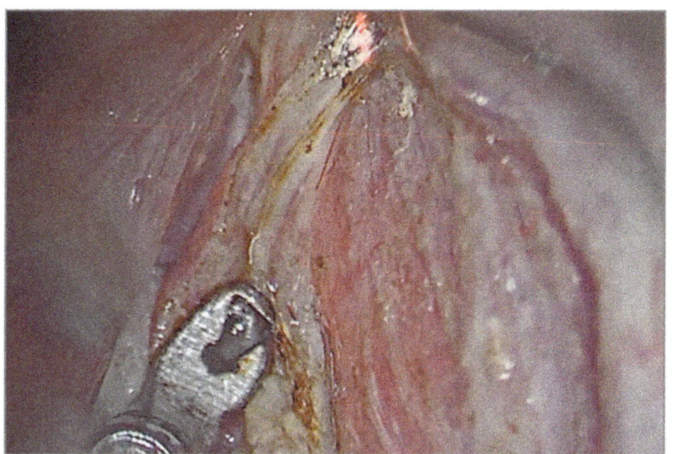

FIG. 22.29: The ligament is now cut anteriorly with the AcuBlade. (M-CC)

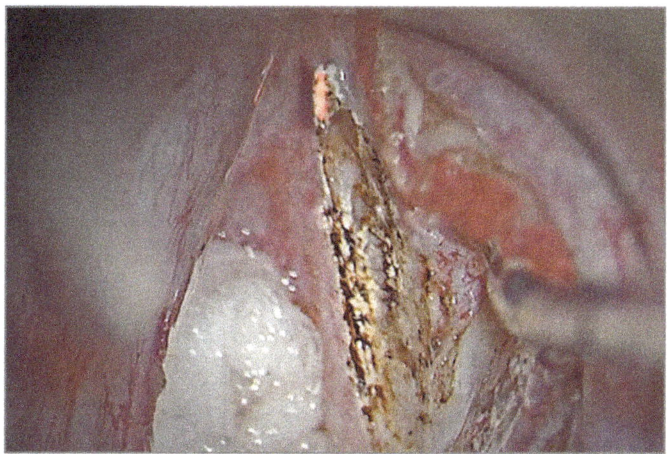

FIG. 22.30: The infraglottic cut has been made up to the anterior commissure to completely free the vocal ligament. (M-CC)

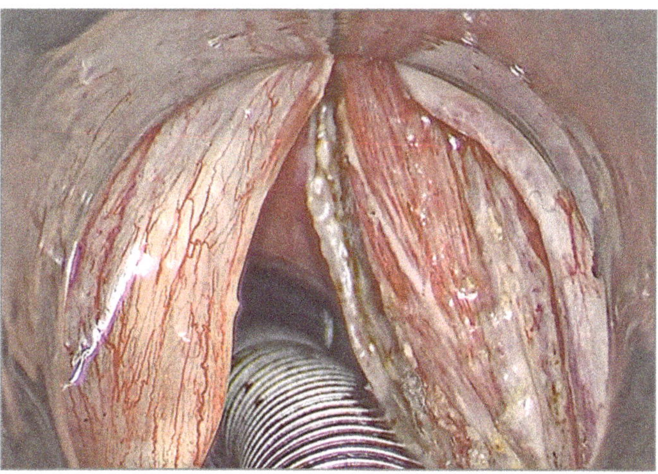

FIG. 22.31: The final postoperative view following the completion of the right type 2 cordectomy. The vocalis muscle fibers can be clearly seen. (E-CC)

CASE 3

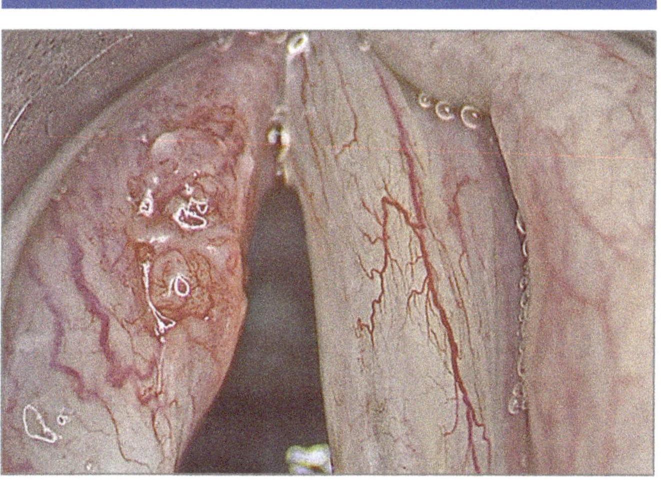

FIG. 22.32: A left mid-membranous invasive squamous cell carcinoma. Both vocal folds are mobile and the computed tomography does not reveal cartilage destruction or paraglottic extension of the tumor which is graded T1aN0M0. (E-CC)

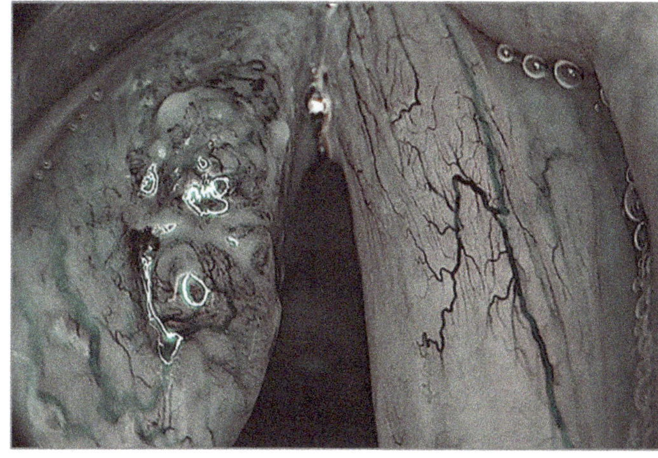

FIG. 22.33: Image of 22.32 in spectra A mode, a type 5b Ni pattern is seen on the left vocal fold. A type 1 Ni pattern is seen on the right vocal fold

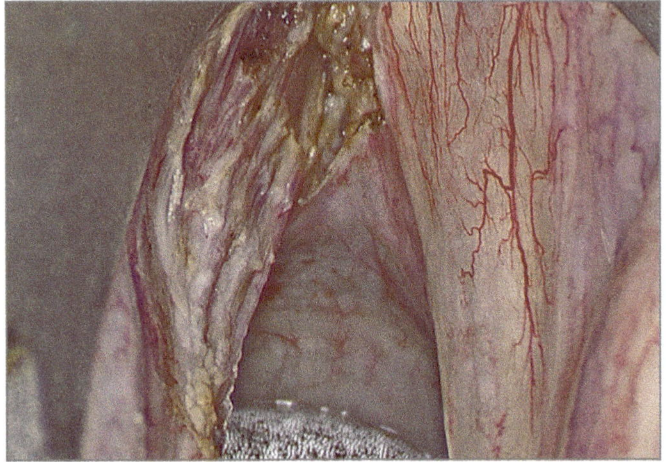

FIG. 22.34: Final postoperative image following a type 2 cordectomy of the left vocal fold. The ligament on frozen was free of cancer

CASE 4

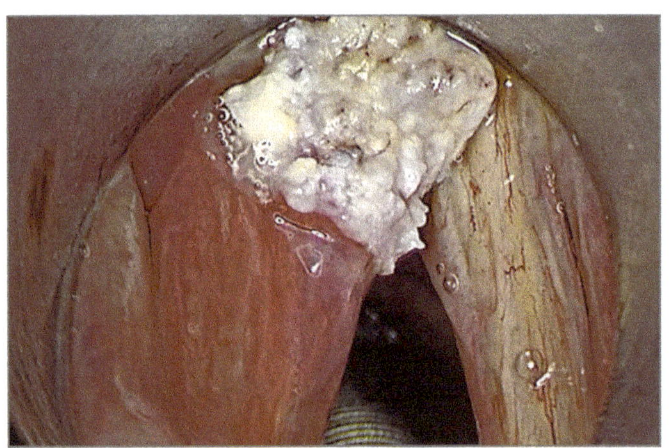

FIG. 22.35: A left keratotic growth with a congested left vocal fold is seen in an adult male patient. Both the vocal folds are mobile. (E-CC)

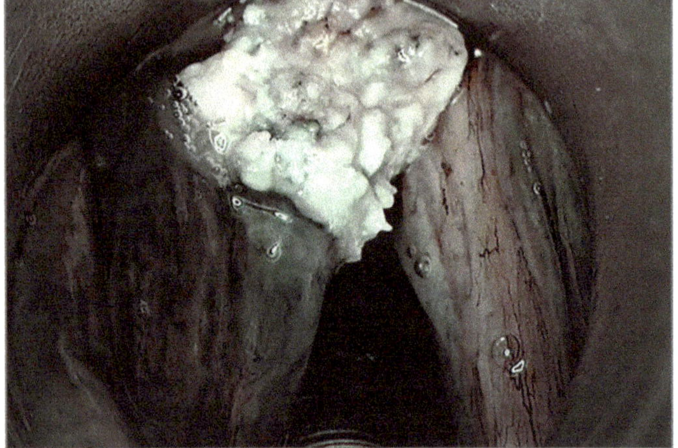

FIG. 22.36: Image of 22.35 in spectra A mode. No abnormal vascularity is observed in this image, though the patient had an invasive squamous cell carcinoma. The thick keratotic surface of the tumor probably hides the neovascularization associated with malignancy. (E-SA)

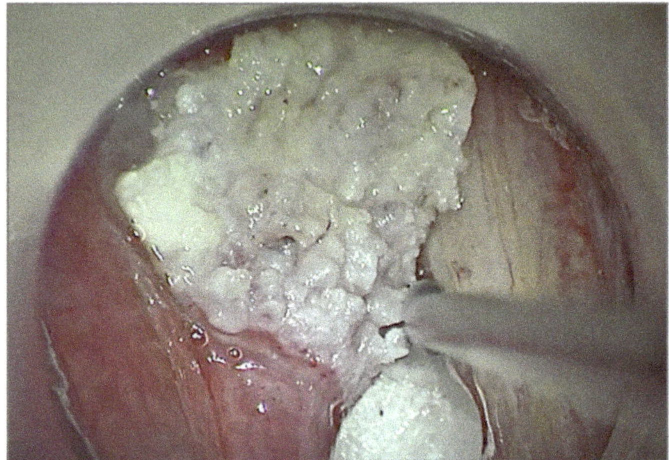

FIG. 22.37: The lesion and both the vocal folds are palpated. (M-CC)

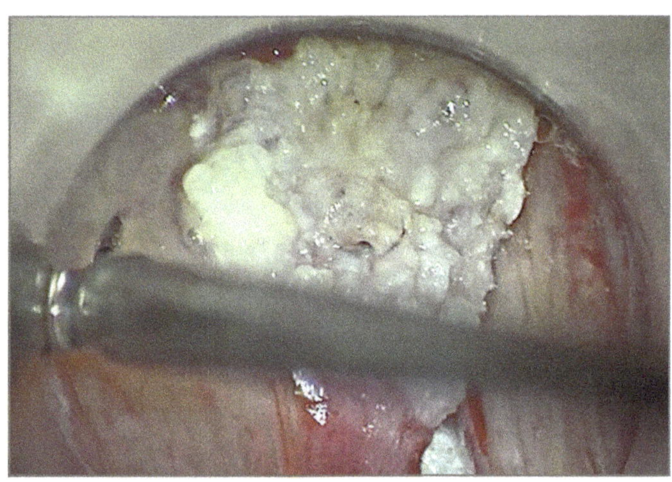

FIG. 22.38: Subepithelial infiltration technique being utilized. No doughnut effect is witnessed. (M-CC)

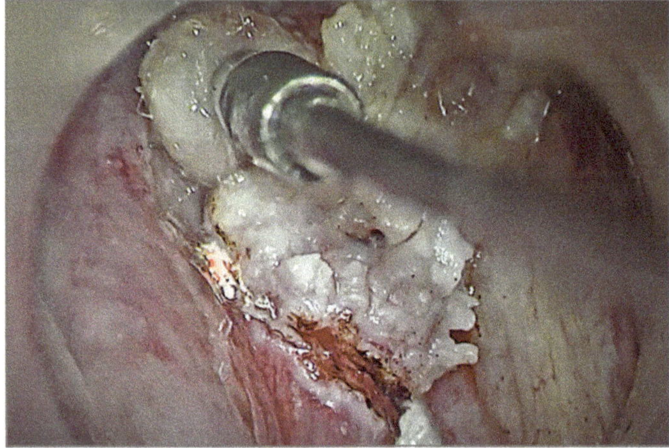

FIG. 22.39: The tumor is being excised by the CO_2 AcuBlade. A cotton pledget is being used to medially retract the lesion to facilitate lateral excision. (M-CC)

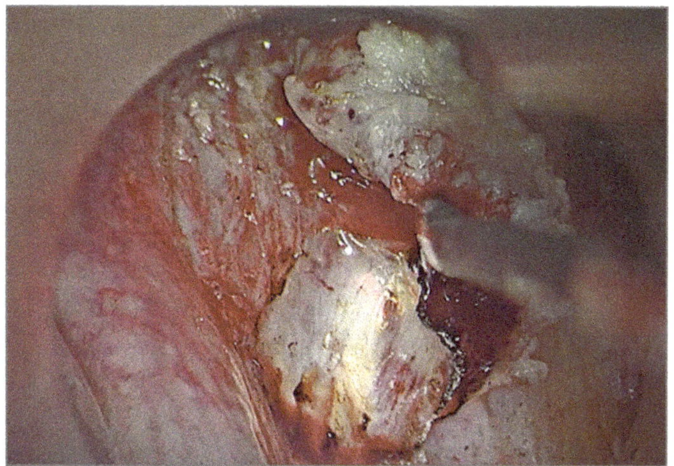

FIG. 22.40: The microflap elevator can also be effectively used to retract the lesion as it is atraumatic. Holding friable lesions is best avoided as far as possible. The white ligament can be seen on the bed following the posterior tumor excision. (M-CC)

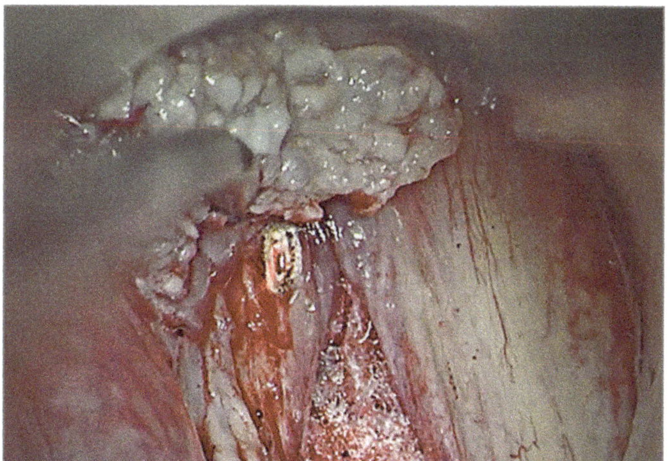

FIG. 22.41: Lateral retraction of the tumor with the microflap elevator helps in placing the infraglottic incision. (M-CC)

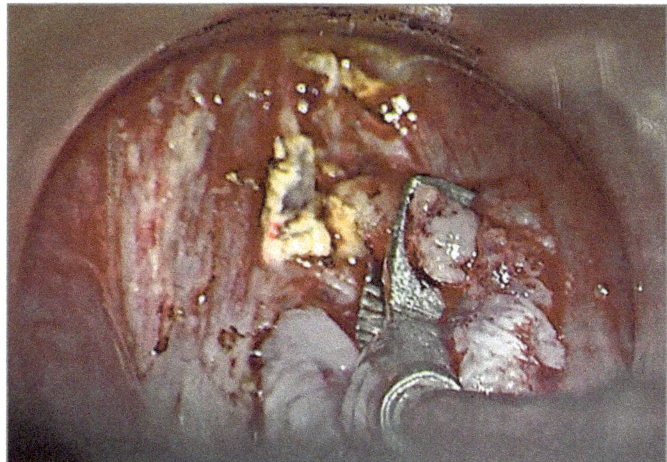

FIG. 22.42: Excision of the final medial attachments of the lesion is performed. The frozen report was invasive squamous cell carcinoma. (M-CC)

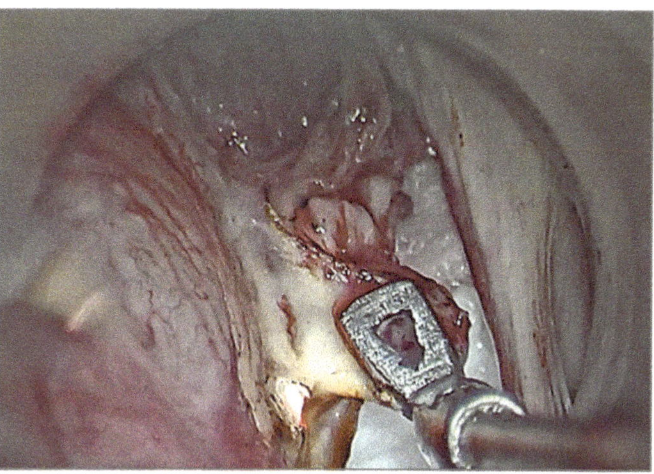

FIG. 22.43: The ligament is now excised, in order to achieve a depth clearance, along with peripheral margin clearance. The posterior part of the ligament is seen held by a Bouchayer forceps. (M-CC)

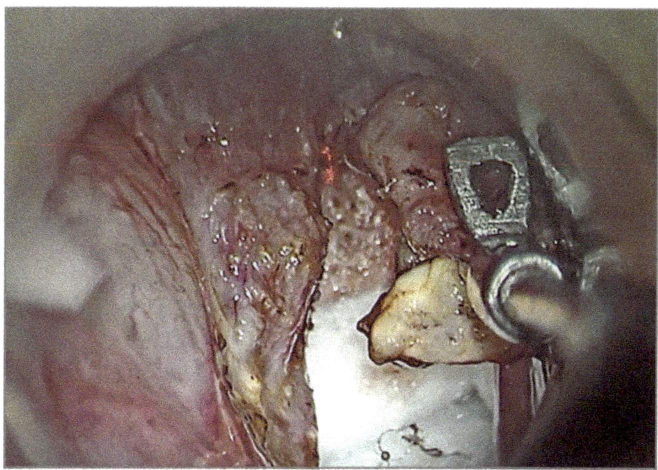

FIG. 22.44: The entire left vocal ligament is excised, leaving behind the muscle. (M-CC)

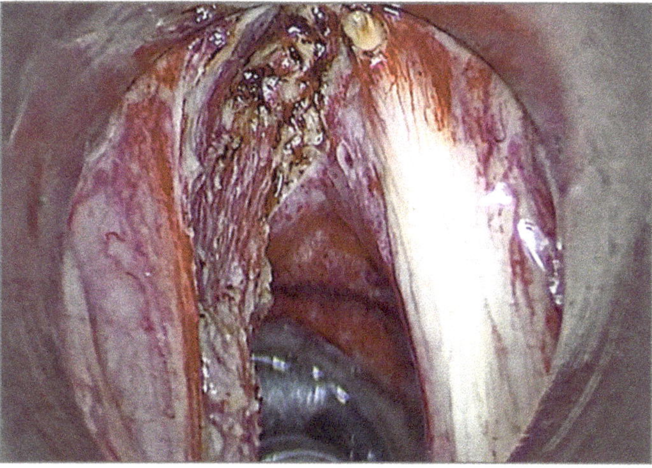

FIG. 22.45: Final postoperative image of 22.35 following left type 2 cordectomy. (E-CC)

CASE 5

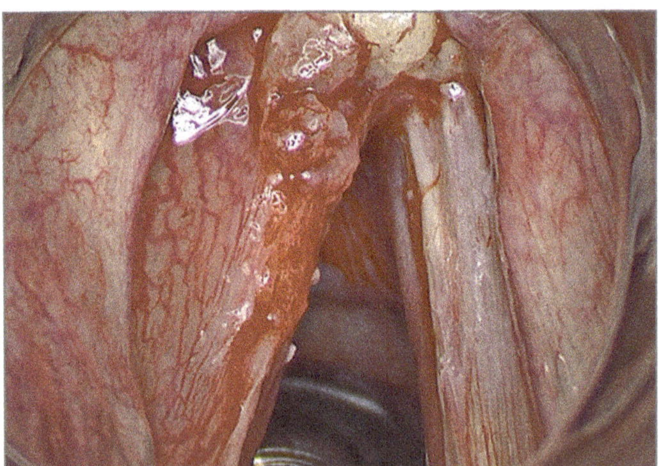

FIG. 22.46: A left Invasive squamous cell carcinoma with crossover to the right at the anterior commissure, T1bN0M0. (E-CC)

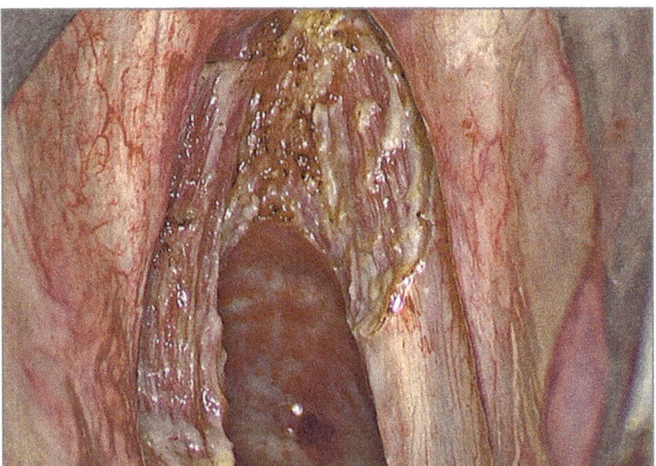

FIG. 22.47: A bilateral type 2 cordectomy was performed; the vocal ligament was free of malignancy on frozen section. The excision on the right vocal fold is not upto the posterior commissure but with 2 mm margins around the periphery of the tumor. The patient is taken up for slough clearance at 7–10 days time, to minimize the anterior glottic web formation. The patient is also encouraged to talk post surgery and not be on voice-rest, again in a bid to minimize the web formation. The other option to prevent a web formation is to stage the surgeries of the two sides with a 4–6 week interval. (E-CC)

CASE 6

A 45-year-old female patient is referred with hoarseness of voice of 4 months duration, and a history of having received radiation therapy 10 years back for right vocal fold squamous cell carcinoma. Stroboscopy revealed a compete loss of mucosal wave of the right vocal fold.

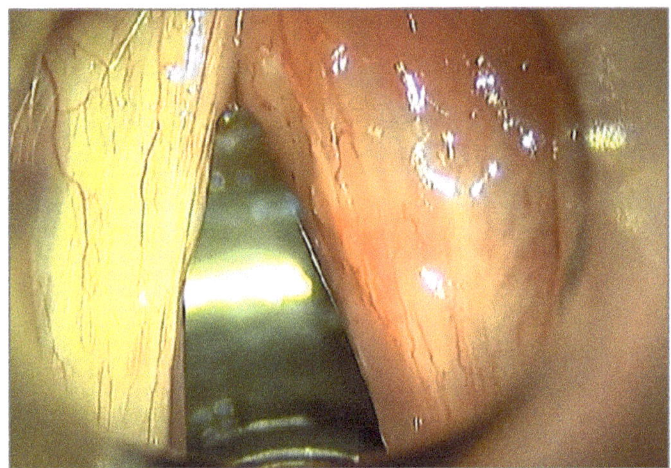

FIG. 22.48: Right congested, thickened and irregular vocal fold. (M-3 chip)

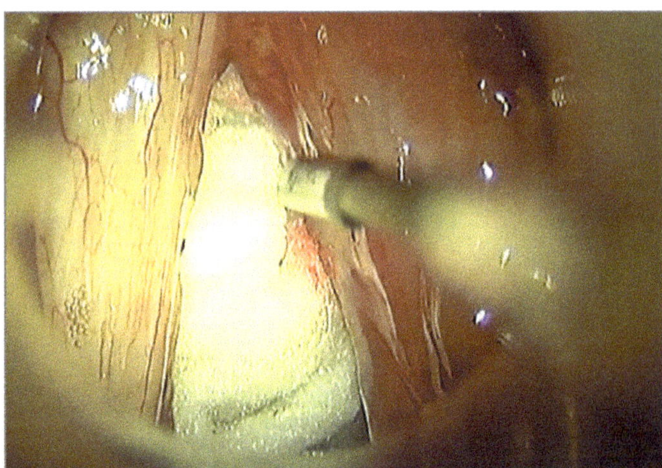

FIG. 22.49: The right vocal fold is firm to hard on palpation. (M-3 chip)

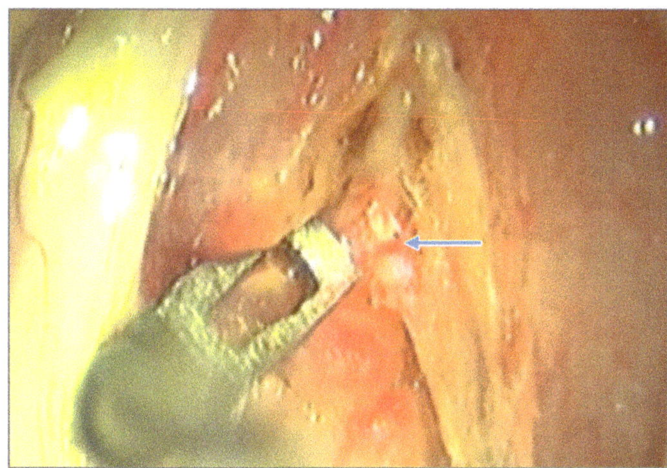

FIG. 22.50: The ligament is found involved with the lesion, which on frozen is invasive squamous cell carcinoma. The involvement of the ligament is seen in this image (blue arrow). (M-3 chip)

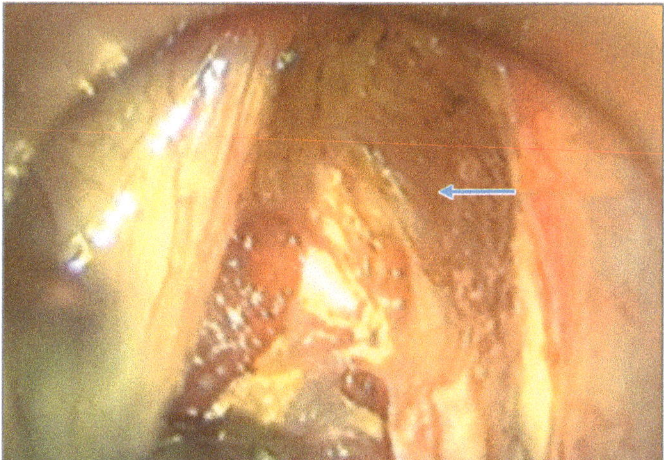

FIG. 22.51: Transmuscular cordectomy (type 3 cordectomy) performed of the anterior 2/3rd of the right vocal fold. The concavity in the thyroarytenoid muscle post excision is present (blue arrow). (M- 3 chip)

A regular follow up of all patients of glottic malignancy treated by TLM is vital for at least 5 years. Imaging tests to rule out local spread and confirm staging is equally important. All patients must be counseled regarding other options of treatment such as radiation therapy and benefits and drawbacks of each and similar possibility of recurrence with either modality. The final choice must lie with the patient.

REFERENCES

1. Vyas MN, Marc R. Lasers in early glottic cancer. In: Nerurkar NK, Roychoudhary A, editors. Textbook of Laryngology. Official Publication of the Association of Phonosurgeons of India. New Delhi: Jaypee Brothers Medical Publichers (P) Ltd.; 2017. pp. 185-99.
2. Greene FL, Page DL, Fleming ID, et al., editors. AJCC Cancer Staging Manual. 6th ed. New York, NY: Springer; 2002.
3. Patel SG, Shah JP. TNM Staging of Cancers of the head and neck: Striving for uniformity among diversity. CA Cancer J Clin. 2005;55:242-58.
4. Remacle M, Eckel HE, Antonelli A, et al. Endoscopic cordectomy. A proposal for a classification by the Working Committee, European Laryngological Society. Eur Arch Otorhinolaryngol. 2000;257(4):227-31.
5. Remacle M, Van Haverbeke C, Eckel H, et al. Proposal for revision of the European Laryngological Society classification of endoscopic cordectomies. Eur Arch Otorhinolaryngol. 2007;264(5):499-504.

APPENDIX

Ni Classification

Diagrammatic representation of the classification of intraepithelial papillary capillary loop features using Narrow Band Imaging is depicted below.

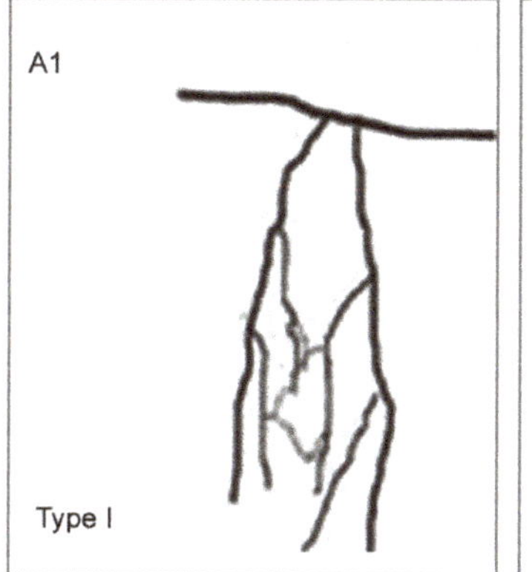

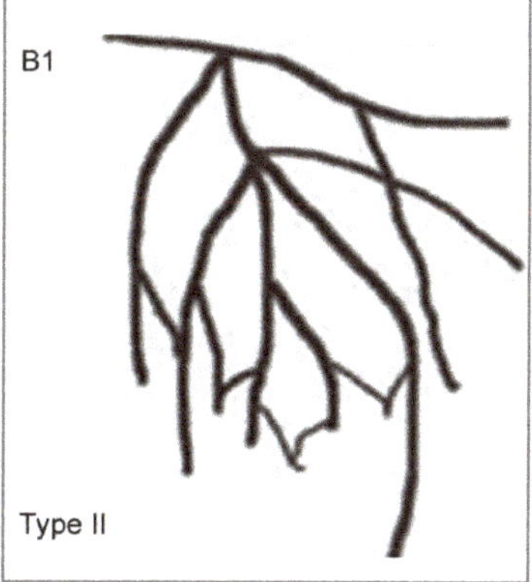

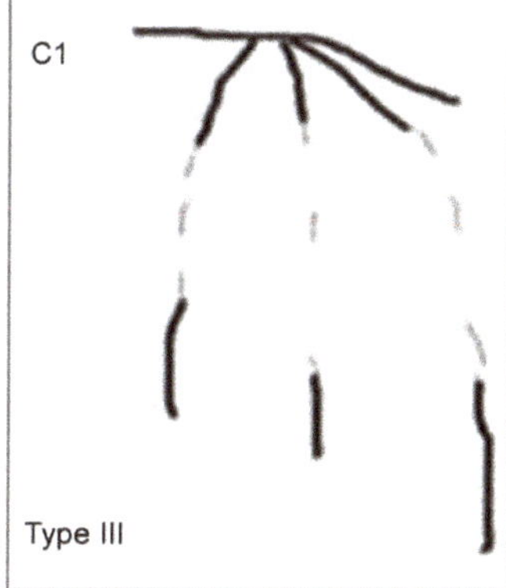

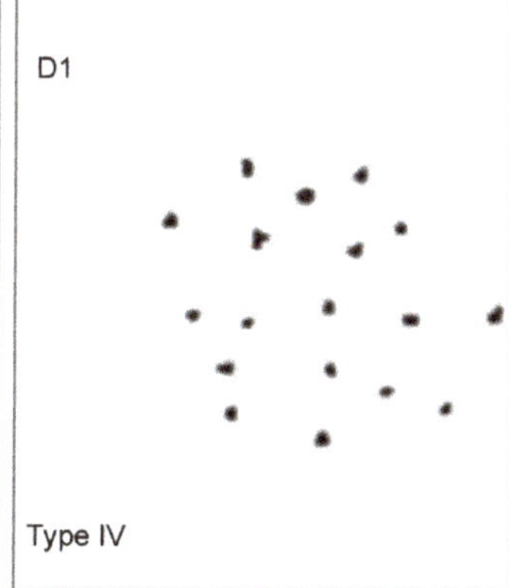

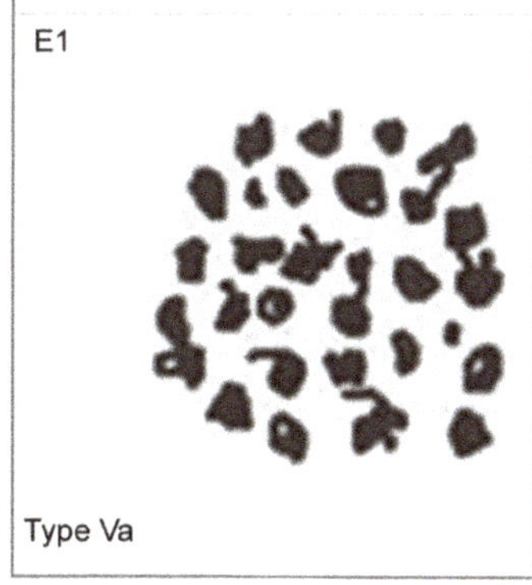

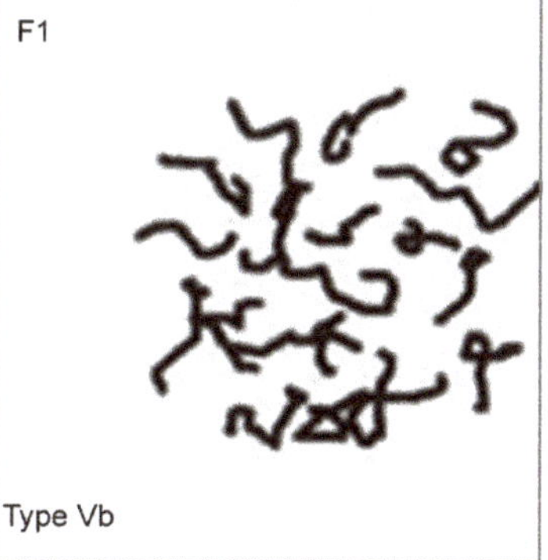

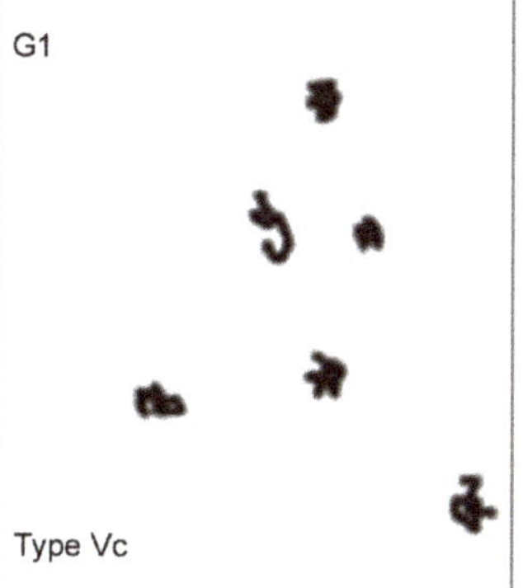

Type I

Thin, oblique, and arborescent vessels are interconnected and intraepithelial papillary loops are almost invisible.

Type II

Diameter of oblique and arborescent vessels is enlarged, and intraepithelial papillary capillary loops are almost invisible.

Type III

Intraepithelial papillary capillary loops are obscured by white mucosa.

Type IV

Intraepithelial papillary capillary loops can be recognized as small brown dots.

Type Va

Intraepithelial papillary capillary loops appear as solid or hollow, with a brownish speckled pattern and various shapes.

Type Vb

Intraepithelial papillary capillary loops appear as irregular, tortuous, line like shapes

Type Vc

Intraepithelial papillary capillary loops appear as brownish speckles or tortuous, line-like shapes with irregular distribution, scattered on the tumor surface.

REFERENCE

Ni XG, He S, Xu ZG, et al. Endoscopic diagnosis of laryngeal cancer and precancerous lesions by narrow band imaging. J Laryngol Otol. 2011;125(3):288-96.

Index

Page numbers followed by *f* refer to figure.

E

F

G

H

I

J

K

L

M

N

P

R

S

T

U

V

W

Z